# DISASTER!

## A COMPENDIUM OF TERRORIST, NATURAL, AND MAN-MADE CATASTROPHES

## MICHAEL I. GREENBERG, MD, MPH

Professor of Public Health
Professor of Emergency Medicine
Drexel University College of Medicine
Medical College Hospital
Department of Emergency Medicine
Division of Toxicology
Philadelphia, PA

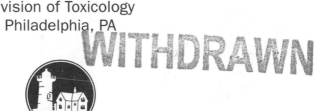

JONES AND BARTLETT PUBLISHERS
*Sudbury, Massachusetts*
BOSTON    TORONTO    LONDON    SINGAPORE

*World Headquarters*
Jones and Bartlett Publishers
40 Tall Pine Drive
Sudbury, MA 01776
978-443-5000
info@jbpub.com
www.jbpub.com

Jones and Bartlett Publishers Canada
6339 Ormindale Way
Mississauga, Ontario L5V 1J2
CANADA

Jones and Bartlett Publishers International
Barb House, Barb Mews
London W6 7PA
UK

Jones and Bartlett's books and products are available through most bookstores and online booksellers. To contact Jones and Bartlett Publishers directly, call 800-832-0034, fax 978-443-8000, or visit our website at www.jbpub.com.

Substantial discounts on bulk quantities of Jones and Bartlett's publications are available to corporations, professional associations, and other qualified organizations. For details and specific discount information, contact the special sales department at Jones and Bartlett via the above contact information or send an email to specialsales@jbpub.com.

**Library of Congress Cataloging-in-Publication Data**

Greenberg, Michael I.
  Compendium of terrorist, natural, and man-made catastrophes / by Michael I. Greenberg.
    p. cm.
  Includes bibliographical references.
  ISBN-13: 978-0-7637-3989-8 (pbk.)
  ISBN-10: 0-7637-3989-8 (pbk.)
  1. Hazardous substances—Accidents—Encyclopedias. 2. Pollution—Encyclopedias. 3. Nuclear accidents—Encyclopedias. 4. Poisoning—Encyclopedias. 5. Explosions—Encyclopedias. 6. Disasters—Encyclopedias. I. Title.
  T55.3.H3G7425 2006
  363.3403—dc22

                                                                                                    2006002402

6048

**Production Credits**
Executive Publisher: Christopher Davis
Production Director: Amy Rose
Associate Editor: Kathy Richardson
Production Editor: Renée Sekerak
Associate Marketing Manager: Laura Kavigian
Manufacturing Buyer: Therese Connell
Composition and Text Design: Auburn Associates, Inc.
Cover Design: Kristin E. Ohlin
Printing and Binding: Malloy Incorporated
Cover printing: Malloy Incorporated

Printed in the United States of America
10 09 08 07 06    10 9 8 7 6 5 4 3 2 1

# CONTENTS

Chapter **2**  **BIOLOGICAL EVENTS** . . . . . . . . . . . . . . . . . . . . . .75

# ACKNOWLEDGMENTS

I would like to gratefully acknowledge the exceptional research and organizational skills of Kate Buchert in bringing this manuscript project together and keeping it on track.

# CONTRIBUTING AUTHORS

**John Curtis, MD**
**Rachel Haroz, MD**
**Ben Roemer, MD**
**Matthew Salzman, MD**

*all from the*
Department of Emergency Medicine
Drexel University College of Medicine
Philadelphia, PA

# PREFACE

H.G. Wells once said, "Human history becomes more and more a race between education and catastrophe" (H.G. Wells, Outline of History, 1920). When one considers the vast numbers of man-made and natural disasters that have befallen this planet over time, the truth in this statement becomes apparent. Learning about disasters of all types is the first step in possibly interfering with and possibly limiting their devastation either by prevention or efficient interventional responses. The study of disasters as to the relevant epidemiology, toxicology, sociology, ethnology, geography, and politics begins with the disaster timeline as has been presented in this book. It is my hope that by studying this timeline and educating readers in this way, a path toward averting catastrophes may be defined.

Michael I. Greenberg, MD, MPH

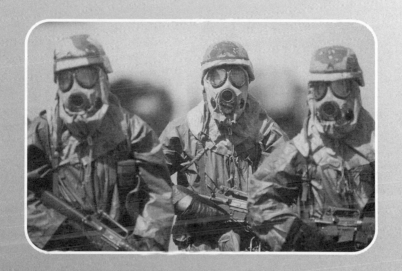

# CHEMICAL EVENTS

# Chapter 1

# CHEMICAL EVENTS

## Acetonitrile (CH₃CN)

### *1988: Utah*

Two cases of pediatric accidental ingestion of a cosmetic containing acetonitrile were reported. One 16-month-old boy died and a 2-year-old boy survived with intensive supportive care.

Caravati EM, Litovitz TL. Pediatric cyanide intoxication and death from an acetonitrile-containing cosmetic. *JAMA* 1988; 260(23):3470–3473.

### *1959*

Sixteen workers exposed to acetonitrile while applying corrosion-resistant material to the inside of tanks, they developed toxicity due to acentonitrile's metabolism to cyanide. Symptoms included nausea, headache, vomiting, abdominal cramps, respiratory depression, and bradycardia.

Hryhorczuk DO, Aks SE, Turk JW. Unusual occupational toxins. *Occup Med* 1992; 7(3):567–586.

## Acrylonitrile

Worker exposure to acrylonitrile in the polymer industry has been related to symptoms including headache, chest discomfort, irritation of the mucous membranes, and a nervous irritability. Acrylonitrile is a suspected human carcinogen and has been associated with lung cancer.

Hryhorczuk DO, Aks SE, Turk JW. Unusual occupational toxins. *Occup Med* 1992; 7(3):567–586.

Delzell E, Monson RR. Mortality among rubber workers: VI. Men with potential exposure to acrylonitrile. *J Occup Med* 1982; 24(10):767–769.

## Air Pollution, Photochemical Smog

### 1997: Indonesia

A widespread forest fire in Indonesia was associated with an increase in mortality and morbidity. The resultant smoke cloud also affected Malaysia, Singapore, Brunei, southern Thailand, and parts of the Philippines. The number of hospital admissions increased, with a high degree of respiratory complaints.

Langford NJ, Ferner RE. Episodes of environmental poisoning worldwide. *Occup Environ Med* 2002; 59:855–860.

### August 1971: Osaka, Japan

An episode of air pollution resulted in 249 school children reporting symptoms of throat pain, headache, coughing, difficulty breathing, eye irritation, and numbness in their limbs.

Fujii T. Studies on air pollution by photochemical reaction. 1. The results of field research of photochemical smog in Osaka, 1971. In: *Proceedings of the Research Section,* Osaka Environmental Pollution Control Centre; 1972; No. 3, pp. 21–34.

### December 1962: London, England, United Kingdom

Air pollution resulted in more than 700 deaths, which was 3,000 fewer than a similar episode in 1952.

Environmental Institute of Houston. *The History of Air Quality.* Available at: http://www.eih.uh.edu/outreach/tfors/history.htm.

### 1961–1982: Armadale, Scotland, United Kingdom

The standardized mortality ratios (SMRs) for lung cancer were high during this time period, and a large cluster of these lung cancer patients were located in a residential zone downwind from a foundry.

Lloyd OL, Williams FL, Gailey FA. Is the Armadale epidemic over? Air pollution and mortality from lung cancer and other diseases, 1961–1982. *Br J Ind Med* 1985; 42(12):815–823.

### 1953: New York City, New York

Smog from air pollution resulted in more than 200 deaths.

Greenburg L, Jacobs MB, Drolette BM, et al. Report of an air pollution incident in New York City. November 1953. *Public Health Rep* 1962; 77:7–16.

### 1952: London, England, United Kingdom

From December 5 to December 9, 1952, London experienced a dense, lethal smog arising from the combination of foggy weather and coal-burning homes, power plants, and factories. This phenomenon resulted in about 3,000 deaths, about three times the normal mortality rate.

Bell ML, Davis DL. Reassessment of the lethal London fog of 1952: novel indicators of acute and chronic consequences of acute exposure to air pollution. *Environ Health Perspect* 2001; 109(Suppl 3):389–394.

Ministry of Health. Mortality and morbidity during the London fog of December 1952. Reports on Public Health and Medical Subjects No 95. London, UK: London Ministry of Health; 1954.

### 1948: Donora, Pennsylvania
Fueled by pollutants from metal works, coal-fired homes, and industrial furnaces, coke ovens, and a zinc retort refinery, an anticyclonic atmospheric inversion settled on the valley, killing 20 people within a 1-week period. The death rate was six times the normal mortality rate.

Schrenk HH, Heimann H, et al. Air pollution in Donora, PA: epidemiology of the unusual smog episode of October 1948, Preliminary Report. Public Health Bulletin No 306. Washington, DC: U.S. Public Health Service; 1949.

Gammage J. *In 1948, a killer fog spurred air cleanup.* The Philadelphia Inquirer; October 28, 1998.

### 1930: Meuse Valley, Liege, Belgium
Over a 5-day period, industrial pollution from steel mills, coke ovens, foundries, and smelters contributed to the accumulation of the air pollutants sulfur dioxide, sulfuric acid mists, and fluoride gases. More than 60 people died during this time, which was 10 times the normal mortality rate.

Nemery BN, Hoet PHM, Nemmar A. The Meuse Valley fog of 1930: an air pollution disaster. *Lancet* 2001; 357(9257):704–708.

Firket J. Fog along the Meuse Valley. *Trans Faraday Soc* 1936; 32:1192–1197.

## Allyl Alcohol Vapor
### April 12, 2004: Dalton, Georgia
Allyl alcohol vapors were released from a chemical manufacturing plant after a chemical reactor overheated. One hundred fifty-four people were hospitalized and nearby residents were evacuated. The vegetation and aquatic life near the plant were destroyed.

U.S. Chemical Safety and Hazard Investigation Board. CSB Investigation Information Page. *MFG Chemical Inc.* Toxic Gas Release Dalton, GA, April 12, 2004. Available at: http://www.csb.gov/index.cfm?folder=current_investigations&page=info&INV_ID=46.

# Aluminum (Al)

### 1991: Pennsylvania

Fifty-nine patients were found to have elevated serum aluminum levels associated with dialysis. Several developed seizures and mental status changes. An electric pump containing aluminum housing, used to deliver acid concentrate, was found to be the cause.

Burwen DR, Olsen SM, et al. Epidemic aluminum intoxication in hemodialysis patients traced to use of an aluminum pump. *Kidney Int* 1995; 48(2):469–474.

# Aluminum Sulfate [Al$_2$(SO$_4$)$_3$]

### 1988: Lowermoor, United Kingdom

Twenty tons of liquid aluminum sulfate were accidentally introduced into the water distribution system at the Lowermoor Water Treatment Works. Gastrointestinal and skin disorders were subsequently reported in the local population.

Lowermoor Incident Health Advisory Group; Department of Health. Water pollution at Lowermoor, North Cornwall. 2nd report. London, UK: HMSO; 1991; pp. 1–51.

Health Stream Report on UK Aluminium Incident. Issue 37. Available at: http://www.waterquality.crc.org.au/hs/pdf/hs37.pdf. Accessed March 2005.

Langford NJ, Ferner RE. Episodes of environmental poisoning worldwide. *Occup Environ Med* 2002; 59:855–860.

# Ammonia (NH$_3$)

### 1989

Two fatalities occurred after a leak during transport.

Singh S, Fadnis P, Sharma BK. Two fatalities following ammonia (NH$_3$) gassing leaked during transport. *J Assoc Physicians India* 1989; 37(7):481–482.

### 1989: Lithuania

An ammonia tank within a fertilizer plant exploded, killing seven people, injuring 57, and resulting in the evacuation of approximately 32,000 people.

Langford NJ, Ferner RE. Episodes of environmental poisoning worldwide. *Occup Environ Med* 2002; 59:855–860.

### January 16, 1976: Port of Landskrona, Sweden

An ammonia spill on the tanker *Rene 16* resulted in the deaths of two crewmen due to pulmonary edema.

Molitor E. HELCOM Manual on Co-operation in Response to Marine Pollution Within the Framework of the Convention on the Protection of the Marine Environment of the Baltic Sea Area (Helsinki Convention), vol 2, Annex 3. Case Histories. (abstract). Available at http://www.coastguard.se/ra/volume2/start.htm. Accessed February 27, 2003.

Ammonia Loading Line Rupture. Report from Supra, 1976, Sweden.

### 1940s: London, England, United Kingdom
A bomb fragment pierced an ammonia-carrying condenser pipe in a World War II bomb shelter, which had been a brewery cellar. Patients developed acute lung injury with a 63% mortality rate.

Caplin M. Ammonia gas poisoning. Forty-seven cases in a London shelter. *Lancet* 1941; 2:95–96.


## Ammonia, Anhydrous
### 2002: Minot, North Dakota
A train derailment caused the rupture of five tank cars carrying anhydrous ammonia. This resulted in a large vapor plume over the area affecting 11,600 people. One death was reported.

National Transportation Safety Board. Safety Recommendation, Washington, DC. Available at: http://www.ntsb.gov/Recs/letters/2004/R04_01_07.pdf. Accessed March 15, 2004.

### July 14, 1993: Truro, Novia Scotia, Canada
A refrigeration leak caused liquid anhydrous ammonia to drain into the Salmon River, causing a major die-off of the aquatic life.

Public Safety and Emergency Preparedness Canada. *Canadian Disaster Database.* Available at: http://www.psepc=sppcc.gc.ca/res/em/cdd/search=en.asp. Accessed September 21, 2005.


## Antimony Pentachloride Gas
### July 29, 2003: Baton Rouge, Louisiana
A release of antimony pentachloride from a gas cylinder killed one worker at the Honeywell refrigerant manufacturing plant.

U.S. Chemical Safety and Hazard Investigation Board. CSB Investigation Information Page. Honeywell Chemical Incidents, Baton Rouge, LA, July 20, 2003. Available at: http://www.csb.gov/index.cfm?folder=current_investigations&page=info&INV_ID=33.

## Arsenate, Chromated Copper

### 2002: Djibouti, East Africa

Two hundred tons of chromated copper arsenate spilled onto the docks of Djibouti after it burnt through plastic drum containers. Standard formulations of the chemical contain 22% arsenic.

Pearce F. Deadly cargo should be shipped back to Blighty. *New Scientist* 2002; 173(2332):8–11.

## Arsenic ($As_2O_3$; $As_4O_6$)

### April 2003: New Sweden, Maine

Multiple people fell ill and one died after a parishioner of a local church placed arsenic in coffee at a church function.

CNN Report. Police: Church poisoner might have had accomplice. Available at: http://www.cnn.com/2003/US/Northeast/05/05/arsenic.killing/index.html. Accessed May 5, 2003.

### 1998: Guizhou Province, China

Three thousand cases of arsenic poisoning occurred due to pollution from a nearby coal mine.

Zheng B, Ding Z, et al. Major ingestion pathways of arsenic in endemic arsenosis in Guizhou Province, China. *Chin Sci Bull* 1999; 44: 69–70.

### 1998: Wakayama, Japan

Sixty-seven people were diagnosed with arsenic toxicity after eating contaminated curry soup at a local festival.

Kishi Y, Sasaki H, et al. An epidemic of arsenic neuropathy from a spiked curry. *Neurology* 2001; 56:1417–1418.

### 1993: Bangladesh

Most of the nine million shallow tube wells dug by the World Health Organization (WHO) in the 1970s to provide "clean water" were found to be heavily contaminated from geological sources of arsenic. Some wells had 400 times the allowable limit. There were approximately 8,500 reported cases of arsenic poisoning from government sources. One study of 10 provinces showed 95% of all hair samples contained high levels of arsenic.

Pearce F. *Bangladesh's arsenic poisoning: who is to blame?* The UNESCO Courier; January 2001; pp. 10–13.

### 1991: Buenos Aires, Argentina

Contaminated meat products resulted in the illness of 718 people. No deaths
were reported. The contamination was a result of vandals breaking into a
butcher's shop and pouring an unspecified amount of 45% sodium arsenite over 200 kg of minced meat.

Roses OE, Garcia-Fernandez JC, et al. Mass poisoning by sodium arsenite. *J Toxicol
Clin Toxicol* 1991; 29(2):209–213.

Sibbald B. Arsenic poisoning rampant in Bangladesh. *CMAJ* 2002; 166(12):1378a.

Zheng B, Ding Z, et al. Major ingestion pathways of arsenic in endemic arsenosis in
Guizhou Province, China. *Chin Sci Bull* 1999; 44:69–70.

### Late 1950s: St. Helena, Italy

The American ambassador to Italy, Clare Boothe Luce, was diagnosed with
arsenic poisoning that may have been caused by paint chips that fell from
stucco roses on her bedroom ceiling. Arsenic as copper arsenide was used
in "Scheele's green," a paint pigment used in wallpaper.

Newman C. Twelve toxic tales. *National Geographic*, May 2005.

### 1900s: Staffordshire, England, United Kingdom

Arsenic-contaminated sugar was used in the manufacturing of beer.

Massey FW, Wold D, Heyman A. Arsenic: homicidal intoxication. *South Med J* 1984;
77:848.

### 1890s: Italy

Arsenic as copper acetoarsenite was used for paint pigments in wallpaper,
both for its color and antifungal properties. The most commonly known
example of this is "Paris Green." Before electricity, the hydrogen released
from coal fires and gas lighting combined with the arsenic in the wallpaper
to form the toxic gas arsine. The fungus *Scopulariopsis breviculis* present in
the damp wallpaper also metabolized arsenic to arsine.

Ratnaike RN. Acute and chronic arsenic toxicity. *Postgrad Med J* 2003;
79(933):391–396.

### 1884: Liverpool, England, United Kingdom

Margaret Higgins and her sister, Catherine Flanagan, were sentenced to death
when they were found guilty of poisoning Thomas Higgins with arsenic.
It was discovered that the two women took part in a series of murders to
receive insurance money.

Brabin A. The black widows of Liverpool. *History Today* October 2002; pp. 40–46.

### 1828: France
Arsenical neuropathy developed in an estimated 40,000 people after wine and bread were unintentionally contaminated by arsenious acid.

Massey EW, Wold D, Heyman A. Arsenic: homicidal intoxication. *South Med J* 1984; 77:848–851.

Leschke E. Clinical toxicology: modern methods. In: *The Diagnosis and Treatment of Poisoning*. Baltimore: William Wood and Co.; 1934.

### 15th Century: Italy
The Borgia family, namely Alexander VI and his son Cesare, were rumored to specialize in faith-based poisonings involving the use of arsenic.

Newman C. Twelve toxic tales. *National Geographic;* May 2005.

## Arsine

### 1975: United Kingdom
Eight sailors aboard the *Asiafreighter* were exposed to arsine, which had escaped from a cylinder into the cargo hold. Four of the sailors experienced severe effects, including fever, weakness, nausea, vomiting, abdominal pain, hemolysis and hemoglobinuria.

Wilkinson SP, McHugh P, Horsley S, et al. Arsine toxicity aboard the *Asiafreighter*. *BMJ* 1975; 6:559–562.

## Asbestos

### 1920s–1990s: Worldwide
Exposure to asbestos resulted in a significant increase in the rate of asbestos-related disease and cancer.

Murray R. Asbestos: a chronology of its origins and health effects. *Br J Indust Med* 1990; 47:361.

## Barium (Ba)

### May 2003: Goiás State, Brazil
Three patients at radiology clinics were hospitalized after ingesting barium-containing contrast solutions, and two of them died within 24 hours. A local and federal investigation showed that 44 people had suspected barium toxicity, nine of whom died. Eight of the nine victims were linked to a single lot of a brand contrast solution. A national recall was initiated, and the manufacturing site was inspected and closed.

Centers for Disease Control and Prevention. Barium toxicity after exposure to contaminated contrast solution–Goiás State, Brazil, 2003. *MMWR Morbid Mortal Wkly Rep* 2003; 52(43):1047–1048.

## Barium, Carbonate (BaCO₃)

### 1989: Taiwan

A family party led to the poisoning of 13 family members, as well as one death. The poisoning resulted from the use of barium carbonate (a pesticide) instead of flour for the food for the party. Symptoms included nausea, vomiting, abdominal colic, and diarrhea.

Langford NJ, Ferner RE. Episodes of environmental poisoning worldwide. *Occup Environ Med* 2002; 59:855–860.

## Benzene (C₆H₆)

### 1993: Canada

Three cases of fatal benzene poisoning were reported as a result of an industrial accident aboard a cargo ship.

Avis SP, Hutton CJ. Acute benzene poisoning: a report of three fatalities. *J Forensic Sci* 1993; 38(3):599–602.

### February 9, 1990: USA

Perrier, a company that distributed bottled water, was forced to recall millions of bottles of water when it was discovered the water was contaminated with benzene.

CNN.com with Reuters. *Probe starts into New York bottled water poisoning fears.* Available at: http://archives.cnn.com/2000/US/09/14/contaminated.water.02/reut. Accessed September 14, 2000.

Food and Drug Administration (FDA )Enforcement Report for February 28, 1990. Available at: http://www.fda.gov/bbs/topics/ENFORCE/ENF00080.html.

### August 1978: Niagara Falls, New York

Benzene and other waste leached into the soil, backyards and basements of homes in the Love Canal area, triggered by rainfalls. Deteriorating drums were hence exposed. There was a high degree of birth defects observed in the community. Eventually the residents had to be relocated.

Beck EC. The Love Canal tragedy. *EPA Journal* January 1979. Available at: http://www.epa.gov/history/topics/lovecanal/01.htm.

Janerich DT, et al. Cancer incidence in the Love Canal area. *Science* 1981; 212:1404.

Paigen B. Controversy at Love Canal. *Hastings Center Rep* 1982; 12:29.

*1916–1928: Newark, New Jersey*

Exposure to benzene among artificial leather manufacturers was associated with aplastic anemia.

Wax PM. Toxicologic plagues and disasters in history. In: Goldfrank LR, ed. *Goldfrank's Toxicologic Emergencies*, 7th ed. New York: McGraw-Hill; 2002; pp. 23–34.

Sharpe WD. Benzene, artificial leather and aplastic anemia: Newark, 1916–1928. *Bull N Y Acad Med* 1993; 69:47–60.

## Benzine, Dinitrobenzene

*April 1986: Ohio*

Exposure to dinitrobenzene resulted in methemoglobinemia in steam-press employees.

Centers for Disease Control and Prevention (CDC). Methemoglobinemia due to occupational exposure to dinitrobenzene–Ohio, 1986. *MMWR Morbid Mortal Wkly Rep* 1988; 37(22):353–355.

## Benzine, Orthodichlorobenzene, Propylene Dichloride, and Ethylene Dichloride

*October 24, 1954: Philadelphia, Pennsylvania*

Philadelphia firefighters were investigating a reported gas leak emanating from a 4,000-gallon aluminum tank that held a mixture of ortho-dichlorobenzene, propylene dichloride, and ethylene dichloride. During the investigation, the tank exploded, releasing 3,000 gallons of the chemical mixture into a 5,000 square-foot area in which 45 personnel were present. The blast killed three men, and 39 others were sent to the hospital.

Conner EH, Dubious AB, Comroe JH. Acute chemical injury of the airway and lungs. Experience with six cases. *Anesthesiology* 1962; 23(4):538–547.

## Benzyl Alcohol

*1981*

Deaths of premature infants due to gasping syndrome characterized by severe metabolic acidosis, respiratory depression, and encephalopathy were linked to benzyl alcohol. The source was traced to contaminated IV solutions. The benzyl alcohol was converted to benzoic acid in the bloodstream.

Gershanik J, Boecler B, et al. The gasping syndrome and benzyl alcohol poisoning. *N Engl J Med* 1982; 307(22):1384–1388.

# Beryllium (Be)

### 1950's–1980s: Rocky Flats, Colorado

Beryllium disease, characterized largely by respiratory symptoms, was diagnosed in more than 200 employees of a ceramics plant that supported a nuclear weapons trigger plant.

Newman LS, Kreiss K, King TE Jr, Seay S, Campbell PA. Pathologic and immunologic alterations in early stages of beryllium disease. Reexamination of disease definition and natural history. *Am Rev Respir Dis* 1989; 139(6):1479–1486.

# Boron Hydrides (B)

Diborane exposure among research engineers produced a syndrome of exhaustion, shortness of breath, chills, fever, and pneumonia. Exposure to pentaborane in these researchers led to dizziness, muscle twitching, generalized seizures, and trouble with concentration and memory.

Hryhorczuk DO, Aks SE, Turk JW. Unusual occupational toxins. *Occup Med* 1992; 7(3):567–586.

# Bromine (Br)

### 1996: Boston, Massachusetts

Seventeen teenagers developed bromine poisoning from a swimming pool when bromine-containing cleaning products were overused.

Woolf A, Shannon M. Reactive airway dysfunction and systemic complaints after mass exposure to bromine. *Environ Health Perspect* 1999; 107(6):507–509.

### 1994

Forty-four people became ill after a bromine-containing disinfectant was used to clean a building's ventilation system.

Sesline D, Ames RG, Howd RA. Irritative and systemic symptoms following exposure to Microban disinfectant through a school ventilation system. *Arch Environ Health* 1994; 49:439–444.

### 1984: Geneva, Switzerland

Ninety-one patients became sick after a liquid bromide spill at a chemical plant produced a noxious vapor cloud. The symptoms included upper respiratory tract irritation, cough, and headache.

Morabia A, Selleger C, et al. Accidental bromine exposure in an urban population: an acute epidemiological assessment. *Int J Epidemiol* 1988; 17:148–152.

Langford NJ, Ferner RE. Episodes of environmental poisoning worldwide. *Occup Environ Med* 2002; 59:855–860.

## Cadmium (Cd)

### 1939–1954: Japan
Water from the Jonzu River used to irrigate rice fields was contaminated with cadmium from local mines and zinc refineries, leading to Itai-Itai disease. The disease is characterized by renal disease and chronic bone pain.

Cadmium pollution and Itai-Itai disease. *Lancet* 1971; 2:382.

Langford NJ, Ferner RE. Episodes of environmental poisoning worldwide. *Occup Environ Med* 2002; 59:855–860.

## Carbon Dioxide (CO₂)

### 1986: Cameroon, West Africa
Approximately 1,700 people died when a large amount of natural gas, including carbon dioxide, was emitted from Lake Nyos, a volcanic crater lake. A similar event had occurred in 1984 at Lake Monoun, Cameroon.

Baxter PJ, Kapila M, Mfonfu D. Lake Nyos disaster, Cameroon, 1986: the medical effects of large emission of carbon dioxide? *BMJ* 1989; 298:1437–1441.

## Carbon Disulfide (CS₂)

### 1950s: Italy
Occupational exposure to carbon disulfide in workers was associated with symptoms of depression and suicide.

World Health Organization. *Neurotoxicity Risk Assessment for Human Health: Principles and Approaches. Environmental Health Criteria 223.* Geneva, Switzerland; 2001. Available at: http://www.inchem.org/documents/ehc/ehc/ehc223.htm#223230000.

Vigliani EC. Carbon disulfide poisoning in viscose rayon factories. *Br J Ind Med* 1954; 11:325–344.

## Carbon Monoxide (CO)

### September 2005: Louisiana, Mississippi, Alabama, and Florida
Hurricane Katrina, a category 4 hurricane, flooded the southern Gulf Coast that resulted in hundreds of deaths and the displacement of thousands of people. Hyperbaric-oxygen facilities reported 51 cases of carbon monoxide poisoning from August 29 (the date Katrina made landfall) to September 24, 2005. Five Louisiana residents died. The cause of all these exposures, both fatal and nonfatal, was traced to exposure to portable-generator exhaust.

Centers for Disease Control and Prevention (CDC). Carbon monoxide poisoning after Hurricane Katrina—Alabama, Louisiana, and Mississippi, August–September 2005. *MMWR Morbid Mortal Wkly Rep* 54(Early release):1–3.

### 2004: Japan

Seven people died from apparent suicide in the Japanese mountains of Saitama. Two women were also found dead south of Tokyo. All had charcoal burners in their vehicles and police believed they died from inhaling carbon monoxide from the charcoal. Authorities believed these people became
acquainted through Internet suicide Web sites.

BBC News. *Nine die in Japan 'suicide pacts'*. Available at: http://newsbbc.co.uk/2/hi/asia-pacific/3735372.stm. Accessed October 12, 2004.

### 2002: Salang Pass, Afghanistan

An avalanche blocked exits of a tunnel, trapping 300 people in their vehicles for 24 hours. Keeping their vehicles running for warmth, 5 people died of carbon monoxide poisoning, including one child.

BBC News, South Asia. *Rescuers fight Afghan blizzard*. February 7, 2002.

### 1996: St. Louis, Missouri

Five hundred sixty-four people were exposed to a CO leak in an elementary school. Of these, 177 children were taken to 3 area hospitals.

Klasner AE, Smith SR, et al. Carbon monoxide mass exposure in a pediatric population. *Acad Emerg Med* 1998; 5(10):992–996.

Gill JR, Goldfeder LB, Stajic M. The happy land homicides: 87 deaths due to smoke inhalation. *J Forensic Sci* 2003; 48(1):161–163.

### 1990–2002: USA

The Centers for Disease Control and Prevention (CDC) reported 17 deaths and 36 nonfatal carbon monoxide poisonings from houseboat and recreational water vehicle exhaust.

Centers for Disease Control and Prevention (CDC). Carbon monoxide poisoning resulting from exposure to ski-boat exhaust. Georgia, June 2002. *MMWR Morbid Mortal Wkly Rep* 2002; 51(37):829–830.

*September 1985: North Carolina*

Twelve employees in a garment-manufacturing plant experienced headaches, nausea, faintness, and dizziness after exposure to carbon monoxide from indoor use of a forklift.

Center for Disease Control and Prevention (CDC). Epidemiologic notes and reports carbon monoxide poisoning in a garment-manufacturing plant—North Carolina. *MMWR Morbid Mortal Wkly Rep* 1987; 36(32):543–545.

## Carbon Monoxide (CO) and Cyanide

*March 25, 1990: Bronx, New York*

Carbon monoxide and cyanide caused 87 deaths from smoke inhalation at the Happy Land Social Club.

CO and Cyanide. March 25, 1990: Bronx, New York.

Gill JR, Goldfeder LB, Stajic M. The Happy Land homicides: 87 deaths due to smoke inhalation. *J Forensic Sci* 2003; 48(1): 161–163.

*November 28, 1942: Boston, Massachusetts*

Carbon monoxide and cyanide released during a fire at the Cocoanut Grove nightclub caused 498 deaths. The fire was started in the Melody Lounge from a lit match.

Faxon NW, Churchill ED. The Cocoanut Grove disaster in Boston. *JAMA* 1942; 120:1385.

Beller D, Sapochetti J. Searching for answers to the Cocoanut Grove Fire of 1942. National Fire Protection Association Journal 2000:85–92. Available at: http://www.nfpa.org/assets/files/PDF/CocoGrove.pdf.

## Carbon Monoxide (CO) and Nitrogen Dioxide (NO₂)

*December 2002: Lehigh Valley, Pennsylvania*

Breathing difficulties, cough, and dizziness in 18 hockey players and their coach resulted when carbon monoxide and nitrogen dioxide leaked from a malfunctioning Zamboni machine at the ice rink.

Ditzen LS. *Ice arenas pose danger of toxic air, officials say.* Philadelphia Inquirer, December 3, 2002.

## Chemical Fumes

*March 26, 1942: Allentown, Pennsylvania*

Thirty-one people died from asphyxiation from fumes at the limestone quarry Sandts Eddy Quarry.

CDC and NIOSH Safety and Health Research. Historical Mining Disasters. Available at: http://www.cdc.gov/niosh/mining/statistics/disall.htm. Accessed September 21, 2005.

### August 15, 1902: Park City, Utah

Fumes from lead, zinc, copper, and silver resulted in 34 deaths at the Park-Utah mine.

CDC and NIOSH Safety and Health Research. *Historical Mining Disasters.* Available at: http://www.cdc.gov/niosh/mining/statistics/disall.htm. Accessed September 21, 2005.

## Chemical Warfare

### 1937: China and Japan

The Japanese army released poisonous gases in their offensive against the Chinese army.

Eckert WG. Mass deaths by gas or poisoning: a historical perspective. *Am J Forens Med Pathol* 1991; 12(2):119–125.

## Chemical Warfare, Chlorine

### 1915–1918: Ypres, France

On April 22, 1915, 150 tons of chlorine gas were released by the Germans around the village of Ypres. Multiple French troops died and approximately 800 soldiers were incapacitated with respiratory distress.

Langford NJ, Ferner RE. Episodes of environmental poisoning worldwide. *Occup Environ Med* 2002; 59:855–860.

Eckert WG. Mass deaths by gas or poisoning: a historical perspective. *Am J Forens Med Pathol* 1991; 12(2):119–125.

## Chemical Warfare, Cyanide, Carbon Monoxide, and Zyklon-B

### 1940s: Europe

During World War II, lethal gases were used in the German concentration camps as agents for extermination, including carbon monoxide, cyanide, and Zyklon-B gas. The Zyklon-B gas pellets released hydrogen cyanide gas upon exposure to the air.

Hanlon V. The centaur's memory. *CMAJ* 2001; 165(9):1238–1239.

Eckert WG. Mass deaths by gas or poisoning: a historical perspective. *Am J Forens Med Pathol* 1991; 12(2):119–125.

## Chemical Warfare, Mustard Gas

### 1980–1988: Iraq and Iran
Mustard gas was used as an agent in the Iraq-Iran War.

Federation of American Scientists. *CW Use in Iran-Iraq War.* Declassified on 2 July
1996. Available at: http://www.fas.org/irp/gulf/cia/960702/72566_01.htm.

### 1985: Baltic Sea
After World War II, approximately 100,000 tons of mustard gas bombs were
deposited into the Baltic Sea. Fishermen have periodically suffered from
mustard gas poisoning as a result of bringing the bombs back up in their
nets. By 1985, 97 fishermen had been affected; 26 required hospital treatment, and two had died.

Langford NJ, Ferner RE. Episodes of environmental poisoning worldwide. *Occup
Environ Med* 2002; 59:855–860.

### 1980: Afghanistan
Mustard gas was allegedly used against Afghani troops during the conflict
with the Soviet Union.

Eckert WG. Mass deaths by gas or poisoning: a historical perspective. *Am J Forens Med
Pathol* 1991; 12(2):119–125.

### 1935: Ethiopia
The Italian army utilized mustard gas during its campaigns in Ethiopia.

Eckert WG. Mass deaths by gas or poisoning: a historical perspective. *Am J Forens Med
Pathol* 1991; 12(2):119–125.

## Chemical Warfare, Phosgene

### 1914–1918: Europe
Phosgene was used as a warfare agent in World War I.

Langford NJ, Ferner RE. Episodes of environmental poisoning worldwide. *Occup
Environ Med* 2002; 59:855–860.

## Chemical Warfare, Picric Acid

### 1899–1902: South Africa
During the Boer War, the British used artillery shells containing picric acid.

Eckert WG. Mass deaths by gas or poisoning: a historical perspective. *Am J Forens Med
Pathol* 1991; 12(2):119–125.

# Chemical Warfare, Sarin

### February 2004: Anniston, Alabama

A small amount of sarin nerve agent leaked from a weapons storage bunker at Anniston Army Depot. No injuries were reported.

Reeves J. The Associated Press. *Ala. weapons furnace shut down.* February 5, 2004.

The Associated Press. *Sarin nerve agent leaks from Ala. bunker.* March 3, 2004.

### 1995: Tokyo, Japan

A sarin attack in a busy subway affected up to 5,500 passengers. Seventeen of these were critically ill, and 12 passengers died. Symptoms were consistent with organophosphate poisoning.

Langford NJ, Ferner RE. Episodes of environmental poisoning worldwide. *Occup Environ Med* 2002; 59:855–860.

Woodall J. Tokyo subway gas attack. *Lancet* 1997; 350:296.

### March 1994: Matsumoto, Japan

A sarin attack in a residential area affected 600 people, resulting in 58 hospital admissions and seven deaths. Symptoms were consistent with organophosphate poisoning.

Langford NJ, Ferner RE. Episodes of environmental poisoning worldwide. *Occup Environ Med* 2002; 59:855–860.

Morita H, Yanagisawa N, Nakajima T, et al. Sarin poisoning in Matsumoto, Japan. *Lancet* 1995; 346:290–293.

# Chemical Warfare, Sulfur Gas

### 1854–1856: Crimean Peninsula

During the Crimean War, the British forces attempted to use sulfur gas against the Russian troops at Sebastopol. The attempt proved ineffective.

Eckert WG. Mass deaths by gas or poisoning: a historical perspective. *Am J Forens Med Pathol* 1991; 12(2):119–125.

# Chemical Warfare, Sulfur and Pitch

### 431 BC: Ancient Greece

During the Athenian and Spartan wars, sulfur and pitch were burned beneath besieged walls in the cities of Platea and Belium.

Eckert WG. Mass deaths by gas or poisoning: a historical perspective. *Am J Forens Med Pathol* 1991; 12(2):119–125.

# Chloramine

### September 2000: Minas Gerais, Brazil

Sixteen patients undergoing hemodialysis treatment experienced hemolytic
  reactions due to chlorine and chloramine water contamination.

Calderaro RV, Heller L. Outbreak of hemolytic reactions associated with chlorine and
chloramine residuals in hemodialysis water. [Portuguese] *Rev Saude Publica* 2001;
35(5):481–486.

### 1998

Seventy-two male soldiers presented with acute inhalation of chloramine gas
  after a "cleaning party" in the barracks. Ten days after the group of male
  soldiers presented, a second group of female soldiers was exposed in a
  similar manner.

Pascizzi TA, Storrow AB. Mass casualties from acute inhalation of chloramine gas. *Mil
Med* 1998; 163(2):102–104.

### 1987

Patients were exposed to chloramine at an outpatient dialysis center when the
  carbon filter failed in a water treatment system. Forty-one patients received
  transfusions to treat hemolytic anemia, and an epidemiologic study
  demonstrated that the mortality rate among the dialysis patients increased
  for the five-month period after the chloramine exposure.

Tipple MA, Shusterman N, et al. Illness in hemodialysis patients after exposure to
chloramine contaminated dialysate. *ASAIO Trans* 1991; 37(4):588–591.

# Chlorhexidine

### 1988

Five newborns were accidentally fed a dilute antiseptic solution containing
  chlorhexidine. The infants developed caustic burns of the lips, mouth, and
  tongue within minutes of feeding. One infant developed acute pulmonary
  edema. No deaths were reported.

Mucklow ES. Accidental feeding of a dilute antiseptic solution (chlorhexidine 0.05%
with cetrimide 1%) to five babies. *Hum Toxicol* 1988; 7(6):567–569.

# Chloride, Stannic

### 1982: Massachusetts

Exposure to stannic chloride led to respiratory symptoms in workers of a
  glass-bottle manufacturing plant.

Levy BS, Davis F, Johnson B. Respiratory symptoms among glass bottle makers exposed to stannic chloride solution and other potentially hazardous substances. *J Occup Med* 1985; 27(4):277–282.

## Chlorine (Cl), Chlorine Gas

### January 6, 2005: Graniteville, South Carolina

A train collision punctured a tanker carrying chlorine gas. The resultant leak killed nine people in the nearby mill town and injured more than 250. Approximately 5,400 residents were evacuated from their homes.

Augusta Chronicle. *Graniteville train accident.* Available at: http://chronicle.augusta. com/train/.

CNN.com. *Some residents returning home after chlorine leak.* Available at: http://www. cnn.com/2005/US/01/07/train.wreck/index.html. Accessed January 13, 2005.

CNN.com/Associated Press. *Train wreck evacuees going home.* Available at: http://www. cnn.com/2005/US/01/15/train.citizens.return.ap/index.html. Accessed January 15, 2005.

### June 2004: San Antonio, Texas

Two freight trains collided, releasing chlorine gas and a small amount of ammonium nitrate. The chlorine gas cloud drifted 10 miles to San Antonio's Sea World amusement park. Three people died and about 40 other people suffered respiratory symptoms.

Badger, T.A. *Three killed by fumes from Texas train crash.* The Associated Press. June 29, 2004.

### April 18, 2004: Chongqing, China

Chlorine gas leaks and ensuing explosions at the Tianyuan plant in southwest China killed nine people and injured three others. About 150,000 residents were evacuated from the local municipality.

Nei Geo. *Chongqing gas leak controlled; nine dead.* China Daily. April 19, 2004. Available at: http://www.chinadaily.com.cn/english/doc/2004-04/19/content_324380.htm.

### November 17, 2003: Glendale, Arizona

At the DPC Enterprises repackaging facility, chlorine vapors from a rail-car unloading operation escaped from the recapture system. Fourteen people, including 10 police personnel, were treated for chlorine exposure.

U.S. Chemical Safety and Hazard Investigation Board. CSB Investigation Page. DPC Enterprises Chlorine Release, Glendale, AZ, November 17, 2003. Available at: http:// www.csb.gov/index.cfm?folder=current_investigations&page=info&INV_ID=45.

*July 20, 2003: Baton Rouge, Louisiana*
A release of chlorine gas from the Honeywell refrigerant manufacturing plant hospitalized four plant workers and forced residents within a half-mile radius to seek shelter in their homes.

U.S. Chemical Safety and Hazard Investigation Board. CSB News Release. CSB Provides Interim Report to Community on Three Honeywell International Accidents at Baton Rouge, LA, Facility. Available at: http:// www.csb.gov/index.cfm?folder= news_releases&pages=news&NEWS_ID=148.

*August 14, 2002: Festus, Missouri*
Forty-eight thousand pounds of chlorine were released when a chlorine-transfer hose ruptured during the unloading of a rail car at the DPC Enterprises chlorine repackaging facility. Sixty-four people sought medical attention.

U.S. Chemical Safety and Hazard Investigation Board. CSB Investigation Information Page. DPC Enterprises Chlorine Release, Festus, MO, August 14, 2002. Available at: http:// www.csb.gov/index.cfm?folder=completed_investigations&page=info&INV_ID=20.

*October 22, 1998: Rome, Italy*
Chlorine gas vapors were released from a chlorinating-maintenance procedures room of a recreational center. Approximately 282 people (including 134 children) inhaled hydrogen chloride and sodium hypochlorite, which resulted in acute respiratory symptoms.

Di Napoli A, Agabiti N, Ancona C, et al. Respiratory effects of exposure to chlorine vapors during a swimming pool accident in a recreational center in Rome. [Italian] *Epidemiol Prev* 2002; 26(5):240–247.

*1978: Youngstown, Florida*
A rail tank car carrying 90 tons of liquid chlorine was punctured, resulting in eight deaths and 23 hospitalizations due to respiratory injuries.

Jones RN, Hughes JM, et al. Lung function after acute chlorine exposure. *Am Rev Respir Dis* 1986; 134(6):1190–1195.

Langford NJ, Ferner RE. Episodes of environmental poisoning worldwide. *Occup Environ Med* 2002; 59:855–860.

*1967: USA*
One hundred fifty longshoremen were accidentally exposed to chlorine when the main valve of a cylinder containing liquid chlorine ruptured. Long-term studies revealed evidence of chronic lung damage.

Hamilton A, Hardy HL, Finkel AJ., eds. *Hamilton and Hardy's Industrial Toxicology*, 4th ed. Boston, MA: J. Wright; 1983.

### 1947: New York City, New York

A leaking cylinder of chlorine (100 lbs.) was mistakenly placed over a ventilation grate in a Brooklyn subway station, exposing 1,000 people. Two hundred eight people were admitted to hospitals. Patients complained of burning of the eyes and throat, respiratory distress, and lacrimation and rhinorrhea.

Hamilton A, Hardy HL, Finkel AJ, eds. *Hamilton and Hardy's Industrial Toxicology*, 4th ed. Boston, MA: J. Wright; 1983.

## Chlordecone

### 1973–1975: James River, Virginia

Exposure to chlordecone (Kepone), an organochlorine insecticide, was associated with the development of tremors, opsoclonus, hepatospleno-megaly, weight loss, pleuritic pain, and arthralgias in workers.

Taylor JR, Selhorst JB, et al. Chlordecone intoxication in man. I. Clinical observations. *Neurology* 1978; 28(7):626–630.

Reich MR, Spong JK. Kepone: a disaster in Hopewell, Virginia. *Intl J Health Services* 1983; 13(2):227–246.

Ferrer A, Cabral R. Recent epidemics of poisoning by pesticides. *Toxicol Lett* 1995; 82–83:55–63.

## 2-Chloro-6 Fluorophenol

### January 5, 2002: Holley, New York

Pent-up pressure in a storage tank containing 2-chloro-6 flurophenol caused approximately 75 gallons to erupt into the air. Local residents reported sore throats, headaches, and skin irritation.

U.S. Safety and Hazard Investigation Board—Incident Reports Center. Available at: http://www.csb.gov/circ. Accessed June 24, 2003.

## Chromium (Cr)

### 1988: Taiwan

Ten enamel workers at a manufacturing plant developed chromium ulcers after exposure to $Cr^{+6}$.

Deng JF, Fleeger AK, Sinks T. An outbreak of chromium ulcer in a manufacturing plant. *Vet Hum Toxicol* 1990; 32(2):142–146.

# Clioquinol

### 1960s: Japan

Chinoform (clioquinol), used extensively throughout Japan as a digestive stabilizer, was associated with subacute myelo-optico-neuropathy (SMON) affecting more than 11,000 people.

Woodall B, Yoshikawa A. *Japan's Failure in Pharmaceuticals: Why Is the World Saying "No" to Japanese Drugs?* (Draft). March 1997. Available at: http://www.ciber. gatech.edu/workingpaper/1997/woodall.html.

Tabira T. Clioquinol's Return: Cautions from Japan. *Science* 2001; 292(5525):2251–2252.

# Coal Mine Gas

### October 23, 1891: Glen Carbon, Pennsylvania

Seven people at the Richardson coal mine were suffocated by gas.

CDC and NIOSH Safety and Health Research. *Historical Mining Disasters.* Available at: http://www.cdc.gov/niosh/mining/statistics/discoal.htm. Accessed September 21, 2005.

### October 1, 1887: Girardville, Pennsylvania

Five workers at the Bast coal mine suffocated from gas.

CDC and NIOSH Safety and Health Research. *Historical Mining Disasters.* Available at: http://www.cdc.gov/niosh/mining/statistics/discoal.htm. Accessed September 21, 2005.

### April 27, 1887: Ashland, Pennsylvania

Five workers at the Tunnel coal mine suffocated from gas.

CDC and NIOSH Safety and Health Research. *Historical Mining Disasters.* Available at: http://www.cdc.gov/niosh/mining/statistics/discoal.htm. Accessed September 21, 2005.

### September 13, 1886: Scranton, Pennsylvania

Eight workers at the Marvine coal mine suffocated from gas.

CDC and NIOSH Safety and Health Research. *Historical Mining Disasters.* Available at: http://www.cdc.gov/niosh/mining/statistics/discoal.htm. Accessed September 21, 2005.

# Cobalt (Co)

### 1996

Four cases of cobalt-chloride poisoning were documented from exposure to a chemistry set.

Mucklow ES. Chemistry set poisoning. *Int J Clin Pract* 1997; 51(5):321–323.

### 1960s–1970s: Quebec City, Canada

A clinical and pathologic study of 28 cases demonstrated that a particular beer processing technique resulted in cobalt-contaminated products from the late 1960s to early 1970s. This led to cobalt-beer cardiomyopathy.

Alexander CS. Cobalt-beer cardiomyopathy: a clinical and pathologic study of twenty-eight cases. *Am J Med* 1972; 53(4):395–417.

Wax PM. Toxicologic plagues and disasters in history. In: Goldfrank LR, ed. *Goldfrank's Toxicologic Emergencies*, 7th ed. New York: McGraw-Hill, 2002; pp. 23–34.

## Copper (Cu)

### 1996

Fourteen cases of copper-sulfate poisoning were documented from exposure to a chemistry set.

Mucklow ES. Chemistry set poisoning. *Int J Clin Pract* 1997; 51(5): 321–323.

## Copper Sulfate (CuSO₄)

### 1969: France

Copper sulfate neutralized with hydrated lime ("Bordeaux mixture") resulted in granulomatous disease in those spraying the mixture.

Pimentel JC, Marques F. Vineyard sprayer's lung. *Thorax* 1969; 24:415.

## Cyanide (KCN)

### January 30, 2000: Baia Mare, Romania

A cyanide spill from the Aurul precious metals recovery plant contaminated the Tisza River in Hungary. The cyanide was sufficiently diluted as not to harm people using the river as a drinking source, but fish along the river were found to contain 2.6 mg/kg of cyanide.

Kovac C. Cyanide spill threatens health in Hungary. *BMJ* 2000; 320:536.

### February 1991: Washington State

Three people developed acute cyanide poisoning after having taken over-the-counter Sudafed® 12-hour capsules for nasal congestion. Two of them died.

Centers for Disease Control and Prevention. Cyanide poisonings associated with over-the-counter medication—Washington State, 1991. *MMWR Morbid Mortal Wkly Rep* 1991; 40(10):161, 167–168.

### 1982: Chicago, Illinois
Seven deaths were reported from cyanide-contaminated Tylenol.

Dunea G. Death over the counter. *BMJ* 1983; 286:211–212.

### 1978: Jonestown, Guyana
A mass suicide of 914 people was carried out with cyanide-contaminated grape Kool-Aid.

*Jonestown suicides shocked world.* The Associated Press. March 27, 1997.

## Cyclohexane

### 1974: Flixborough, United Kingdom
An explosion of cyclohexane killed 28, injured 104, and forced the evacuation of 3,000 people.

UNEP-APELL Disasters Database. Available at: http://www.uneptie.org/pc/apell/disasters/disasters.html. Accessed September 21, 2005.

## Daconil, Chlorothalonil

### 1982: Arlington, Virginia
While playing golf at the Army-Navy Country Club, a Navy lieutenant was exposed to Daconil, an FDA-approved fungicide. He developed a fever and rash and died 10 days later.

Attorney General of New York, Office of the Attorney General, Environmental Protection Bureau. *Toxic Fairways: Risking Groundwater Contamination from Pesticides on Long Island Golf Courses.* July 1991 (Revised December 1995). Available at: http://www.oag.state.ny.us/environment/golf95.html.

## Dexfenfluramine/Fenfluramine

### 1997: USA
The so-called "fen-phen" diet regimen led to the development of cardiac valvulopathy and pulmonary hypertension in patients prescribed this drug combination.

Wax PM. Toxicologic plagues and disasters in history. In: Goldfrank LR, ed. *Goldfrank's Toxicologic Emergencies*, 7th ed. New York: McGraw-Hill; 2002; pp. 23–34.

Shively BK, Roldan CA, Gill EA, et al. Prevalence and determinants of valvopathy in patients treated with dexfenfluramine. *Circulation* 1999; 100:2161–2167.

Connolly HM, Crary JL, McGoon MD, et al. Valvular heart disease associated with fenfluramine-phentermine. *N Engl J Med* 1997; 337:581–588.

# 1,2-Dibromo-3-Chloropropane (DBCP)

### 1970s: California

DBCP, which was injected into soil to act as a nematocide, resulted in increased infertility, azoopsermia, and oligospermia.

Whorton MD, et al. Infertility in male pesticide workers. *Lancet* 1977; 2:1259.

# 2,4-Dichlorophenol

### 1980–1998: USA and England, United Kingdom

Multiple case reports describe seizures, respiratory failure and cardiac arrest from direct exposure to 2,4-dichlorophenol.

U.S. Chemical Safety and Hazard Investigation Board. Incident Reports Center. Available at: http://www.csb.gov/circ. Accessed June 24, 2003.

Centers for Disease Control and Prevention (CDC). Occupational fatalities associated with 2,4-dichlorophenol (2,4-DCP) exposure, 1980–1998. *MMWR Morbid Mortal Wkly Rep* 2000; 49(23):516–518.

# Diethylene Glycol

### 1998: Guragon, India

Thirty-six children developed acute renal failure from diethylene-glycol contaminated cough syrup. Thirty-three of the children died.

Singh J, Dutta AK, et al. Diethylene glycol poisoning in Guragon, India 1998. *Bull WHO* 2001; 79(2):88–100.

### 1995–1996: Port-au-Prince, Haiti

At least 68 children were poisoned and 30 died from an over-the-counter cough syrup that was contaminated with diethylene glycol.

Wax P. It's happening again—another diethylene glycol mass poisoning. *J Toxicol Clin Toxicol* 1996; 34(5):517–520.

O'Brien KL, Selanikio JD, et al. Epidemic of pediatric deaths from acute renal failure caused by diethylene glycol poisoning. *JAMA* 1998; 279(15):1175.

### 1990–1992: Bangladesh

Three hundred thirty-nine children developed acute renal failure and 236 died from diethylene-glycol–contaminated paracetamol acetaminophen elixirs.

Hanif M, Mobarak M, et al. Fatal renal failure caused by diethylene glycol in paracetamol elixir. The Bangladesh epidemic. *BMJ* 1995; 311:88–91.

**1990: Jos University Hospital, Nigeria**

Forty-seven children died from diethylene-glycol–contaminated acetaminophen syrup.

Okuonghae HO, Ighogboja IS, et al. Diethylene glycol poisoning in Nigerian children.
*Ann Trop Paediatr* 1992; 12(3):235–238.

**1986: Bombay, India**

Fourteen deaths were documented from diethylene glycol contamination after
treatment for head injuries and glaucoma.

Pandys SK. An unmitigated tragedy. *BMJ* 1988; 297:117–199.

**1969: Capetown, South Africa**

Seven deaths resulted from diethylene-glycol–contaminated sedative elixirs.

Bowie MD, McKenzie D. Diethylene glycol poisoning in children. *South Afr Med J*
1972; 46:931–934.

**1937: Oklahoma, Illinois, and South Carolina**

Diethylene glycol was used as a solvent in the formulation of sulfanilamide,
an early antibiotic. Three hundred fifty-three people took the drug and 105
died (34 children, 71 adults).

Calvary HO, Klumpp TG. The toxicity for human beings of diethylene glycol with
sulfanilamide. *South Med J* 1939; 32:1105–1109.

## N,N-Diethyl-m-Toluamide (DEET)

**August 1989: New York City, New York**

Four young boys, aged 3–7 years, as well as a 29-year-old male, experienced
generalized seizures temporarily associated with the topical use of DEET as
an insect repellant.

Ferrer A, Cabral R. Recent epidemics of poisoning by pesticides. *Toxicol Lett* 1995;
82–83:55–63.

## Diethylstilbestrol (DES)

**1940–1971: USA**

DES was used to treat threatened or habitual abortions; as many as 10 million
American received DES during pregnancy or were exposed in utero. Adverse health effects associated with DES exposure included increased risk
of breast cancer (in DES mothers) and reproductive anomalies (in DES
daughters). Use of DES during pregnancy was prohibited in 1971.

Giusti RM, Iwamoto K, Hatch EE. Diethylstilbestrol revisited: a review of the long-term health effects. *Ann Intern Med* 1995; 122(10):778–788.

## Diethyltin Diiodide

### *1950s*

Diethyltin diiodide was used in the treatment of staphylococcal skin infections, which resulted in an epidemic of neurologic disease. One hundred two people died and hundreds of patients suffered permanent sequelae.

Raffle PAB, Lee WR, McCallum RI, Murray R, eds. *Hunter's Diseases of Occupations*, 7th ed. Boston: Little, Brown; 1987; pp. 310–311.

## Dimethylaminopropionitrile (DMAPN)

### *1980*

Exposure to dimethylaminopropionitrile in employees working in the manufacture of polyurethane foam was associated with neurogenic bladder dysfunction.

Hryhorczuk DO, Aks SE, Turk JW. Unusual occupational toxins. *Occup Med* 1992; 7(3):567–586.

Kreiss K, Wegman DH, et al. Neurological dysfunction of the bladder in workers exposed to dimethylaminopropionitrile. *JAMA* 1980; 243(8):741–745.

## Dimethylformamide (DMF)

### *1992: E.I. DuPont Plants, USA*

Exposure to dimethylformamide in workers has been related to hepatotoxicity, dermatitis, and disulfiram-like reactions to alcohol.

Hryhorczuk DO, Aks SE, Turk JW. Unusual occupational toxins. *Occup Med* 1992; 7(3):567–586.

## Dioxins

### *September 2004: Ukraine*

Dioxin poisoning is believed to be the cause of the disfiguring illness that afflicted Ukrainian opposition presidential candidate Viktor Yushchenko. Whether the poisoning was intentional or not, Yushchenko ingested the dioxins that led to a serum concentration 1,000 times above normal.

Dougherty, J. *Doctors: Yushchenko was poisoned.* CNN.com. December 1, 2004. Available at: http://www.cnn.com/2004/WORLD/europe/12/11/yushchenko.austria/.

### 1983: Times Beach, Missouri

Soil contamination after roadway work led to the evacuation of Times Beach's residents. There were no discernable health effects.

U.S. Environmental Protection Agency (EPA). *Superfund Redevelopment Program: Times Beach One-Page Summary 1988.* Available at: http://www.epa.gov/superfund/ programs/recycle/success/1-pagers/timesbch.htm.

### July 10, 1976: Seveso, Italy

An exothermic reaction initiated a factory explosion, releasing a cloud of chemicals into the air. The dispersion cloud included the dioxin 2,3,7,8-tetrachlorodibenzo-p-dioxin (TCDD), and affected a local population of roughly 40,000 people. At least two kg of TCDD were released from the factory, forcing the human evacuation of 80.3 hectares of land within the fallout zone. Demolition and earth scarification were performed on 53 hectares. Health effects have ranged from early to long-term: contact dermatitis and chloracne were reported within days of the incident, and cancer and reproductive effects have been observed in long-term studies on the Seveso population.

Pesatori AC, Consonni D, Bachetti S, et al. Short- and long-term morbidity and mortality in the population exposed to dioxin after the "Seveso accident." *Ind Health* 2003; 41(3):127–138.

Signorini S, Gerthoux PM, Dassi C, et al. Environmental exposure to dioxin: the Seveso experience. *Andrologia* 2000; 32:263–270.

Garagna S, Rubini PG, Redi CA. Recovering Seveso [letters]. *Science* 1999; 283(5406):1265.

### 1962–1971: Vietnam

Spraying Agent Orange may have exposed many to dioxins—95% of the blood samples from 43 residents of Bin Hoa City showed elevated levels of dioxin, used as a marker for Agent Orange. Dioxin was a contaminant of Agent Orange and was present in an average three parts per million.

Rhem KT. *Air Force Study Suggests Agent Orange, Diabetes Link.* American Forces Press Service. March 29, 2000. Available at: http://www.dod.mil/news/Mar2000/n03292000_20003294.html.

Schecter A, Pavuk M, et al. A follow-up: high level of dioxin contamination in Vietnamese from Agent Orange, three decades after the end of spraying. *J Occup Environ Med* 2002; 44(3):218–220.

### March 8, 1949: Nitro, West Virginia

Workers at the Monsanto Company were exposed to tetrachlorodibenzo-p-dioxin (TCDD) after an explosion of the trichlorophenol reactor. Approximately 121 workers developed chloracne. Other adverse health effects were reported.

Zack JA, Suskind RR. The mortality experience of workers exposed to tetra-chlorodibenzodioxin in a trichlorophenol process accident. *J Occup Med* 1980; 22(1):11–14.

Sweeney MH, Mocarelli P. Human health effects after exposure to 2,3,7,8-TCDD. *Food Addit Contam* 2000, 17(4):303–316.

## Dioxins and Polychlorinated Biphenyls (PCBs)

### January 1999: Belgium

Five hundred tons of PCB- and dioxin-contaminated feed were distributed to Belgian poultry farms and a lesser number of French, German, and Netherlands farms from the Flemish fat-melting company Verkest. Chicken edema disease was noted a month later; the health impact of exposure or ingestion to the Belgian human population is still under investigation.

van Larebeke N, Hens L, Schepens P, et al. The Belgian PCB and dioxin incident of January-June 1999: Exposure data and potential impact on health. *Environ Health Perspect* 2001; 109:265–273.

## Endosulfan

### March 1991: Sudan

Three hundred fifty villagers were affected and 31 people died when they ate bread made from contaminated maize flour at a local funeral. The flour had been treated with endosulfan as part of an anti-bird campaign in 1983.

Ferrer A, Cabral R. Recent epidemics of poisoning by pesticides. *Toxicol Lett* 1995; 82–83:55–63.

### 1988: Um Badda, Sudan

Sorghum coated with pesticide was baked into bread and served at a local funeral, resulting in the acute poisoning of 87 attendees.

Ferrer A, Cabral R. Recent epidemics of poisoning by pesticides. *Toxicol Lett* 1995; 82–83:55–63.

# Epichlorohydrin

### July 18, 1989: Germany

Adverse weather caused the cargo of the ship *Oostzee*, including 975 tons of epichlorohydrin, to shift and leak. The leak caused inhalation poisoning among the crew. All 14 of the crewmembers were hospitalized for 10 days.

Loostrom B (abstract). HELCOM Manual on Co-Operation in Response to Marine Pollution Within the Framework of the Convention on the Protection of the Marine Environment of the Baltic Sea Area (Helsinki Convention), vol 2, Annex 3. Case Histories. Last updated February 27, 2003.

*The OOSTZEE Case July/August 1989.* Waterways and Shipping Directorate North, Special Federal Unit for Marine Pollution Control, Deichstrasse 12, D-2190, Cuxhaven, Germany.

# Epinephrine, Racemic

### 1983

Racemic epinephrine was administered in a nursery instead of vitamin E, producing an epidemic that resembled neonatal sepsis.

Solomon SL, Ford-Jones EL, Baker WM. Medication errors with inhalant epinephrine mimicking an epidemic of neonatal sepsis. *N Engl J Med* 1984; 310:166–170.

# Ergonovine

Accidental administration of ergonovine maleate (ergometrine) to newborns resulted in encephalopathy, seizures, vascular disturbances, and respiratory failure.

Dargaville PA, Campbell NT. Overdose of ergometrine in the newborn infant: acute symptomatology and long-term outcome. *J Paediatr Child Health* 1998; 34(1):83–89.

Whitfield MF, Salfield SA. Accidental administration of Syntometrine in adult dosage to the newborn. *Arch Dis Child* 1980; 55(1):68–70.

Edwards WM. Accidental poisoning of newborn infants with ergonovine maleate. *Clin Pediatr* 1971; 12:257–260.

# Ethyldichlorosilane

### 1990: London, England, United Kingdom

An overturned truck resulted in a spill of ethyldichlorosilane, which forms hydrochloric acid and polysiloxane products when it comes into contact with water. Twelve people were hospitalized.

Thanabalasingham T, Beckett MW, Murray V. Hospital response to a chemical incident: report on casualties of an ethyldichlorosilane spill. *BMJ* 1991; 302:101–102.

# Ethylene Dibromide

### 1984

Two workers exposed to ethylene dibromide died after developing metabolic acidosis and hepatic and renal failure.

Letz GA, Pond SM, et al. Two fatalities after acute occupational exposure to ethylene dibromide. *JAMA* 1984; 252(17):2428–2431.

# Ethylene Dichloride (EDC)

### May 1994: Lake Charles, Louisiana

An ethylene dichloride spill from the Condea Vista facility led to widespread groundwater contamination.

Fairley P. Louisiana jury finds against Condea Vista in EDC leak. Week 0/29/97 159(41):19. State of Louisiana Department of Environmental Quality. Available at: http://www.deq.state.la.us/news/2000/n000601.pdf.

# Ethylene Glycol

### 1985–1987: New York and North Dakota

Two cases of ethylene glycol intoxication were related to contamination of water systems. One death resulted from exposure from a session of hemodialysis. The second case resulted from antifreeze contamination at a local firehall event.

Centers for Disease Control and Prevention (CDC). Schultz S, Kinde M, et al. Ethylene glycol intoxication due to contamination of water systems. *MMWR Morbid Mortal Wkly Rep* 1987; 36(36):611–614.

# 2-Ethylhexanol

### July 10, 1999: Shreveport, Louisiana

Approximately 19,000 gallons of 2-ethylhexanol leaked from railroad cargo into the Red River.

NOAA National Oceanic and Atmospheric Administration. Oil and Hazardous Materials Spill Reports–May 2001. Available at: http://archive.orr.noaa.gov/oilaids/spillreps/OHMRRF99.pdf.

# Fentanyl-Laced Heroin

### 1990: New York City, New York

An epidemic of deaths resulted from fentanyl-laced heroin labeled "Tango & Cash."

Fernando D. Fentanyl laced heroin. *JAMA* 1991; 265:2962.

## Fentanyl, 3-Methylfentanyl

### October 1988: Pittsburgh, Pennsylvania
An epidemic of increased deaths in intravenous drug users was associated with the use of "China White," 3-methylfentanyl.

Hibbs J, Perper J, Winek CL. An outbreak of designer drug-related deaths in Pennsylvania. *JAMA* 1991; 265(8):1011–1013.

### 1979: Orange County, California
An epidemic of deaths resulted secondary to heroin substitute, 3-methylfentanyl, known as "China White."

Kram TC, Cooper DA, Allen AC. Behind the identification of China White. *Anal Chem* 1981; 53(12):1379A–1386A.

## Fluoride

### June 2000: Karbi Anglong, India
Excessive fluoride levels were reported in local groundwater, affecting approximately 100,000 villagers in the remote region. Many suffered from severe anemia, stiff joints, restricted movements, mottled teeth, and kidney failure.

Times of India. UNI, June 2, 2000.

### August 1993: Mississippi
A faulty feed pump at one of the town's treatment plants allowed saturated fluoride solution to siphon into the ground reservoir. A large bolus of the overfluorinated water had been accidentally pumped into the town water supply, resulting in acute fluoride poisoning in more than 50 individuals.

Penman AD, Brackin BT, Embrey R. Outbreak of acute fluoride poisoning caused by a fluoride overfeed, Mississippi, 1993. *Public Health Rep* 1997; 112(5):403–409.

### May 1992: Alaska
As a result of excess fluoride in one of two public water systems in an Alaskan village, there was an outbreak of acute fluoride poisoning. An estimated 296 people were poisoned; one person died. Symptoms included nausea, vomiting, diarrhea, and/or numbness or tingling of the face or extremities.

Gessner BD, Beller M, et al. Acute fluoride poisoning from a public water system. *N Engl J Med* 1994; 330(2):95–99.

### 1977–1985: North Africa; Turkey to China
This area, including the Ethiopian Rift Valley system, has very high concentrations of fluoride in the drinking water and has led to fluoride poisoning of local residents.

Langford NJ, Ferner RE. Episodes of environmental poisoning worldwide. *Occup Environ Med* 2002; 59:855–860.

Haimanot RT, Fekadu A, Bushra B. Endemic fluorosis in the Ethiopian Rift Valley. *Trop Geogr Med* 1987; 39(3):209–217.

## Fluoride and Arsenic

### Xinjiang, China

Studies on the 102 water wells containing high levels of fluoride and arsenic in the Kuitun area indicated that the high content was associated with the environment. Drinking the water for a long period of time may be the cause of fluorosis and arsenism seen in the local population.

Wang G, Xiao B, Huang Y. Epidemiological studies on endemic fluorosis and arsenism in Xinjiang. [Chinese] *Zhonghua Yu Fang Yi Xue Za Zhi* 1995; 29(1):30–33.

## Fluoride, Sodium Fluoride

### 1942: Oregon

Approximately 263 patients became ill after eating scrambled eggs made with sodium fluoride instead of powdered milk. The pesticide was kept in the kitchen as an insecticide. Symptoms included nausea, vomiting, and bloody diarrhea, followed by collapse, paralysis, and muscle spasm. Forty-seven people died.

Ferrer A, Cabral R. Recent epidemics of poisoning by pesticides. *Toxicol Lett* 1995; 82–83:55–63.

## Gas Blast

### February 2004: Jixi, China

Twenty-four Chinese coal miners were found dead after a gas blast that occurred in a coal mine.

Reuters. *Twenty-four of 37 trapped Chinese miners found dead.* February 23, 2004.

## Gas, Liquified Natural (LNG)

### 1973: Staten Island, New York

A fire inside an empty LNG storage tank led to the deaths of 37 construction crewmen.

California Energy Commission. *LNG Safety.* Available at: http://www.energy.ca.gov/lng/safety.html.

### 1944: Cleveland, Ohio

A liquified natural gas (LNG) tank at the Cleveland peak-shaving plant failed
and spilled its contents into the street and storm sewer system. The fire and
explosion from the spillage resulted in 128 deaths.

California Energy Commission. *Liquified Natural Gas Safety.* Available at: http://www.
energy.ca.gov/lng/safety.html.

## Heroin, Pyrolysate

### 1980s: Amsterdam, Netherlands

Forty-seven patients developed spongiform leukoencephalopathy. Eleven
deaths were reported. Epidemiological studies traced the source to the
inhalatory use of heroin vapors.

Wolters EC, van Wijngaarden GK, et al. Leucoencephalopathy after inhaling 'heroin'
pyrolysate. *Lancet* 1982; 2:1233–1237.

## Hexachlorobenzene

### 1956: Turkey

Wheat seed treated with fungicide intended for planting was inadvertently
used for human consumption. As a result, 4,000 cases of porphyria cutanea
tarda were reported. Other symptoms, including hepatomegaly and hyper-
trichosis, were also reported.

Schmid R. Cutaneous porphyria in Turkey. *N Engl J Med* 1960; 263:397–398.

Peters HA, Johnson SAM, et al. Hexachlorobenzene-induced porphyria: effect of chela-
tion on the disease, porphyrin, and metal metabolism. *Am J Med Sci* 1966; 251:314–322.

## Hexachlorophene

### 1971–1972: USA and France

Disinfectant contaminated with hexachlorophene was associated with central
nervous system edema and demyelination.

World Health Organization. *Neurotoxicity Risk Assessment for Human Health: Principles and Approaches. Environmental Health Criteria 223.* Geneva, Switzerland, 2001.
Available at: http://www.inchem.org/documents/ehc/ehc/ehc223.htm#223230000.

Klaassen CD, Amdur MO, Doull J, eds. *Casarett and Doull's Toxicology: The Basic
Science of Poisons,* 3rd ed. New York: Macmillan; 1986.

Martin-Bouyer G, Lebreton R, et al. Outbreak of accidental hexachlorophene poisoning
in France. *Lancet* 1982; 1(8263):91–95.

# Hexane, n-Hexane

### 1980s: Taipei, Taiwan
Polyneuropathy among 59 press-proofing workers was related to exposure to n-hexane.

Wang JD, Chang YC, Kao KP. An outbreak of n-hexane induced polyneuropathy among press proofing workers in Taipei. *Am J Indust Med* 1986; 10:111–118.

### 1973: USA
Workers at a coated fabrics factory, exposed to n-hexane for more than six months, developed peripheral neuropathy.

World Health Organization. *Neurotoxicity Risk Assessment for Human Health: Principles and Approaches. Environmental Health Criteria 223.* Geneva, Switzerland, 2001. Available at: http://www.inchem.org/documents/ehc/ehc/ehc223.htm#223230000.

Billmaier D, Yee HT, Allan N, et al. Peripheral neuropathy in a coated fabrics plant. *J Occup Med* 1974; 16:665–671.

### 1969: Japan
Occupational exposure to n-hexane was related to central and peripheral neuropathy.

World Health Organization. *Neurotoxicity Risk Assessment for Human Health: Principles and Approaches. Environmental Health Criteria 223.* Geneva, Switzerland, 2001. Available at: http://www.inchem.org/documents/ehc/ehc/ehc223.htm#223230000.

Spencer PS, Schaumburg HH, Ludolph AC, eds. *Experimental and Clinical Neurotoxicology*, 6th ed. New York: Oxford University Press; 2000.

# Hexane, n-Hexane, and Methyl n-Butyl Ketone

### 1975–1977: Germany
Twenty-five cases of exposure to glue (sniffing) containing n-hexane and methyl n-butyl ketone were related to central and peripheral neuropathies.

World Health Organization. *Neurotoxicity Risk Assessment for Human Health: Principles and Approaches. Environmental Health Criteria 223.* Geneva, Switzerland, 2001. Available at: http://www.inchem.org/documents/ehc/ehc/ehc223.htm#223230000.

Spencer PS, Schaumburg HH, Ludolph AC, eds. *Experimental and Clinical Neurotoxicology*, 6th ed. New York: Oxford University Press; 2000.

## Hexane, 2-t-Butylazo-2-Hydroxy-5-Methylhexane
### 1979–1980: USA
Occupational exposure to lucel-7 containing 2-t-butylazo-2-hydroxy-5-methylhexane was associated with central, peripheral, and optic neuropathy in seven workers employed in the manufacture of reinforced plastic bathtubs.

World Health Organization. *Neurotoxicity Risk Assessment for Human Health: Principles and Approaches. Environmental Health Criteria 223.* Geneva, Switzerland, 2001. Available at: http://www.inchem.org/documents/ehc/ehc/ehc223.htm#223230000.

Horan JM, Kurt TL, et al. Neurologic dysfunction from exposure to 2-t-butylazo-2-hydroxy-5-methylhexane (BHMH): a new occupational neuropathy. *Am J Public Health* 1985; 75:513–517.

## Hexogen
### 1960–1970: Vietnam
During the Vietnam War, American soldiers intentionally ingested cyclotri-methylenetrinitramine (RDX) powder because it had presumed psychotropic effects. Neurotoxicity was reported.

Testud F, Glanclaude J-M, Descotes J. Acute hexogen poisoning after occupational exposure. *J Toxicol Clin Toxicol* 1996; 34(1):109–112.

Ketel WB, Hughes JR. Toxic encephalopathy with seizures secondary to ingestion of composition C-4. A clinical and electroencephalographic study. *Neurology* 1972; 22:871–876.

### 1962: USA
Five cases of hexogen intoxication were reported in an American explosive plant.

Testud F, Glanclaude J-M, Descotes J. Acute hexogen poisoning after occupational exposure. *J Toxicol Clin Toxicol* 1996; 34(1):109–112.

Kaplan AS, Berghout CF, Peczenik A. Human intoxication from RDX. *Arch Environ Health* 1965; 10:877–883.

### 1951: Germany
Seizures were reported in 56 workers of a German ammunitions plant related to their exposure to hexogen.

Testud F, Glanclaude J-M, Descotes J. Acute hexogen poisoning after occupational exposure. *J Toxicol Clin Toxicol* 1996; 34(1):109–112.

Vogel W. Hexogen poisoning in human beings. *Abl Arbeitsmed* 1951; 1:51–54.

### 1939–1942: Italy
Seventeen cases of hexogen poisoning were described in an Italian factory. Seizures and loss of consciousness were reported preceded by sleeplessness, confusion, and vertigo.

Testud F, Glanclaude J-M, Descotes J. Acute hexogen poisoning after occupational exposure. *J Toxicol Clin Toxicol* 1996; 34(1):109–112.

Barsotti M, Crotti G. Epileptic attacks as manifestations of industrial intoxication caused by trimethylenetrinitroamine (T4) [Italian]. *Med Lavoro* 1949; 40.

## Hydrazine (N$_2$H$_4$)
### 1970s–1980s
Exposure to hydrazine and its methylated derivatives has been related to respiratory, central nervous system, and liver toxicity.

Hryhorczuk DO, Aks SE, Turk JW. Unusual occupational toxins. *Occup Med* 1992; 7(3):567–586.

Sotaniemi E, Hirvonen J, Isomaki H, et al. Hydrazine toxicity in the human. Report of a fatal case. *Ann Clin Res* 1971; 3:30–33.

Dhennin C, Vesin L, Feauveaux J. Burns and the toxic effects of a derivative of hydrazine. *Burns* 1988; 14:130–134.

## Hydrocarbon
### February 28, 2004: Virginia
Three crew members were reported dead, and 18 others were missing after the explosion of a tanker off the coast of Virginia. The tanker was carrying 3.5 million gallons of ethanol, 200,000 gallons of fuel oil, and 53,000 gallons of diesel fuel.

CNN.com. *At least three dead in tanker explosion off Virginia.* February 29, 2004.

### July 23, 1984: Romeoville, Illinois
A monoethanolamine column ruptured, resulting in 17 deaths from the vapor cloud.

Mogul MG. Reduced corrosion in amine gas absorption column. *Hydrocarbon Processing: Plant Safety and Reliability: A Special Report.* October 1999.

Novokshchenov V. Proceedings of Fifth Middle East Corrosion Conference, Oct. 28–30, 1991, Manama, Bahrain; pp. 209–223.

**1955: Whiting, Indiana**

A refinery blast occurred, releasing hydrocarbons.

Riecher A. Whiting, Indiana. August 27, 1955. *Industrial Fire World.* Mar–Apr 2001.

## Hydrocarbon, Chlorinated Hydrocarbon Pesticide (Endrin)

### March 1988: Orange County, California

Five people experienced grand mal seizures 30 minutes to 1 hour after eating taquitos, a commercially prepared food bought at the same discount store within a 5-day period. Analysis revealed endrin contamination.

Centers for Disease Control and Prevention (CDC). Endrin poisoning associated with taquito ingestion—California. *MMWR Morbid Mortal Wkly Rep* 1989; 38(19):345–347.

### 1984: Pakistan

Sugar contaminated with endrin resulted in seizures in 192 people, with a 10% case-fatality rate.

Centers for Disease Control and Prevention (CDC). International notes: acute convulsions associated with endrin poisoning—Pakistan. *MMWR Morbid Mortal Wkly Rep* 1984; 33(49):687–688, 693.

### 1967: Doha, Qatar, Hofuf, and Saudi Arabia

Four outbreaks stemmed from the mixing and contamination of flour with endrin. A total of 874 people were admitted to the hospital, and 36 died.

Langford NJ, Ferner RE. Episodes of environmental poisoning worldwide. *Occup Environ Med* 2002; 59:855–860.

## Hydrocarbon, Polycyclic Aromatic Hydrocarbons (PAHs)

### 1910: Manchester, England, United Kingdom

Polycyclic aromatic hydrocarbons were associated with increased incidents of scrotal cancer in cotton textile mulespinners and tar and paraffin workers.

Goldblatt MW. Vesical tumours induced by compounds. *Br J Indust Med* 1949; 6:65.

Lee WR, McCann JK. Mulespinners cancer and the wool industry. *Br J Indust Med* 1967; 24:148.

### 1700s: England, United Kingdom

Exposure to polycyclic aromatic hydrocarbons led to an increase rate of scrotal cancer in chimney sweeps.

Goldberg ED. *Black Carbon in the Environment.* New York: Wiley-Interscience; 1985.

# Hydrochloric Acid (HCl)

### July 18, 2001: Baltimore, Maryland

A train carrying multiple hazardous chemicals including hydrochloric acid, glacial acetic acid, hydrofluoric acid, propylene glycol, tripropylene, and ethyl hexyl phthalate derailed and caught fire, blocking all major highways into Baltimore. There were several reported injuries and major evacuations and disruption of normal activities.

Effects of Catastrophic Events on Transportation System Management and Operations: Howard Street Tunnel Fire; Baltimore City, Maryland, July 18, 2001. Final report: Findings. Prepared by SAIC for USDOT, ITS Joint Program Office. Available at: http://www.itsdocs.fhwa.dot.gov/JPODOCS/REPTS_TE/13754.html.

### March 28, 2000: Oresund, Sweden

A collision of the tanker *Martina* and the cargo ship *Werder Bremen* resulted in 600 tons of 30% hydrochloric acid sinking a few hours later. Five crewmen died.

Molitor E. HELCOM Manual on Co-operation in Response to Marine Pollution Within the Framework of the Convention on the Protection of the Marine Environment of the Baltic Sea Area (Helsinki Convention), vol 2, Annex 3. Case Histories [abstract]. Last updated February 27, 2003.

# Hydrofluoric Acid

### October 1987: Texas

A leak from a petrol plant caused the evacuation of 3,000 people, with more than 1,000 people seeking medical attention. One hundred people were hospitalized. No deaths were reported.

Wing JS, et al. Acute health effects in a community after a release of hydrofluoric acid. *Arch Environ Health* 1991; 46:155.

# Hydrogen Cyanide

### 1990: Buenos Aires, Argentina

Thirty-five prisoners died in a polyurethane-mattress fire from the inhalation of hydrogen cyanide.

Ferrari LA, Arado MG, Giannuzzi L, et al. Hydrogen cyanide and carbon monoxide in blood of convicted dead in a polyurethane combustion: a proposition for the data analysis. *Forensic Sci Int* 2001; 121(1-2):140–143.

# Hydrogen Sulfide (H$_2$S)

### January 16, 2002: Pennington, Alabama
Several people were exposed to hydrogen sulfide gas from a hydrogen-sulfide leak in a sewer manway at the Georgia-Pacific Naheola mill. Two construction contractors were killed. Eight others were injured.

U.S. Chemical Safety and Hazard Investigation Board. Investigation Digest. Georgia-Pacific Hydrogen Sulfide Release. Available at: http://www.csb.gov/completed_investigations/docs/CSB_GeorgiaPacificFINAL.pdf.

### 1993: Japan
Three men died after falling into an artificial lake contaminated with hydrogen sulfide. A fourth survived. High levels of hydrogen sulfide were detected in the victims' tissues at autopsy.

Kimura K, Hasegawa M, et al. A fatal disaster case based on exposure to hydrogen sulfide—an estimation of the hydrogen sulfide concentration at the scene. *Forens Sci Int* 1994; 66:111–116.

### 1978: Chicago, Illinois
Sodium sulfide was released from a tannery tank, dispelling hydrogen sulfide gas. Seven people died.

Langford NJ, Ferner RE. Episodes of environmental poisoning worldwide. *Occup Environ Med* 2002; 59:855–860.

### April 12, 1971: Rosiclare, Illinois
Seven people died from hydrogen-sulfide asphyxiation at the Barnett Complex Mine, a flurospar plant.

CDC and NIOSH Safety and Health Research. *Historical Mining Disasters*. Available at: http://www.cdc.gov/niosh/mining/statistics/discoal.htm. Accessed September 21, 2005.

# Intralipid

### 1979
Three patients died after receiving intravenous nutrition with fat emulsions (20% Intralipid). Postmortem studies revealed milky white, shiny, clotted lumps in the heart with a fatty acid composition resembling fat emulsions.

Hessov I, Melsen F, Haug A. Postmortem findings in three patients treated with intravenous fat emulsions. *Arch Surg* 1979; 114(1):66–68.

# Isoniazid, Isonicotinic Acid Hydrazide (INH)

### 1970: Washington, D.C.

Approximately 2,321 Capitol Hill employees were started on isoniazid therapy after converting their PPD status (purified protein derivative). Nineteen of these patients developed hepatitis and two died of fulminant hepatic failure.

Garibaldi RA, Drusin RE, et al. Isoniazid-associated hepatitis: report of an outbreak. *Am Rev Respir Dis* 1972; 106:357–365.

# Lead

### 1998: Australia

Lead poisoning occurred in a married couple who drank Kombucha tea from a ceramic pot. It was postulated the tea acids eluted the lead from the glaze pigment.

Phan TG, Estell J, et al. Lead poisoning from drinking Kombucha tea brewed in a ceramic pot. *Med J Aust* 1998; 169(11-12):644–646.

### 1994: Hungary

Ingestion of lead-contaminated paprika led to symptoms, including anemia and colic, in 53 patients.

Kakosy T, Hudak A, Naray M. Lead intoxication epidemic caused by ingestion of contaminated ground paprika. *J Toxicol Clin Toxicol* 1996; 34(5):507–511.

### 1975: El Paso, Texas and Kellogg, Idaho

Children living close to smelters were found to have elevated blood lead levels.

Landrigan PJ, et al. Epidemic lead absorption near an ore smelter: the role of particulate lead. *N Engl J Med* 1975; 292:123.

### 1846: Canada

Lead from soldered cans contaminated foodstuffs in the Franklin expedition to the Canadian Arctic, and may have contributed to the failure of the expedition.

Was the ill-fated Franklin expedition a victim of lead poisoning? *Nutr Rev* 1989; 47(10):322–323.

Beattie O, Geiger J. *Frozen in Time: The Fate of the Franklin Expedition*. Vancouver, BC, Canada: Greystone Books; 2000.

### 18th and 19th Centuries: England, United Kingdom

Lead poisoning has been implicated as the cause of gout in the noble and
aristocratic social classes. Consumption of port during this time period
was paralleled by a high incidence of gout. Lead levels in fortified wines
bottled between 1770 and 1820 were as high as 300 to 1,900 μg/L.

Phan TG, Estell J, et al. Lead poisoning from drinking Kombucha tea brewed in a
ceramic pot. *Med J Aust* 1998; 169(11-12):644–646.

### 1767: Devonshire, England, United Kingdom

Cider contaminated with lead caused colic, and was later found to be associated
with gout in the same episode.

Waldron HA. The Devonshire colic. *J Hist Med* 1970; 25:38.

### AD 193 : Rome, Italy and Europe

During the reign of the Roman Empire, gout pandemics were reported
among the aristocrats. These outbreaks have been linked to chronic lead
poisoning from contaminated wines. The Roman wines contained a
boiled-down grape syrup called sapa that was simmered in a lead pot or
a lead-lined copper kettle. Modern attempts to prepare sapa according to
ancient recipes have produced lead levels of 240 to 1000 mg/L.

Phan TG, Estell J, et al. Lead poisoning from drinking Kombucha tea brewed in a
ceramic pot. *Med J Aust* 1998; 169(11-12):644–646.

Nriagu JO. Saturnine gout among Roman aristocrats. Did lead poisoning contribute to
the fall of the Empire? *N Engl J Med* 1983; 308(11):660–663.

## Lead, Tetraethyl

### 1946: England, United Kingdom

Exposure to tetraethyl lead in workers cleaning gasoline tanks was related to
encephalopathy.

World Health Organization. *Neurotoxicity Risk Assessment for Human Health: Principles and Approaches. Environmental Health Criteria 223.* Geneva, Switzerland, 2001.
Available at: http://www.inchem.org/documents/ehc/ehc/ehc223.htm#223230000.

Cassells DAK, Dodds EC. Tetra-ethyl lead poisoning. *BMJ* 1946; 2:4479–4483.

### 1924: USA

Occupational exposure to tetraethyl lead resulted in psychosis.

World Health Organization. *Neurotoxicity Risk Assessment for Human Health: Principles and Approaches. Environmental Health Criteria 223.* Geneva, Switzerland, 2001. Available at: http://www.inchem.org/documents/ehc/ehc/ehc223.htm#223230000.

Rosner D, Markowitz G. A "gift of God"? The public health controversy over leaded gasoline during the 1920s. *Am J Publ Health* 1985; 75:344–352.

## Lead, Tetraethyl, and Tetramethyl

### July 14, 1974: Strait of Otranto, Italy

A collision between the *Cavtat* and the *Lady Rita* resulted in 400 drums of tetraethyl and tetramethyl lead sinking to the seafloor. In 1977, salvage commenced to recover the drums.

Loostrom B. HELCOM Manual on Co operation in Response to Marine Pollution Within the Framework of the Convention on the Protection of the Marine Environment of the Baltic Sea Area (Helsinki Convention), vol 2, Annex 3. Case Histories [abstract]. Last updated February 27, 2003.

Tiravanti G, Boari G. Potential pollution of a marine environment by lead alkyls: the *Cavtat* incident. *Environ Sci Tech* 1979; 13(7):849–854.

## L-Tryptophan Contamination (Eosinophilia-Myalgia Syndrome)

### 1989: USA

Several thousand cases of eosinophilia-myalgia syndrome and 36 deaths were linked to the ingestion of l-tryptophan produced by the Japanese company Showa Denko.

Stutsker L, Hoesly FC, et al. EMS associated with exposure to tryptophan from a single manufacturer. *JAMA* 1990; 264:213–217.

Hertzman PA, Blevins WL, et al. Association of the eosinophilia-myalgia syndrome with the ingestion of tryptophan. *N Engl J Med* 1990; 322(13):869–873.

## Magnesium (Mg)

### December 2003: Garfield Heights, Ohio

A magnesium fire at the Garfield Alloys industrial plant forced the evacuation of 30 to 40 local residents within a quarter-mile of the plant.

Milicia J. The Associated Press. *Magnesium fire in Ohio diminishing.* December 30, 2003.

## Manganese (Mn)

### 1950s: Morocco

Exposure to manganese was associated with a Parkinsonian-like syndrome in miners.

World Health Organization. *Neurotoxicity Risk Assessment for Human Health: Principles and Approaches. Environmental Health Criteria 223*. Geneva, Switzerland, 2001. Available at: http://www.inchem.org/documents/ehc/ehc/ehc223.htm#223230000.

Spencer PS, Schaumburg HH, Ludolph AC, eds. *Experimental and Clinical Neurotoxicology*, 6th ed. New York: Oxford University Press; 2000.

## Mercurous Nitrate

### 1800s: New Jersey

Mercurous nitrate, used in the felting process of the hatting industry, led to mercurialism in exposed workers.

Wedeen RP. Were the hatters of New Jersey "mad?" *Am J Indust Med* 1989; 16:225.

## Mercury (Hg)

### Amazon Basin

The Brazilian Amazon basin is a major site of gold mining and refining, which uses elemental mercury. The use of mercury has led to a significant increase of mercury concentrations in miners and the local fishing population.

Langford NJ, Ferner RE. Episodes of environmental poisoning worldwide. *Occup Environ Med* 2002; 59:855–860.

Epstein PR. Mercury poisoning. *Lancet* 1991; 337:1344.

### 2000: New York City, New York

Nine children and their mother were exposed to mercury vapors that were traced to a vial of metallic mercury that was associated with the practice of Santeria, an Afro-Caribbean religion.

Forman J, Moline J, Cernichiari E, et al. A cluster of pediatric metallic mercury exposure cases treated with meso-2, 3-dimercaptosuccinic acid (DMSA). *Environ Health Perspect* 2000; 108(6):575–577.

### 1980: Buenos Aires, Argentina

A large outbreak of acrodynia (mercury poisoning) occurred in children exposed to commercially laundered diapers containing a mercurial antibacterial agent.

Boyd A, Seger D, et al. Mercury exposure and cutaneous disease. *J Am Acad Dermatol* 2000; 43:81–90.

Astalfi A, Goello C. Monitereo Biologico: Proceedings of Academia Nacional de Medicino de Buenos Aires Conference: November 3, 1981; Buenos Aires, Argentina.

### 1950s: Minimata Bay, Japan

Mercuric compounds were used as catalysts by the Chisso Corporation, and subsequently dumped into the bay. The factory effluent contained mercuric chloride, which was concentrated and biotransformed within the Bay's fish population. Local villagers ingested these fish and developed symptoms of ataxia, and impairment of speech, hearing, and gait. More than 2,000 patients were diagnosed with "Minamata disease."

Langford NJ, Ferner RE. Episodes of environmental poisoning worldwide. *Occup Environ Med* 2002; 59:855–860.

### 1920s–1950s: England, United Kingdom; Australia; and USA

Calomel, or "sweet mercury," was recognized to cause mercury poisoning in the 1940s, when calomel-based teething powders caused "pink disease" (acrodynia) among infants and children. Although banned in the United States, they are still used in parts of the world such as southeast Asia.

Wooltorton E. Facts on mercury and fish consumption. *CMAJ* 2002; 167(8):897.

Dally A. The rise and fall of pink disease. *Soc Hist Med* 1997; 10(2):291–304.

Boyd A, Seger D, et al. Mercury exposure and cutaneous disease. *J Am Acad Dermatol* 2000; 43:81–90.

Chopra A, Doiphide VV. Ayurvedic medicine: core concept, therapeutic principles, and current relevance. *Med Clin North Am* 2002; 86(1):75–89.

## Metam-Sodium

### 1991: Mount Shasta, California

A train derailment led to a release of 75,700 liters of a 37% aqueous solution of metam-sodium (sodium methyl dithiocarbamate, a soil fumigant) into the Sacramento River.

Wang PF, Mill T, et al. Fate and transport of metam spill in Sacramento River. *J Environ Engineer* 1997; 123(7):704–712.

# Methanol

### June 2005: Machakos District, Kenya
At least 48 people died from drinking home-distilled alcohol laced with methanol. The methanol may have been added to the alcohol to make it more potent. An additional 84 cases of suspected methanol poisoning were reported. Three of the patients lost their eyesight and another five developed eye complications. Approximately 105 liters of the alcohol were confiscated by officials and four people arrested.

International Society for Infectious Diseases. ProMED-mail. *Methanol Poisoning, Fatal—Kenya.* Available at: http://www.escribe.com/medicine/occenvmed/m21623. html. Accessed August 4, 2002.

*KENYA: Contaminated alcohol kills 48 near Nairobi.* IRINnews.org: UN Office for the Coordination of Humanitarian Affairs. Available at: http://www.irinnews.org/report. asp?ReportID=47830&SelectRegion=East_Africa&SelectCountry=KENYA.

### 2000: Kenya
More than 100 people died after drinking alcohol contaminated with methanol. The alcohol was called "Kumi Kumi" because it cost 10 Kenyan shillings. This was the largest outbreak of methanol poisoning to date.

International Society for Infectious Diseases. ProMED-mail. *Methanol Poisoning, Fatal—Kenya.* Available at http://www.escribe.com/medicine/occenvmed/m21623. html. Accessed August 4, 2002.

### 1998: Cambodia
Rice wine contaminated with methanol led to 60 deaths and more than 400 illnesses. Fomepizole was emergently imported in the area to treat the victims.

Wax PM. Toxicologic plagues and disasters in history. In: Goldfrank LR, ed. *Goldfrank's Toxicologic Emergencies,* 7th ed. New York: McGraw-Hill; 2002; pp. 23–34.

*Cambodian mob kills two Vietnamese in poisoning hysteria.* Deutsche Presse-Agentur, September 4, 1998.

### October 17, 1994: Lethbridge, Alberta, Canada
Six railroad cars containing methanol derailed, releasing the methanol into the local environment. Two hundred residents were evacuated.

Public Safety and Emergency Preparedness Canada. *Canadian Disaster Database.* Available at: http://www.psepc=sppcc.gc.ca/res/em/cdd/search=en.asp. Accessed September 21, 2005.

### 1992: Cuttack, India
One hundred sixty-two people died and an additional 228 were hospitalized after ingesting liquor contaminated with methanol.

Wax PM. Toxicologic plagues and disasters in history. In: Goldfrank LR, ed. *Goldfrank's Toxicologic Emergencies*, 7th ed. New York: McGraw-Hill; 2002; pp. 23–34.

*Tainted liquor kills 162, sickens 228.* Los Angeles Times; May 10, 1992.

### 1991: New Delhi, India
Antidiarrhea medication contaminated with methanol led to more than 200 deaths.

Wax PM. Toxicologic plagues and disasters in history. In: Goldfrank LR, ed. *Goldfrank's Toxicologic Emergencies*, 7th ed. New York: McGraw-Hill; 2002; pp. 23–34.

Coll S. *Tainted foods, medicine make mass poisonings rife in India: Critics press for tougher inspection, more accurate labels.* Washington Post; December 8, 1991; p. A36.

### 1989: Baroda, India
One hundred deaths and two hundred illnesses occurred as a result of contaminated moonshine.

Wax PM. Toxicologic plagues and disasters in history. In: Goldfrank LR, ed. *Goldfrank's Toxicologic Emergencies*, 7th ed. New York: McGraw-Hill; 2002; pp. 23–34.

### 1979: Michigan
One hundred fifty inmates of a southern Michigan prison stated that they drank moonshine contaminated with methanol; 50 samples were confirmed by laboratory analysis.

Swartz RD, Millman RP, et al. Epidemic methanol poisoning: clinical and bio analysis of a recent episode. *Medicine* 1981; 60:373–382.

### 1951: Atlanta, Georgia
Bootleg whiskey contaminated with methanol resulted in 3,232 poisonings and 41 deaths.

Bennet IL, Pary FH, et al. Acute methanol poisoning: a review based on experiences in an outbreak of 323 cases. *Medicine* 1953; 32:431–436.

Swartz RD, et al. Epidemic methanol poisoning: clinical and biochemical analysis of a recent episode. *Medicine (Baltimore)* 1981; 60(15):373–382.

## Methomyl and Propanil

Eleven workers at a pesticide factory were hospitalized after they showed signs of methomyl intoxication. Their symptoms included blurred vision or papillary constriction. Five of the hospitalized workers were in the packaging department and worked the most with methomyl. In addition, 17 production workers at the plant developed chloracne after exposure to propanil and dichloroaniline.

Morse DL, Baker EL Jr, Kimbrough RD, Wisseman CL III. Propanil-chloracne and methomyl toxicity in workers of a pesticide manufacturing plant. *Clin Toxicol* 1979; 15(1):13–21.


## Methyl Alcohol

### *March 2005: Istanbul, Turkey*

At least 19 people died after ingesting fake Turkish raki, and an additional 29 were treated for poisoning. Raki, a national drink in Turkey, is a strong aniseed-flavored alcohol served in bars and restaurants. The imitation raki was thought to have come from a makeshift distillery; it contained 57% to 97% methyl alcohol, whereas genuine raki contains 0.15% methyl alcohol.

CNN.com and Reuters Ltd. *More Killed by Fake Turkish Liquor.* March 6, 2005. Available at: http://www.cnn.com/2005/WORLD/europe/03/06/turkey.raki.reut/index.html.


## Methylenedianiline

### *1965: Epping, England, United Kingdom*

Food products contaminated with methylenedianiline led to liver damage in 84 people. Biopsies revealed both parenchymal and biliary damage.

Koppelman H, Robertson MH, Saunders PG. The Epping jaundice. *BMJ* 1966; 1:514.


## Methyl Isocyanate (MIC)

### *December 1984: Bhopal, India*

Forty tons of methyl isocyanate were released from the Union Carbide plant. A reported 3,849 people were killed and 20,000 injured. The injuries included eye damage, pulmonary edema, spontaneous abortions, stillbirths, and fetal abnormalities.

U.S. News and World Report 1994; 117(22):14.

Union Carbide Chronology Web site. Copyrighted 2001; Nov. 16, 1990. Available at: http://www.bhopal.com/review.htm.

Hryhorczuk DO, Aks SE, Turk JW. Unusual occupational toxins. *Occup Med* 1992; 7(3):567–586.

## Methylmercury

### *1971–1972: Iraq*

Approximately 6,530 people were hospitalized, 459 died, and 49 children developed neurological symptoms including ataxia, weakness, and visual and sensory changes when they ingested bread contaminated with methylmercury.

Amin-zaki L, Majeed MA, et al. Methylmercury poisoning in Iraqi children: clinical observations over two years. *Br Med J* 1978; 1(6113):613–616.

Bakir F, et al. Methylmercury poisoning in Iraq. *Science* 1973; 181:230.

### *1969: USA*

Grain contaminated with methylmercury led to multiple central and peripheral nervous system effects.

World Health Organization. *Neurotoxicity Risk Assessment for Human Health: Principles and Approaches. Environmental Health Criteria 223.* Geneva, Switzerland, 2001. Available at: http://www.inchem.org/documents/ehc/ehc/ehc223.htm#223230000.

Pierce PE, Thompson JF, Hikaskcy WH, Nickey LN, Barthel WF, Hinman AR. Alkyl mercury poisoning in humans. Report of an outbreak. *JAMA* 1972; 220:1439–1442.

## Methyl-4-Phenyl-1,2,5,6-Tetrahydropyridine (MPTP)

### *1982: San Jose, California*

Four people developed marked parkinsonism after using the illicit drug MPTP intravenously. The drug contained small amounts of l-methyl-4-phenyl-propionoxy-piperidine (MPPP). Severe bradykinesia caused these patients to be labeled "frozen addicts." MPTP is a potent neurotoxin.

Uhl GR, Javitch JA, et al. Normal MPTP binding in Parkinsonian substantial nigra: evidence for extraneuronal toxin conversion in human brain. *Lancet* 1985; 1(8435): 956–957.

Langston JW, Ballard P, et al. Chronic Parkinsonism in humans due to a product of meperidine-analog synthesis. *Science* 1983; 219(4587):979–980.

## Methyl Tert-Butyl Ether (MTBE)

### November 1992: Fairbanks, Alaska

Two hundred residents experienced symptoms of headache, dizziness, eye irritation, burning of the nose and throat, disorientation, and nausea possibly related to the use of MTBE in the gasoline.

U.S. Geological Survey. *Occurrence of MTBE Fact Sheet.* Available at: http://sd.water. usgs.gov/nawqa/pubs/factsheet/fs114.95/fact.html.

Gordian ME, Huelsman MD, Brecht ML, Fisher DG. Health effects of methyl tertiary butyl ether (MTBE) in gasoline in Alaska. *Alaska Med* 1995; 37(3):101–103, 119.

## B-Naphthylamine

### 1900s: USA and India

B-Naphthylamine, used in the dye industry, resulted in an increase in bladder cancer in exposed workers.

Goldblatt MW. Vesical tumours induced by compounds. *Br J Indust Med* 1949; 6:65–81.

## Natural Gas Explosion

### June 2, 2003: Tyler County, Texas

A spark from a tanker truck caused a natural gas storage facility to explode. Thirteen storage tanks were involved in the fire. No deaths were reported.

U.S. Chemical Safety and Hazard Investigation Board. Incident Reports Center. Available at: http://www.csb.gov/circ. Accessed June 24, 2003.

## Nickel

### 1997

Twenty-three dialysis patients suffered nickel intoxication when leaching of a nickel-plated stainless-steel water-heater tank contaminated the dialysate. Symptoms included nausea, vomiting, weakness, headache, and palpitations. There was spontaneous symptom remission approximately 3 to 13 hours after dialysis.

Webster JD, Parker TF, et al. Acute nickel intoxication by dialysis. *Ann Intern Med* 1980; 92(5):631–633.

### 1980s

Contamination of drinking water in an electroplating plant resulted in the ingestion of drinking water contaminated with nickel sulfate and chloride by 32 workers. Twenty employees developed symptoms that included nausea, vomiting, diarrhea, headache, and cough.

Sunderman FW Jr, Dingle B, Hopfer SM, Swift T. Acute nickel toxicity in electroplating workers who accidentally ingested a solution of nickel sulfate and nickel chloride. *Am J Ind Med* 1988; 14(3):257–266.

### January 1969: Nagoya, Japan

Approximately 156 people at the Toa Gosei chemical plant were exposed to nickel carbonyl, with 137 of the exposed workers displaying symptoms of intoxication. Ninety-six of them were hospitalized, and four developed encephalopathy that resolved within three to five weeks without long-term sequalae.

Sunderman FW. A pilgrimage into the archives of nickel toxicology. *Ann Clin Laboratory Sci* 1989; 19(1):1–19.

### April 1953: Port Arthur, Texas

More than 100 workers at the Gulf oil refinery were exposed to nickel carbonyl during the repair of a reactor in one of the chemical plants. Thirty-one patients had to be hospitalized, and two of the workers died.

Sunderman FW. A pilgrimage into the archives of nickel toxicology. *Ann Clin Laboratory Sci* 1989; 19(1):1–19.

## Nicotine

### January 2003: Michigan

Approximately 1,700 pounds of nicotine-contaminated ground beef were recalled, prompted by complaints from people who became ill after ingesting the beef. A total of 92 people had symptoms of burning of the mouth, nausea, vomiting, and dizziness. A supermarket employee was arrested for poisoning the beef with Black Leaf 40, a pesticide containing nicotine.

Centers for Disease Control and Prevention (CDC). Nicotine poisoning after ingestion of contaminated ground beef—Michigan. *MMWR Morbid Mortal Wkly Rep* 2003; 52(18):413–416.

### 1992: Kentucky

Dermal exposure to nicotine caused "green tobacco sickness" in 47 tobacco workers in a five-county region. "Green tobacco sickness" is a form of nicotine poisoning that is related to direct nicotine contact (e.g., harvesting). Symptoms included weakness, nausea, vomiting, dizziness, abdominal cramps, headache, and difficulty breathing.

Ballard T, Ehlers J, Freund E, et al. Green tobacco sickness: occupational nicotine poisoning in tobacco workers. *Arch Environ Health* 1995; 50(5):384–390.

# Nitrogen (N)

### March 27, 1998: Hahnville, Louisiana

One worker at the Union Carbide Corp.'s Taft/Star manufacturing plant was
killed and another seriously injured when they were asphyxiated by nitrogen.

U.S. Safety and Hazard Investigation Board. CSB Investigation Information Page.
Union Carbide Corp. Nitrogen Asphyxiation Incident, Hahnville, LA, March 27, 1998.
Available at: http://www.csb.gov/index.cfm?folder=completed_investigations&page=
info&INV_ID=5.

# Nitrogen Tetroxide

### 1995: Bogalusa, Louisiana

An accidental tank-car implosion containing nitrogen tetroxide affected
4,000 people. Delayed development of severe pulmonary inflammation
was reported.

Lee C, Ryan M, et al. Nitrogen tetroxide abstract #99. *J Toxicol Clin Toxicol* 1996; 34(5).

# 2-Nitropropane

### 1987

Dermal exposure to 2-nitropropane in two construction workers resulted in
elevated serum hepatic aminotransferases and fulminant hepatic failure.

Hryhorczuk DO, Aks SE, Turk JW. Unusual Occupational Toxins. *Occup Med* 1992;
7(3):567–586.

Harrison R, Letz G, Pasternak G, Blanc P. Fulminant hepatic failure after occupational
exposure to 2-nitropropane. *Ann Intern Med* 1987; 107(4):466–468.

# Organophosphates

### 1989: California

Thirty-five workers became ill after harvesting a cauliflower field for approximately one hour. The field had been sprayed 20 hours earlier with the
organophosphate insecticides mevinphos and oxydemeton-methyl as well
as the carbamate methomyl. All members presented with cholinergic signs
and symptoms.

Ferrer A, Cabral R. Recent epidemics of poisoning by pesticides. *Toxicol Lett* 1995;
82–83:55–63.

Romero P, Barnett PG, Midtling JE. Congenital anomalies associated with maternal exposure to oxydementon-methyl. *Environ Res* 1989; 50(2):256–261.

## Organophosphates, Carbamates and Aldicarb

### 1992: Ireland
Thirty people became ill after eating cucumbers contaminated with aldicarb.

Ferrer A, Cabral R. Recent epidemics of poisoning by pesticides. *Toxicol Lett* 1995; 82–83:55–63.

### 1985: California and Oregon
Aldicarb, found in watermelons, resulted in cholinergic symptoms in more than 1,000 cases reported to state health departments. Symptoms included diarrhea, vomiting, lacrimation, salivation, miosis, and convulsions.

Green MA, et al. An outbreak of watermelon-borne pesticide toxicity. *Am J Public Health* 1987; 77:1431.

Langford NJ, Ferner RE. Episodes of environmental poisoning worldwide. *Occup Environ Med* 2002; 59:855–860.

## Organophosphates, Carbamates and Chloropyrifos

### 1986: California
Five office occupants developed symptoms after application of chlorpyrifos. The patients' symptoms were consistent with organophosphate intoxication.

Ferrer A, Cabral R. Recent epidemics of poisoning by pesticides. *Toxicol Lett* 1995; 82–83:55–63.

Hodgson MJ, Block GD, Parkinson DK. Organophosphate poisoning in office workers. *J Occup Med* 1986; 28(6):434–437.

## Organophosphates, Carbamates and Fonofos

### March 11, 1994: Cadiz, Spain
Nine attendees at a family dinner celebration developed vomiting, nausea, and visual problems from exposure to fonofos used on the hunting estate where the dinner birds originated.

Pena Gonzalez P, Perez-Rendon Gonzalez J, et al. Epidemic outbreak of acute food poisoning caused by pesticides. [Spanish] *Aten Primaria* 1996; 17(7):467–470.

## Organophosphates, Carbamates and Malathion

### 1994: Spain
Three members of a Spanish family became sick and died after ingesting
  fish coated with malathion instead of bread. Symptoms included nausea,
  vomiting, sweating, hypotension, and convulsions.

Ferrer A, Cabral R. Recent epidemics of poisoning by pesticides. *Toxicol Lett* 1995,
82–83:55–63.

### 1976: Pakistan
During the peak of the Pakistan malaria-control spraying program, there were
  2,800 reported cases of illness and five deaths associated with malathion
  formulations. The epidemic stemmed from exposure during a malaria
  eradication program.

Ferrer A, Cabral R. Recent epidemics of poisoning by pesticides. *Toxicol Lett* 1995;
82–83:55–63.

Spencer PS, Schaumburg HH, Ludolph AC, eds. *Experimental and Clinical Neurotoxicology*, 6th ed. New York: Oxford University Press; 2000.

World Health Organization. *Neurotoxicity Risk Assessment for Human Health: Principles and Approaches. Environmental Health Criteria 223.* Geneva, Switzerland, 2001.
Available at: http://www.inchem.org/documents/ehc/ehc/ehc223.htm#223230000.

## Organophosphates, Carbamates and Parathion

### 1986: Sierra Leone
Flour contaminated with parathion, a pesticide, led to the deaths of 21 people.

Langford NJ, Ferner RE. Episodes of environmental poisoning worldwide. *Occup
Environ Med* 2002; 59:855–860.

### August 1984: Tunica County, Mississippi
Seven siblings became ill and one died after the interior of their home was
  sprayed with methyl parathion. It was likely the children were exposed via
  ingestion and by inhalational and dermal contact.

Centers for Disease Control and Prevention (CDC). Epidemiologic notes and reports
organophosphate insecticide poisoning among siblings—Mississippi. *MMWR Morbid
Mortal Wkly Rep* 1984; 33(42):592–594.

### 1975: Jamaica

Flour used to make dumplings was found to be contaminated with parathion, leading to 17 deaths and 62 illnesses.

Langford NJ, Ferner RE. Episodes of environmental poisoning worldwide. *Occup Environ Med* 2002; 59:855–860.

## Organotin Compound

### 1954: France

Accidental oral intoxication of nearly 1,000 people occurred with an organotin compound.

World Health Organization. 1980. *Tin and organotin compounds: a preliminary review. Environmental Health Criteria 15.* WHO, Geneva, Switzerland. June 6, 2003. Available at: http://www.inchem.org/documents/ehc/ehc.ehc015.htm.

## Pancuronium

### 1975: Ann Arbor, Michigan

Deliberate administration of pancuronium resulted in an epidemic of respiratory and cardiac arrests.

Stross JK, Shasby M, Harlan WR. An epidemic of mysterious cardiopulmonary arrests. *N Engl J Med* 1976; 295:1107.

## Pentachlorophenol

### April–August 1967: St. Louis, Missouri

Nine infants became ill in a hospital nursery when diapers and bedding materials were washed with an antimildew agent that contained a high amount of sodium pentachlorophenate, which is the sodium salt of pentachlorophenol. The pentachlorophenol poisoning may have resulted from skin absorption of the salt residues. Two of the cases were fatal.

Robson AM, Kissane JM, et al. Pentachlorophenol poisoning in a nursery for newborn infants. *J Pediatr* 1969; 75:309–316.

Centers for Disease Control and Prevention (CDC). Pentachlorophenol poisoning in newborn infants—St. Louis, Missouri, April–August 1967. *MMWR Morbid Mortal Wkly Rep* 1999; 48(LMRK):91–94.

## Petroleum

### 1989: Avila Beach, California

In 1998, Unocal Oil Co. began an $18 million project to clean up a major oil spill that had been occurring for years. A business developer tested the soil in 1989 and found it to be contaminated. Underground pipeline leaks had saturated Avila Beach with approximately 400,000 gallons of crude oil, gasoline, and diesel over several decades. Many of the local residents had to be relocated.

Phuong Le. *Beach town forced to scrape away oil leak—and a chunk of its past.* Seattle Post-Intelligencer Reporter. August 10, 1999.

## Phenobarbital (Luminal)

### 1997: Rancho Santa Fe, California

Thirty-nine members of the cult Heaven's Gate committed suicide by ingesting alcohol and phenobarbitol and then placing plastic bags over their heads.

Drummond Ayres B Jr. *Families learn of 39 who died willingly.* New York Times. March 29, 1997.

### 1940–1941: USA

At least 82 people died from the therapeutic use of sulfathiazole that had been contaminated with phenobarbital. The contamination was attributed to an error during the tabletting process.

Wax PM. Toxicologic plagues and disasters in history. In: Goldfrank LR, ed. *Goldfrank's Toxicologic Emergencies*, 7th ed. New York: McGraw-Hill; 2002; pp. 23–34.

Swann JP. The 1941 sulfathiazole disaster and the birth of good manufacturing practices. *PDA J Pharm Sci Technol* 1999; 53:148–153.

## Phenol

### 1974–1991: USA, Wales, and Korea

Inadvertent spills of phenol into the local water supply were noted; the spills led to gastrointestinal symptoms such as nausea, vomiting, diarrhea, and abdominal pain.

Langford NJ, Ferner RE. Episodes of environmental poisoning worldwide. *Occup Environ Med* 2002; 59:855–860.

## Phenylpropanolamine (PPA)

### 2000: USA

PPA was withdrawn from the over-the-counter (OTC) market in 2000, after being available in many OTC cold and cough medications for decades. PPA production was halted after a case-control study showed that PPA use was an independent risk factor for hemorrhagic stroke.

Wax PM. Toxicologic plagues and disasters in history. In: Goldfrank LR, ed. *Goldfrank's Toxicologic Emergencies*, 7th ed. New York: McGraw-Hill; 2002; pp. 23–34.

Kernan WN, Viscoli CM, Brass LM, et al. Phenylpropanolamine and the risk of hemorrhagic stroke. *N Engl J Med* 2000; 343:1826–1832.

## Phosgene

### September 20, 1994: Yokohama, Japan

Phosgene was introduced into journalist Shouko Egawa's apartment by the Aum Shinrikyo cult through the mail slot while she slept. She was hospitalized for respiratory distress.

CBWInfo. *Factsheets on Chemical and Biological Warfare Agents*. Available at: http://www.cbwinfo.com//Pulmonary/CG.html.

## Phosphine (PH$_3$)

### August 1996: Los Angeles, California

Phosphine gas produced in association with methamphetamine production led to the deaths of 3 individuals.

Willers-Russo LJ. Three fatalities involving phosphine gas, produced as a result of methamphetamine manufacturing. *J Forensic Sci* 1999; 44(3):647–652.

### 1980

Two children and 29 crew members riding aboard a grain freighter became ill after inhaling the toxic fumigant phosphine over a 4-day period. Symptoms included headache, fatigue, nausea, vomiting, cough, and shortness of breath. One child died.

Hryhorczuk DO, Aks SE, Turk JW. Unusual Occupational Toxins. *Occup Med* 1992; 7(3):567–586.

Wilson R, Lovejoy FH, Jaeger RJ, Landrigan PL. Acute phosphine poisoning aboard a grain freighter. Epidemiologic, clinical, and pathological findings. *JAMA* 1980; 244(2):148–150.

### 1980s: India

Eight cases of phosphine poisoning were reported after patients ingested aluminum phosphide tablets as a suicide attempt. Symptoms included gastritis, change in mental status, respiratory failure, and hypotension. The patients ranged in age from 14 to 25 years. Six of the patients died.

Hryhorczuk DO, Aks SE, Turk JW. Unusual occupational toxins. *Occup Med* 1992; 7(3):567–586.

Misra UK, Tripathi AK, Pandey R, Bhargwa B. Acute phosphine poisoning following ingestion of aluminum phosphide. *Hum Toxicol* 1988; 7(4):343–345.

### India

Twenty-two workers responsible for the fumigation of stored grains reported symptoms that included cough, dyspnea, tightness of the chest, headache, numbness, and lethargy, as well as anorexia and epigastric pain after fumigation. Abnormal physical findings included bilateral diffuse rhonchi and absent ankle reflexes.

Hryhorczuk DO, Aks SE, Turk JW. Unusual occupational toxins. *Occup Med* 1992; 7(3):567–586.

Misra UK, Bhargava SK, et al. Occupational phosphine exposure in Indian workers. *Toxicol Lett* 1988; 42(3)257–263.

## Phosphine, Aluminum Phosphide

### July 27, 1984: Houston, Texas

During unloading of the Rio Neuquen, a container of aluminum phosphide exploded, killing one worker due to phosphine-gas exposure.

Loostrom B (abstract). HELCOM Manual on Co-operation in Response to Marine Pollution Within the Framework of the Convention on the Protection of the Marine Environment of the Baltic Sea Area (Helsinki Convention), vol 2, Annex 3. Case Histories. Last updated February 27, 2003.

Mark CG, et al. 1986 Hazardous Material Spills Conference: Proceeding: May 5–8, 1986; St. Louis, Missouri, USA; pp. 19–24.

## Phosphorus, Yellow

### 1999: Philippines

Health officials in the Philippines have been trying to place a ban on "watusi"— a popular Christmas firework—because it has caused the deaths of hundreds of children by phosphorus poisoning. Children are disabled or killed after mistaking the fireworks for candy and ingesting them. Watusi is made of yellow phosphorus, potassium chlorate, potassium nitrate, and trinitrotoluene. Watusi ingestion may also cause hepatotoxicity.

Wallerstein C. Christmas firework "sweets" kill hundreds of children. *BMJ* 1999; 319 (7219):1222.

Fernandez OU, Canizares LL. Acute hepatotoxicity from ingestion of yellow phosphorus-containing fireworks. *J Clin Gastroenterol* 1995; 21(2):139–142.

### 1800s: Europe

Yellow phosphorus, used in the production of matches, led to necrosis of the jaw termed "phossy jaw" in exposed workers.

Hughes JP, et al. Phosphorus necrosis of the jaw: a present day study. *Br J Indust Med* 1962; 19:83.

## Photochemical Smog (see Air Pollution)

## Polybrominated Biphenyls (PBBs)

### 1973: Michigan

Several hundred pounds of hexabrominated biphenyl flame retardant (Fire-master BP-6) were accidentally introduced into cattle feed. Thousands of animals died, and there was widespread human exposure from contact with contaminated feed and consumption of PBBs in dairy products. Ninety-five percent of all breast milk samples from the lower Michigan peninsula subsequently contained PBBs.

Carter LJ. Michigan's PBB incident: mix-up leads to disaster. *Science* 1976; 192:240–243.

Wolff MS, Anderson HA, Selikoff IJ. Human tissue burdens of halogenated aromatics in Michigan. *JAMA* 1982; 247:2112.

## Polychlorinated Biphenyls (PCBs)

### 1979: Yucheng, Taiwan

More than 2,000 people were sickened when cooking oil that was made from rice bran was contaminated with PCBs.

Guo YL, Yu ML, et al. Chloracne, goiter, arthritis, and anemia after polychlorinated biphenyl poisoning: 14-year follow up of the Taiwan Yucheng cohort. *Environ Health Perspect* 1999; 107(9):715–719.

Guo, YL, Ryan JJ, Lau BP, et al. Blood serum levels of PCBs and PCDFs in Yucheng women fourteen years after exposure to a toxic rice oil. *Arch Environ Contam Toxicol* 1997; 33(1):104–108.

Jones GRN. Polychlorinated biphenyls: where do we stand now? *Lancet* 1989; 2:791–794.

### 1968: Japan

The contamination of a particular lot of rice oil caused an illness called "Yusho" (rice oil disease). This occurred when heat exchange fluid that contained PCBs leaked from a heating pipe into the rice oil. Over 1,600 people developed chloracne, hyperpigmentation, increased liver cancer, and adverse reproductive effects.

Kuratsune M, Yoshimura T, et al. Epidemiologic study on Yusho, a poisoning caused by ingestion of rice oil contaminated with a commercial brand of polychlorinated biphenyls. *Environ Health Perspect* 1972; 1:119.

Buser HR, Rappe C, Gara A. Polychlorinated dibenzofurans (PCDFs) found in Yusho oil and in used Japanese PCB. *Chemosphere* 1978; 5:439.

## Polysorbate 80

A fatal syndrome characterized by acute tubular necrosis (ATN) with oxalate chrystallopathy and progressive intralobar cholestasis of the liver was seen in low birth-weight infants given total parenteral nutrition (TPN) containing polysorbate 80. Thirty-eight infants died.

Alade SL, Brown RE, Paquet A. Polysorbate 80 and E-ferol toxicity. *Pediatrics* 1986; 77(4):593–597.

Balistreri WF, Farrell MK, Bove KE. Lessons from the E-Ferol tragedy. *Pediatrics* 1986; 78(3):503–506.

## Polyvinyl Chloride (PVC)

### August 9, 1979: USA

Exposure to PVC resin fumes led to respiratory symptoms, headache, nausea, and syncope in 63 workers at a PVC-fabricating plant.

Froneberg B, Johnson PL, Landrigan PJ. Respiratory illness caused by overheating of polyvinyl chloride. *Br J Indust Med* 1982; 39:239–243.

### 1973, 1975: USA

PVC fumes have been implicated in "meat packers' " or "meat wrappers' asthma." The respiratory effects are caused by thermal degradation of PVC film, which releases chemical fumes.

Seaton A, Morgan WKC. Toxic Gases and Fumes. In: Morgan WKC, Seaton A, eds. *Occupational Lung Diseases*, 2nd ed. Philadelphia: Saunders; 1984; p. 629.

## Potassium Bromate

Approximately 816 people were affected in a food-poisoning outbreak associated with the use of potassium bromate as a flour additive.

Stewart TN. An outbreak of food-poisoning due to a flour improver, potassium bromate. *S Afr Med J* 1969; 43(8):200–202.

## Propofol

### June 1990–February 1993

Seven hospitals reported outbreaks of infection (both blood-borne and surgical-site) and acute febrile occurrences. The complications were traced to propofol exposure, a lipid-based anesthetic agent.

Bennet SN, McNeil MM, Bland LA, et al. Postoperative infections traced to contamination of an intravenous anesthetic, propofol. *N Engl J Med* 1995; 333(3):147–154.

## Quartz

### 1970s: Scotland, United Kingdom

Exposure to quartz at a Scottish colliery during drilling into sandstone resulted in rapid radiographic pulmonary changes. The colliery was closed in 1981.

Buchanan D, Miller BG, Soutar CA. Quantitative relations between exposure to respirable quartz and risk of silicosis. *Occup Environ Med* 2003; 60:159–164.

## Quinine-Adulterated Heroin

### 1979–1982: Washington, D.C.

Approximately 266 heroin-related deaths were associated with heroin preparations cut with quinine.

Centers for Disease Control and Prevention (CDC). Heroin-related deaths, District of Columbia, 1980–1982. *MMWR Morbid Mortal Wkly Rep* 1983; 32(25):321–324.

Ruttenber AJ, Luke JL. Heroin-related deaths: new epidemiologic insights. *Science* 1984; 226(4670):14–20.

### 1950–1960: New York City and Chicago

Users of quinine-adulterated heroin showed a significant increase in tetanus.

Cherubin CE. Epidemiology of tetanus in narcotic addicts. *N Y State J Med* 1970; 70(2):267–271.

Levinson AK, Marske RL, Shein MK. Tetanus in heroin addicts. *JAMA* 1955; 157: 658–660.

# Ricin

### July 28, 2004: Irvine, California

Two jars of baby food were found to be contaminated with trace amounts of ricin, a component naturally found in castor beans. This is a less toxic form of ricin than the purified, lethal form. The Food and Drug Administration analyzed the substance and concluded that it appeared to be the ground-up remnants of castor beans. It was not purified ricin, but the incident still raised concerns about food tampering. No injuries were reported and the contamination appeared to be confined to the Irvine area.

U.S. Food and Drug Administration. FDA Statement: *FDA Analyses Finds Ground Castor Beans—Not Purified Ricin—In Two Tampered Baby Food Jars in Irvine, California Case.* Department of Health and Human Services; 2004. Available at: http://www.fda.gov/bbs/topics/news/2004/NEW01097.html.

### 1978: London, England, United Kingdom

Georgi Markov was assassinated when ricin pellets were injected into him with the end of an umbrella. Markov was a Bulgarian dissident.

Newman C. Twelve toxic tales. *National Geographic*; May 2005.

# Scopolamine-Adulterated Heroin

### 1995–1996: New York City, Newark, Philadelphia, and Baltimore

Health departments and poison-control centers reported more than 325 cases of patients who developed anticholinergic manifestations after using heroin contaminated with scopolamine.

Centers for Disease Control and Prevention (CDC). Perrone J, Hamilton R, et al. Scopolamine poisoning among heroin users—New York City, Newark, Philadelphia, and Baltimore, 1995 and 1996. *MMWR Morbid Mortal Wkly Rep* 1996; 45(22):457–460.

# Selenium (Se)

### 1961–1964: Hubei Province, China

Endemic human selenosis was discovered in parts of the local population of Enshi County. At its peak, the morbidity was almost 50% in the 248 inhabitants of the five most heavily affected areas. This particular outbreak was precipitated by a drought that caused the rice crop to fail, forcing the residents to eat high-selenium vegetables and maize.

Yang GQ, Wang SZ, et al. Endemic selenium intoxication of humans in China. *Am J Clin Nutr* 1983; 37(5):872–881.

# Silica

### 1930s: West Virginia

An acute epidemic of silicosis occurred after the blasting of rock near Gauley Bridge, West Virginia (the Hawk's Nest Disaster). Four hundred drillers died, and disabilities were reported in the majority of surviving workers. Federal hearings determined that the blasting was conducted through rock that was more than 90% pure silica.

Cherniak MG. Historical perspectives in occupational medicine. Pancoast and the image of silicosis. *Am J Ind Med* 1990; 18(5):599–612.

# Sodium (Na)

### December 5, 1987: Northwestern Spain

A fire among the sodium freight containers aboard the *Cason* left 23 crew members dead.

Loostrom B (abstract). HELCOM Manual on Co-operation in Response to Marine Pollution Within the Framework of the Convention on the Protection of the Marine Environment of the Baltic Sea Area (Helsinki Convention), vol 2, Annex 3. Case Histories. Last updated February 27, 2003.

# Sodium Hypochlorite

### October 2001: Rhode Island

A bomb placed in an empty classroom by a student released chlorine gas upon explosion. Twenty-three people located in the vicinity had to be treated at a local hospital for respiratory irritation.

Centers for Disease Control and Prevention (CDC). Homemade chemical bomb events and resulting injuries—Selected states, January 1996–March 2003. *MMWR Morbid Mortal Wkly Rep* 2003; 52(28):622–664.

# Sodium Nitrite

### 2002: New York City, New York

Five members of the same family developed methemoglobinemia after sprinkling the contents from an imported bag labeled 'iodized table salt' on their food. The bag contained 100% pure sodium nitrite.

Centers for Disease Control (CDC). Methemoglobinemia following unintentional ingestion of sodium nitrite. *MMWR Morbid Mortal Wkly Rep* 2002; 51(29):639–642.

# Sodium Peroxide

### January 10, 1977: Bremerhaven, Germany
During cargo loading of the *Burgenstein*, a sodium peroxide spill resulted in a fire that killed three crewmen.

Loostrom B (abstract). HELCOM Manual on Co-operation in Response to Marine Pollution Within the Framework of the Convention on the Protection of the Marine Environment of the Baltic Sea Area (Helsinki Convention), vol 2, Annex 3. Case Histories. Last updated February 27, 2003.

*The BURGENSTEIN Case*, Waterways and Shipping Directorate North, Special Federal Unit for Marine Pollution Control. Deichstrasse 12, D-2190. Cuxhaven, Germany.

# Sulfur Dioxide

### November 16, 1995: Sudbury, Ontario, Canada
A cloud of sulfur dioxide was released accidentally from a copper refinery that passed over the nearby city. Hundreds of residents reported minor irritations, and a local hospital and clinic were evacuated.

Public Safety and Emergency Preparedness Canada. *Canadian Disaster Database*. Available at: http://www.psepc=sppcc.gc.ca/res/em/cdd/search=en.asp. Accessed September 21, 2005.

# Sulfuric Acid

### January 21, 1995: Hervey Junction, Quebec, Canada
Twenty-eight rail cars derailed, spilling sulfuric acid into Masketi Lake and the Towachiche River. All the vegetation and wildlife were destroyed, the lake was closed for recreation for eight years, and the river was closed for five years.

Public Safety and Emergency Preparedness Canada. *Canadian Disaster Database*. Available at: http://www.psepc=sppcc.gc.ca/res/em/cdd/search=en.asp. Accessed September 21, 2005.

# Tear Gas

### 1933: New York City, New York
Tear gas was released into the New York Stock Exchange's ventilation system.

Aguilera K. *Financial History*. Museum of American Financial History. Available at: http://www.financialhistory.org/fh/2002/74-1.htm.

# Tellurium

### 1940s

A group of foundry workers developed symptoms that included garlic odor of the breath and sweat, dry mouth, metallic taste, nausea, gastrointestinal disturbances, itchy skin, and decreased sweating after exposure to tellurium fumes.

Hryhorczuk DO, Aks SE, Turk JW. Unusual occupational toxins. *Occup Med* 1992; 7(3):567–586.

### 1920

Electrolytic lead refiners were exposed to fumes containing tellurium when the "slime" from the tanks was treated to recover silver. Symptoms included garlic odor of the breath and sweat, dry mouth, metallic taste, nausea, gastrointestinal disturbances, itchy skin, and decreased sweating.

Hryhorczuk DO, Aks SE, Turk JW. Unusual occupational toxins. *Occup Med* 1992; 7(3):567–586.

# Tetramethylenedisulfotetramine

### 2004: Tongchuan City, China

More than 70 students became ill after eating pancakes that had been intentionally poisoned with tetramethylenedisulfotetramine.

Whitlow KS, Belson M, Barrueto F, et al. Tetramethylenedisulfotetramine: old agent and new terror. *Ann Emerg Med* 2005; 45(6):609–613.

### December 2003: Yizhou, China

Seventy-six students were sickened from ingesting food that had been contaminated with tetramethylenedisulfotetramine.

Whitlow KS, Belson M, Barrueto F, et al. Tetramethylenedisulfotetramine: old agent and new terror. *Ann Emerg Med* 2005; 45(6):609–613.

### November 2003: Jiangsu Province, China

More than 30 students were sickened from ingesting food that had been contaminated with tetramethylenedisulfotetramine.

Whitlow KS, Belson M, Barrueto F, et al. Tetramethylenedisulfotetramine: old agent and new terror. *Ann Emerg Med* 2005; 45(6):609–613.

### 2003: Yueyang, China
More than 200 students were sickened from ingesting food that had been
contaminated with tetramethylenedisulfotetramine. The food had been
prepared at the school's dining hall.

Whitlow KS, Belson M, Barrueto F, et al. Tetramethylenedisulfotetramine: old agent
and new terror. *Ann Emerg Med* 2005; 45(6):609–613.

### 2002: Huangpo, China
Seventy children in Guangdong Province became ill after eating porridge that
had been intentionally poisoned with tetramethylenedisulfotetramine.

Whitlow KS, Belson M, Barrueto F, et al. Tetramethylenedisulfotetramine: old agent
and new terror. *Ann Emerg Med* 2005; 45(6):609–613.

### 2002: Nanjing, China
Approximately 400 people were sickened after ingesting food that was contaminated with tetramethylenedisulfotetramine. Thirty-eight of the poisoned individuals died as a result.

Whitlow KS, Belson M, Barrueto F, et al. Tetramethylenedisulfotetramine: old agent
and new terror. *Ann Emerg Med* 2005; 45(6):609–613.

### September 2002: Xi'an, China
A 17-year-old female restaurant worker poisoned the food with tetramine because her boss had withheld her wages. Five people died as a result of ingesting contaminated food.

Croddy E. Rat poison and food security in the People's Republic of China: focus on
tetramethylene disulfotetramine (tetramine). *Arch Toxicol* 2004; 78(1):1–6.

### August 2002: Tongchuan City, China
A man purchased tetramine in order to kill his wife and marry his mistress.
He poisoned the milk the couple had delivered to their residence, and
managed to administer a lethal dose a couple months later. However, the
man also poisoned 15 other residents via secondary contamination.

Croddy E. Rat poison and food security in the People's Republic of China: focus on
tetramethylene disulfotetramine (tetramine). *Arch Toxicol* 2004; 78(1):1–6.

### July 1991: Heibei Province, China
Seventy-eight people were sickened after ingesting rice contaminated with
tetramethylenedisulfotetramine, an odorless, tasteless rodenticide agent.

Guan FY, Liu YT, Luo Y, et al. GC/MS identification of tetramine in samples from
human alimentary intoxication and evaluation of artifical carbonic kidneys for the
treatment of the victims. *J Anal Toxicol* 1993; 17(4):199–201.

# Thalidomide

### 1960s–1970s: Worldwide

Thalidomide, used by pregnant women to treat morning sickness, led to more than 10,000 babies being born worldwide with serious birth defects. These defects were primarily limb malformations such as phocomelia and radial aplasia but also included heart, gastrointestinal, neurologic, genital, and facial abnormalities.

NTP Center for the Evaluation of Risks to Human Reproduction (CERHR). *Thalidomide.* May 20, 2002. Available at: http://cerhr.niehs.nih.gov/genpub/topics/thalidomide2-ccae.html. Accessed May 17, 2005.

Annas GJ, Elias S. Thalidomide and the *Titanic:* reconstructing the technology tragedies of the 20th century. *Am J Public Health* 1999; 89(1):98–101.

McFadyen RE. Thalidomide in America: a brush with tragedy. *Clin Med* 1976; 11:79.

# Thallium

### 1994: New York City, New York

Four people were poisoned with thallium-laced marzipan. All 4 patients recovered.

Meggs WJ, Hoffman RS, et al. Thallium poisoning from maliciously contaminated food. *J Toxicol Clin Toxicol* 1994; 32(6):723–730.

### 1992–1995: Iraq

More than 80 cases of confirmed thallium poisoning inflicted by the Iraqi government on dissidents was reported. In January 1995, former Iraqi officer Major Safa al-Battat was flown to the United Kingdom to receive treatment for thallium poisoning.

United Nations Commission of Human Rights: Report on the situation of human rights in Iraq. Submitted by the Special Rapporteur, Mr. Max van der Stoel, in accordance with Commission resolution 1995/76. March 4, 1996. E/CN.4/1996/61.

### 1988: Florida

Five members of a family were poisoned with thallium that was put in a soda can by a neighbor. One family member died.

Desenclos JC, Wilder MH, et al. Thallium poisoning: an outbreak in Florida, 1988. *South Med J* 1992; 85(12):1203–1206.

### 1931: California

The thallium-containing pesticide "Thalgrain" was dispersed over 10 California counties in order to curb ground-squirrel infestation, resulting in an outbreak of thallotoxicosis in humans.

Chamberlain PH, Stavinoha WB, Davis H, et al. Thallium poisoning. *Pediatrics* 1958; 22(6):1170–1182.

### 1920s–1930s: USA

Thallium used to treat ringworm in the 1920s to 1930s and resulted in 692 cases of thallium toxicity and 31 deaths.

Wax PM. Toxicologic plagues and disasters in history. In: Goldfrank LR, ed. *Goldfrank's Toxicologic Emergencies*, 7th ed. New York: McGraw-Hill; 2002; pp. 23–34.

Munch JC. Human thallotoxicosis. *JAMA* 1934; 102:1929–1934.

## Toxic Oil Syndrome

### May 1981: Spain

More than 20,000 people became ill and over 340 died from what became known as the "toxic oil syndrome," which linked the symptoms to consumption of contaminated cooking oil. The toxic agent has never been identified, but a derivative of analine has been purported.

Terracini B, ed. *Toxic Oil Syndrome: Ten Years of Progress*. World Health Organization Europe with Instituto de Salud Carlos III: Denmark; 2004.

Langford NJ, Ferner RE. Episodes of environmental poisoning worldwide. *Occup Environ Med* 2002; 59:855–860.

Baxter PJ. Major disasters: Britain's health services are poorly prepared. *BMJ* 1991; 302:61–62.

## Trichloroethylene (TCE)

### July 1979: Montgomery County, Pennsylvania

Approximately 1,900 gallons of TCE were released into ground and surface water from a pipe manufacturing plant. Of the 9 exposed workers, 7 reported symptoms of drowsiness, dizziness, or mental confusion.

Landrigan PJ, Kominsky JR, et al. Common-source community and industrial exposure to trichloroethylene. *Arch Environ Health* 1987; 42(6):327–332.

# Triethyltin Iodide

### 1954: France

An oral antibiotic, Stalinon, containing diethyltin diiodide for the treatment of superficial staphylococcal skin infections, was contaminated with triethyltin iodide. Two hundred seventeen cases were reported and more than 100 deaths occurred, largely due to complications from cerebral edema.

Stalinon: a therapeutic disaster. *BMJ* 1958; 1:515.

Hryhorczuk DO, Aks SE, Turk JW. Unusual occupational toxins. *Occup Med* 1992; 7(3):567–586.

# Triorthocresylphosphate (TOCP)

### 1988: Sri Lanka

Oil contaminated with TOCP was associated with peripheral neuropathies.

World Health Organization. *Neurotoxicity Risk Assessment for Human Health: Principles and Approaches. Environmental Health Criteria 223*. Geneva, Switzerland, 2001. Available at: http://www.inchem.org/documents/ehc/ehc/ehc223.htm#223230000.

Spencer PS, Schaumburg HH, Ludolph AC, eds. *Experimental and Clinical Neurotoxicology*, 6th ed. New York: Oxford University Press; 2000.

### 1959: Meknes, Morocco

TOCP-contaminated cooking oil caused more than 10,000 cases of induced paralysis.

Smith HV, Spalding JM. Outbreak of paralysis in Morocco due to ortho-cresyl phosphate poisoning. *Lancet* 1959; 2:1019–1021.

### 1937: South Africa

Contaminated cooking oil led to central and peripheral neuropathy.

World Health Organization. *Neurotoxicity Risk Assessment for Human Health: Principles and Approaches. Environmental Health Criteria 223*. Geneva, Switzerland, 2001. Available at: http://www.inchem.org/documents/ehc/ehc/ehc223.htm#223230000.

Spencer PS, Schaumburg HH, Ludolph AC, eds. *Experimental and Clinical Neurotoxicology*, 6th ed. New York: Oxford University Press; 2000.

### *1930s: Europe*

A drug contaminated with TOCP led to 60 cases of central and peripheral neuropathy.

World Health Organization. Neurotoxicity Risk Assessment for Human Health: Principles and Approaches. Environmental Health Criteria 223. Geneva, Switzerland, 2001. Available at: http://www.inchem.org/documents/ehc/ehc/ehc223.htm#223230000.

Spencer PS, Schaumburg HH, Ludolph AC, eds. *Experimental and Clinical Neurotoxicology*, 6th ed. New York: Oxford University Press; 2000.

### *1930–1931: USA, Europe, and South Africa*

During the Prohibition, an ethanolic extract of the Jamaican ginger plant containing TOCP was sold. A potent neurotoxin, TOCP initiated an upper and lower extremity weakness termed the "ginger jake paralysis" in more than 50,000 people.

Morgan JP. The Jamaican ginger paralysis. *JAMA* 1982; 248:1864–1867.

Langford NJ, Ferner RE. Episodes of environmental poisoning worldwide. *Occup Environ Med* 2002; 59:855–860.

World Health Organization. *Neurotoxicity Risk Assessment for Human Health: Principles and Approaches. Environmental Health Criteria 223.* Geneva, Switzerland, 2001. Available at: http://www.inchem.org/documents/ehc/ehc/ehc223.htm#223230000.

Spencer PS, Schaumburg HH, Ludolph AC. *Experimental and Clinical Neurotoxicology*, 6th ed. New York: Oxford University Press; 2000.

## Vanadium

Worker exposure to vanadium-pentoxide dust concentrations greater than 0.5 $mg/m^3$ in workers resulted in burning of the eyes, sore throat, and a nonproductive cough. Other signs included wheezing, pulmonary rales, pharyngitis, and conjunctivitis.

Hryhorczuk DO, Aks SE, Turk JW. Unusual occupational toxins. *Occup Med* 1992; 7(3):567–586.

## Vinyl Chloride

### *1960–1970: Louisville, Kentucky*

The use of vinyl chloride in PVC polymerization resulted in an increased rate of hepatic angiosarcomas in exposed workers.

Falk H, et al. Hepatic disease among workers at a vinyl chloride polymerization plant. *JAMA* 1974; 230:59.

# Vinyl Chloride, Monomer

### 1997: Porto Marghera, Italy

Exposure to vinyl chloride monomer resulted in the deaths of 116 employees and injuries to an additional 400 workers.

Chemical Week Editorial Staff. Italian VCM trial looms. *Week* 1997; 159(10):6.

# Volcanic Gas

### AD 79: Pompeii, Italy

An eruption from Mount Vesuvius caused thousands of deaths. It is thought that heat, particulates, and oxide gases played a significant part in these deaths.

Bosch X. Scientists solve mystery of volcano's "natural deaths." *BMJ* 2001; 322:946.

# Warfarin

### 1981: Vietnam

Talc contaminated with a dicoumarin-type anticoagulant resulted in an epidemic characterized by a hemorrhagic syndrome. Seven hundred forty-one cases were recorded, with 177 deaths.

Ferrer A, Cabral R. Recent epidemics of poisoning by pesticides. *Toxicol Lett* 1995; 82-83:55–63.

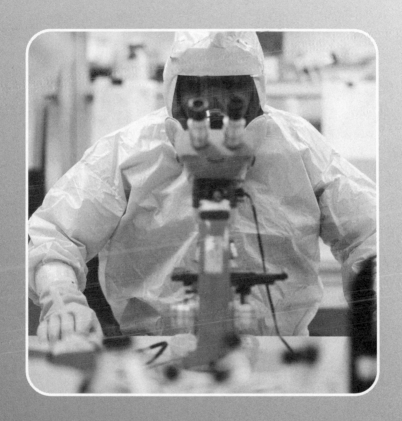

# BIOLOGICAL EVENTS

Chapter **2**

# BIOLOGICAL EVENTS

## Aflatoxin

### October 1988: Perak, Malaysia

An outbreak of food poisoning during the Chinese Festival of the Nine
   Emperor Gods resulted in the deaths of 13 children. The cause was found
   to be the Chinese noodle called 'Loh See Fun' (LSF). The LSF noodles had
   been traced to a Kampar town factory that used a preservative in its recipe
   that had been banned. The food poisoning was attributed to aflatoxins and
   boric acid.

Chao TC, Maxwell SM, Wong SY. An outbreak of aflatoxicosis and boric acid poisoning in Malaysia: a clinicopathological study. *J Pathol* 1991; 164(3):225–233.

Lye MS, Ghazali AA, Mohan J, Alwin N, Nair RC. An outbreak of acute hepatic
encephalopathy due to severe aflatoxicosis in Malaysia. *Am J Trop Med Hyg* 1995;
53(1):68–72.

Cheng CT. Perak, Malaysia, mass poisoning: tale of the nine emperor gods and
rat-tail noodles. *Am J Forensic Med Pathol* 1992; 13:261–263.

### 1981: Kenya

Twenty cases of acute aflatoxicosis were identified in the Makueni district of
   Kenya's Eastern Province among family members who consumed maize
   contaminated with aflatoxins. Aflatoxins are produced by *Aspergillus flavus*.

Ngindu A, Johnson BK, et al. Outbreak of acute hepatitis caused by aflatoxin poisoning
in Kenya. *Lancet* 1982; 1(8285):1346–1348.

**77**

### 1975: Western India

Areas in western India experienced an outbreak of hepatitis that appeared to be a result of aflatoxicosis, which was characterized by jaundice, rapidly developing ascites, portal hypertension, and a high mortality rate. The disease was linked to the consumption of maize contaminated with *Aspergillus flavus*. The victims may have ingested between 2 and 6 mg of aflatoxins on a daily basis for over a month.

Krishnamachari KA, Bhat RV, Nagarajan V, Tilak TB. Hepatitis due to aflatoxicosis. An outbreak in Western India. *Lancet* 1975; 1(7915):1061–1063.

### 1970s: Western India

Cases of acute hepatitis were caused by the consumption of aflatoxin-contaminated maize. The symptoms of aflatoxicosis included jaundice, rapidly developing ascites, portal hypertension, as well as a high mortality rate. Aflatoxins are produced by *Aspergillus flavus*.

Krishnamachari K, Bhat RV, Nagarajan V, Tilak TB. Hepatitis due to aflatoxicosis. An outbreak in Western India. *Lancet* 1975; 1(7915):1061–1063.


## Anthrax

### October–November 2001: Florida

After a man died from anthrax exposure, investigators confirmed that anthrax bacteria were present in the building where the man worked. A second case was also reported, and anthrax was later sent to New York television networks and the Washington office of Senate Majority Leader Tom Daschle.

U.S. Army Timeline of Terrorism: 2004–2000. Last updated September 8, 2004. Available at: http://www.army.mil/terrorism/2004–2000/index.html.

### 1991: Iraq

Weapons Inspectors for the United Nations (UN) discovered that the Iraqi government grew large amounts of anthrax during the first Gulf War, presumably to use as agents of biologic warfare.

Hoff B, Smith C III. *Mapping Epidemics: A Historical Atlas of Disease.* C.H. Calisher, ed. New York: Franklin Watts; 2000.

### April 2, 1979: Soviet Sverdlovsk (Ekaterinburg)

An anthrax outbreak affected 94 people, 64 of whom died. The former Soviet government initially claimed the deaths were due to intestinal anthrax from tainted meat. In 1992, President Boris Yeltsin admitted the outbreak was the result of an explosion at a plant that had been conducting anthrax biological-warfare research.

Hoff B, Smith C III. *Mapping Epidemics: A Historical Atlas of Disease.* C.H. Calisher, ed. New York: Franklin Watts; 2000.

PBS Frontline. *Plague War: The 1979 Anthrax Leak in Sverdlovsk.* Available at: http://www.pbs.org/wgbh/pages/frontline/shows/plague/sverdlovsk/.

Meselon M, Guillemin J, et al. The Sverdlovsk anthrax outbreak of 1979. *Science* 1994; 266(5188):1202–1208.

### 1868: Massachusetts

A local physician described the course of disease for eight patients connected to an animal hair factory. These patients exhibited very possible manifestation of anthrax-related illness, including cutaneous, gastrointestinal, mediastinal, and neurologic disease.

Macher A. Industry-related outbreak of human anthrax, Massachusetts, 1868. *Emerg Infect Dis* 2002; 8(10):1182.

## Atropine, Harmine, and Scopolamine

### June 2001: Prague, Czechoslovakia

Thirty people participated in a mediation session during which they ingested herbal tea allegedly prepared with the South American plant(s) "Ikitos" or "Toe." The participants were admitted to the hospital with clinical features that included impaired perception, hallucinations, aggression, agitation, amnesia, hyperthermia, collapse, coma, and respiratory depression. Analysis revealed atropine, harmine, and scopolamine in the herbal infusion.

Balikova M. Collective poisoning with hallucinogenous herbal tea. *Forensic Sci Int* 2002; 128:50–52.

## Bacillus cereus

### 2002: Canada

Thirty-five partygoers developed gastroenteritis after eating a salad dressed with contaminated mayonnaise.

Gaulin C, Viger YB, Fillion L. An outbreak of *Bacillus cereus* implicating a part-time banquet caterer. *Can J Public Health* 2002; 93(5):353–355.

## Botulism

### July 2002: Western Alaska

Residents of a native Yup'ik village in Alaska found a carcass of a beached beluga whale and collected the tail fluke for consumption. A total of 14 people ate the raw muktuk (skin and a thin blubber layer from whales). Eight of the 14 people who ate the muktuk were affected by botulinum toxin type E.

McLaughlin JB, Sobel J, Lynn T, Funk E, Middaugh JP. Botulism type E outbreak associated with eating a beached whale, Alaska. *Emerg Infect Dis* 2004; 10(9):1685–1687.

### April 1998: Thailand

An outbreak of 13 cases of food-borne botulism occurred in two villages in Thailand. Symptoms included dysphagia, dry mouth, vomiting, dysphonia, diarrhea, symmetrical paralysis, dysarthria, and ptosis. Two patients died. All 13 patients had eaten home-canned bamboo shoots.

Centers for Disease Control and Prevention (CDC). Food-borne botulism associated with home-canned bamboo shoots—Thailand, 1998. *MMWR Morbid Mortal Wkly Rep* 1999; 48(21):437–439.

### February 1989: Kingston, New York

Three cases of botulism were identified in persons who ate garlic bread made from a garlic-in-oil product. The garlic-in-oil tested positive for *Clostridium botulinum*. This led to the Food and Drug Administration (FDA) requiring microbial inhibitors or acidifying agents be added to such products.

Morse DL, Pickard LK, Guzewich JJ, et al. Garlic-in-oil associated botulism: episode leads to product modification. *Am J Public Health* 1990; 80(11):1372–1373.

### September 1985: Vancouver, Canada

The positive identification of type B *botulinum* toxin in the serum of a teenage girl led to the discovery of a cluster of botulism cases caused by chopped garlic in soybean oil, served on sandwiches at a single Vancouver restaurant. Thirty-six identified patients all ate at the restaurant and presented with one or more of the following symptoms: diplopia, opthalmoplegia, or ptosis, and dysphagia or dysarthria.

Michael E, Shaun HS, Peck MB, et al. Botulism from chopped garlic: delayed recognition of a major outbreak. *Ann Int Med* 1998; 108:363–368.

### 1971: Bedford, New York

A man died of botulinum poisoning after he ate vichyssoise soup manufactured by the Bon Vivant Company. This led to the recall of over a million cans of soup, in case of underprocessing. Soon after, the company filed for bankruptcy.

Newman C. Twelve toxic tales. *National Geographic;* May 2005.

## Burkholderia pseudomallei

### 2000: China

Cases of melioidosis were reported in the Chinese provinces of Hainan Island, Guangding, and Guangxi. Melioidosis is an important public health problem, and is a potential bioweapon. Potable water has been a source of recent outbreaks. It may present as pneumonia with skin and soft-tissue abscesses.

Dance DAB. Melioidosis. *Curr Opin Infect Dis* 2002; 15:127–132.

## Campylobacter jejuni

### June 1978: Bennington, Vermont

*Campylobacter jejuni*, which contaminated the community water supply, caused a typhoid-like sickness in more than 3,000 people.

Vogt RL, Sours HE, Barrett T, et al. *Campylobacter enteritis* associated with contaminated water. *Ann Intern Med* 1982; 96(3):292–296.

## Carchaotoxin-A and -B

### November 1993: Manakara, Madagascar

One hundred eighty-eight people were admitted to the hospital after eating the meat of a single shark (*Carcharhinus leucas*). Symptoms, appearing 5 to 10 hours after ingestion, were almost exclusively neurological. Two liposoluble toxins, carchaotoxin A and B were isolated from the shark liver. Mortality was close to 30%.

Boisier P, Ranaivoson G, Rasolofonirina N, et al. Fatal mass poisoning in Madagascar following ingestion of a shark (*Carcharhinus leucas*): clinical and epidemiological aspects and isolation of toxins. *Toxicon* 1995; 33(10):1359–1364.

## Ciguatoxin

### March 6, 1982: Miami, Florida

The U.S. Coast Guard provided medical assistance to an Italian freighter off the coast of Freeport, Bahamas. A total of 14 crew members developed nausea, vomiting, and muscle weakness within six hours of eating a barracuda that had been caught a few days prior. Their symptoms were consistent with ciguatera fish poisoning.

Centers for Disease Control and Prevention (CDC). Epidemiologic notes and reports ciguatera fish poisoning—Bahamas, Miami. *MMWR Morbid Mortal Wkly Rep* 1982; 31(28):391–392.

## Cotton Dust

### 1700s: Italy and Europe

The Italian physician Ramazzini, now regarded as the father of occupational medicine, observed respiratory complaints (brown lung; byssinosis) in workers who handled cotton dust, flax, and soft hemp. His observations were noted along with other occupational exposures in his book, *De Morbis Artificum Diatriba.*

Ramazzini B. *De morbis artificum Berardini Ramazzini diatriba [Diseases of workers].* The Latin text of 1713, revised with translation and notes by Wilmer Cave Wright. Chicago: University of Chicago Press; 1940.

## Cryptosporidiosis

### March 2000: Lancashire, England, United Kingdom

An outbreak of cryptosporidiosis resulted in 58 cases of diarrhea that had positively identified *Cryptosporidium* in stool specimens. Oocysts were also identified in water treatment works and domestic tap samples, and the probable factor common to all the cases was the ingestion of unboiled, contaminated tap water.

Howe AD, Forster S, et al. *Cryptosporidium* oocysts in a water supply associated with a cryptosporidiosis outbreak. *Emerg Infect Dis* 2002; 8(6):619–624.

### April 1993: Milwaukee, Wisconsin

Widespread outbreak of acute, watery diarrhea (cryptosporidiosis) occurred among the residents of Milwaukee, with the source traced to *Cryptosporidium* oocysts that had passed through the filtration system in one of the city's water treatment plants. This was one of the largest documented outbreaks of a waterborne disease in the United States affecting 350,000 people.

Mac Kenzie WR, Hoxie NJ, et al. A massive outbreak in Milwaukee of *cryptosporidium* infection transmitted through the public water supply. *N Engl J Med* 1994; 331(3):161–167.

Morris RD, Naumova EN, Griffiths JK. Did Milwaukee experience waterborne cryptosporidiosis before the large documented outbreak in 1993? *Epidemiology* 1998; 9(3): 264–270.

## Cycad Plant (*Cycas*)

### 1950s: Guam

It has been noted that the Chamorro people of Guam have a high incidence of fatal, paralyzing, neurodegenerative disease (amyotrophic lateral sclerosis and parkinsonism dementia). These people depended heavily on flour made from the starch extracted from cycad seeds. The compounds BMAA and cycasin are found in cycad plants, which are thought to be neurotoxic.

World Health Organization. *Neurotoxicity Risk Assessment for Human Health: Principles and Approaches. Environmental Health Criteria 223.* Geneva, Switzerland, 2001. Available at: http://www.inchem.org/documents/ehc/ehc/ehc223.htm#223230000.

Charlton TS, Marini AM, Markey SP, Norstog K, Duncan MW. Quantification of the neurotoxin 2-amino-3-(methylamino)-propanoic acid (BMAA) in Cycadales. *Phytochemistry* 1992; 31:3429–3432.

Spencer PS, Nunn PB, Hugon J, Ludolph AC, et al. Guam amyotrophic lateral sclerosis-Parkinsonism-dementia linked to a plant excitant neurotoxin. *Science* 1987; 237:517–522.

## Cyclosporiasis

### June 2000: Philadelphia, Pennsylvania

Fifty-five out of 89 wedding guests developed cyclosporiasis, with five of the cases confirmed by the presence of *Cyclospora cayetanensis* in the patients' stools. The source of contamination was traced to the raspberries used in the wedding cake icing, which tested positive for the *Cyclospora* DNA. The raspberries were imported from Guatemala.

Ho AY, Lopez AS, et al. Outbreak of cyclosporiasis associated with imported raspberries, Philadelphia, PA, 2000. *Emerg Inf Dis* 2002; 8(8):783–788.

### May 2000: Fulton County, Georgia

Attendees of a bridal brunch became ill after eating fresh raspberries imported from Guatemala.

Murrow LB, Blake P, Kreckman L. Outbreak of cyclosporiasis in Fulton County, Georgia. *Georgia Epidemiol Rep* 2002; 18:1–2.

### 1996: North America

A total of 1,465 cyclosporiasis cases were reported. Nine hundred and seventy-eight were laboratory-confirmed and traced to the consumption of Guatemalan raspberries. The mode of contamination was not found.

Herwaldt B, Acker ML. An outbreak in 1996 of cyclosporiasis associated with imported raspberries. *N Engl J Med* 1997; 336(22):1548–1556.

**84**  CHAPTER 2

## *Datura suaveolens*

### October 18, 1983: Canada

A husband and wife were poisoned after eating hamburger patty contaminated with Angels' Trumpets (*Datura suaveolens*) seeds. The wife prepared the meat with what she initially thought was seasoning, but soon realized it was *Datura* seed that had been drying over the stove for planting purposes. Most of the seeds were then removed from the meat, but the couple collapsed after eating one patty each. Other symptoms included hallucination, tachycardia, and diarrhea.

Centers for Disease Control and Prevention (CDC). Datura poisoning from hamburger—Canada. *MMWR Morbid Mortal Wkly Rep* 1984; 33(20):282–283.

## Dengue Fever

### January–April 2004: Indonesia

From January to April 2004, the Indonesian Ministry of Health registered 58,301 cases of dengue fever and dengue hemorrhagic fever (DHF). The case-fatality rate was 1.1%, which was lower than that of previous years.

World Health Organization. Epidemic and Pandemic Alert and Response (EPR): Disease Outbreak News. *Dengue fever in Indonesia—update 4.* Available at: http://www.who.int/csr/don/2004_05_11a/en/.

### 2002: Bangladesh

More than 5,000 cases of dengue fever were documented, with two reported deaths.

Rahman M, Rahman K, et al. First outbreak of Dengue fever, Bangladesh. *Emerg Inf Dis* 2002; 8(7):738–740.

### 2002: Brazil

Approximately 555,000 cases of dengue fever were reported. There were 2,000 cases of the hemorrhagic form, which resulted in 80 deaths.

Dengue fever; Outbreak reaching epidemic proportions, WHO says. *TB & Outbreaks Weekly;* August 27, 2002; p. 8.

### 1998: Latin America

Brazil reported 530,578 cases of dengue fever, Venezuela reported 37,586 cases, Suriname reported 1,151 cases, and Guyana reported 42 cases.

Palmer CJ, Validum L, et al. Dengue in Guyana. *Lancet* 1999; 354:304.

### 1998: Southern Vietnam

Officials reported 119,429 cases of dengue hemorrhagic fever, causing 342 deaths.

Ha DQ, Tien NT, Huong VT, Loan HT, Thang CM. Dengue epidemic in Southern Vietnam, 1998. *Emerg Inf Dis Dispatch* 2000; 6(4):422–425.

### Indonesia

Officials reported 20,000 people infected with, and 439 people dead from, dengue fever.

Henderson C. Indonesia public health dengue epidemic adds to economic burden. *Blood Wkly*, May 11, 1998.

### 1981: Puerto Rico

An outbreak of 7,000 cases of dengue fever occurred in the late summer and fall of 1981. The highest number of cases occurred in the districts outside San Juan.

Centers for Disease Control and Prevention (CDC). Epidemiologic notes and reports dengue fever in Puerto Rico—1981. *MMWR Morbid Mortal Wkly Rep* 1982; 31(8):103–104.

### 1826–1828: Savannah, Georgia

An outbreak of dengue fever spread from Savannah to other cities up and down the Atlantic seaboard.

Hoff B, Smith C III. *Mapping Epidemics: A Historical Atlas of Disease.* C.H. Calisher, ed. New York: Franklin Watts; 2000.

## Diphtheria (*Corynebacterium diphtheriae*)

### 1925: Nome, Alaska

An epidemic of diphtheria occurred in Alaska. Cases subsided once dogsleds were utilized to transport antitoxin serum 600 miles during a blizzard.

Hoff B, Smith C III. *Mapping Epidemics: A Historical Atlas of Disease.* C.H. Calisher, ed. New York: Franklin Watts; 2000.

### 1853: Great Britain, United Kingdom

An epidemic of diphtheria began in Great Britain and became a worldwide pandemic by 1856.

Hoff B, Smith C III. *Mapping Epidemics: A Historical Atlas of Disease.* C.H. Calisher, ed. New York: Franklin Watts; 2000.

### 1583–1618: Seville, Spain

Outbreaks of diphtheria ravaged Seville for 35 years.

Hoff B, Smith C III. *Mapping Epidemics: A Historical Atlas of Disease.* C.H. Calisher, ed. New York: Franklin Watts; 2000.

### 1576: France and Europe

Diphtheria swept throughout Paris and other major European cities. It is believed that the source of *C. diphtheriae* was Catholic soldiers housed in Paris.

Hoff B, Smith C III. *Mapping Epidemics: A Historical Atlas of Disease.* C.H. Calisher, ed. New York: Franklin Watts; 2000.

## Diphtheria (*Corynebacterium diphtheriae*) and Scarlett Fever (Group A *Streptococcus*)

### 1735–1740: New England

Both diphtheria and scarlet fever spread throughout the New England area, killing hundreds of residents. Most of the victims were children.

Hoff B, Smith C III. *Mapping Epidemics: A Historical Atlas of Disease.* C.H. Calisher, ed. New York: Franklin Watts; 2000.

## Domoic Acid

### 1991: Monterey Bay, California

The first reported occurrence of domoic acid in shellfish in the United States was in Monterey Bay in the summer of 1991. In October 1991, domoic acid was found in razor clams (*Siliqua patula*) and in the viscera of Dungeness crab (*Cancer magister*) along the Washington and Oregon coasts. The levels peaked in December 1991 and slowly declined to lower levels.

Wekell JC, Gauglitz EJ Jr, Barnett HJ, et al. Occurrence of domoic acid in Washington state razor clams (*Siliqua patula*) during 1991–1993. *Nat Toxins* 1994; 2(4):197–205.

### 1987: Prince Edward Island, Canada

Domoic acid, an excitatory amino acid, from contaminated mussels caused gastrointestinal symptoms, headache, and memory loss in 107 patients. Twelve patients developed seizures and four patients died.

Perl TM, Bedard L, et al. An outbreak of toxic encephalopathy caused by eating mussels contaminated with domoic acid. *N Engl J Med* 1990; 322:1775–1780.

## Dysentery (*Shigella dysenteriae*)

### October–November 1996: Texas

Twelve laboratory workers fell ill with gastrointestinal symptoms (diarrhea, fever, headache, or vomiting) after eating unmarked muffins and doughnuts from the staff's break room. After comparing cultures from the food and cultures from the laboratory's own stock, it was determined that the food was deliberately contaminated with *S. dysenteriae* type 2 from the stock culture located in the medical center's storage freezer.

Kolavic SA, Kimura A, Simons AL, et al. An outbreak of *Shigella dysenteriae* type 2 among laboratory workers due to intentional food contamination. *JAMA* 1997; 278 (5):396–399.

### 1346: France

The English troops at the Battle of Crecy were stricken with an outbreak of dysentery. The soldiers were so ill that the enemy troops teased them with taunts of "the bare-bottomed army."

Hoff B, Smith C III. *Mapping Epidemics: A Historical Atlas of Disease.* C.H. Calisher, ed. New York: Franklin Watts; 2000.

### 480 BC: Ancient Greece

The plague of Xerxes affected the Persian army and helped contribute to their defeat by the Greek forces. The epidemic, probably dysentery, was described by the historian Herodotus, becoming the first epidemic to be described in detail.

Hoff B, Smith C III. *Mapping Epidemics: A Historical Atlas of Disease.* C.H. Calisher, ed. New York: Franklin Watts; 2000.

## Ebola Hemorrhagic Fever

### June 11, 2004: Yambio County, Sudan

As of June 10, 2004, local health authorities had reported a total of 30 cases, with seven fatalities, of Ebola hemorrhagic fever in Yambio, Western Equatoria, Sudan.

World Health Organization. Epidemic and Pandemic Alert and Response (EPR): Disease Outbreak News. *Ebola haemorrhagic fever in south Sudan—update 5.* Available at: http://www.who.int/csr/don/2004_06_11/en.

### February 2003: Congo
An outbreak of Ebola killed 128 people.

World Health Organization. Epidemic and Pandemic Alert and Response (EPR): Disease Outbreak News. *Ebola haemorrhagic fever in the Republic of the Congo–Update 12.* Available at: http://www.who.int/csr/don/2003_05_07/en/index.html.

### March 1997: Gabon
A total of 60 cases and 45 deaths due to Ebola were recorded between July 1996 and January 1997.

World Health Organization. Epidemic and Pandemic Alert and Response (EPR): Disease Outbreak News. *Ebola haemorrhagic fever in Gabon (new outbreak).* Available at: http://www.who.int/csr/don/1997_03_02/en/.

### 1995: Kikwit, Democratic Republic of Congo
This region was the epicenter of a severe Ebola hemorrhagic fever outbreak, in which 317 people were affected and 245 people died.

Muyembe-Tamfun JJ, Kipasa M, et al. Ebola outbreak in Kikwit, Democratic Republic of the Congo: discovery and control measures. *J Infect Dis* 1999; 179(Suppl 1):S259–S262.

Hoff B, Smith C III. *Mapping Epidemics: A Historical Atlas of Disease.* C.H. Calisher, ed. New York: Franklin Watts; 2000.

## Encephalitis, Japanese

### 2002: Assam, India
One hundred forty people were treated for encephalitis. Eighty of these patients died despite treatment efforts.

*Japanese Encephalitis; Indian state seeks federal help to tackle outbreak after 80 die.* TB & Outbreaks Weekly; September 3, 2002; p. 14.

### October–November 1999: Andhra Pradesh, India
An outbreak of Japanese encephalitis killed 178 people. Approximately 87% of the cases were children aged one to nine years.

Rao JS, et al. Japanese Encephalitis epidemic in Anantapur district, Andhra Pradesh (October–November, 1999). *J Commun Dis* 2000; 32(4):306–312.

# Endotoxin

### 1996: Roraima, Brazil

A total of 36 neonates died in a hospital nursery. Endotoxin was found in unopened vials of parenteral medication that had been administered to these infants, which strongly suggested intrinsic contamination of these medications. Twenty of the deaths were attributed to sepsis.

Centers for Disease Control and Prevention (CDC). Clinical sepsis and death in a newborn nursery associated with contaminated parenteral medications—Brazil, 1996. *MMWR Morbid Mortal Wkly Rep* 1998; 47(29):610–612.

Garrett DO, McDonald C, Wanderley A, et al. An outbreak of neonatal deaths in Brazil associated with contaminated intravenous fluids. *J Infect Dis* 2002; 186:81–86.

# Enterobacter sakazakii

### 2002

Contaminated infant formula resulted in seven *Enterobacter-sakazakii*–colonized infants, nine sickened infants, and one infant death due to meningitis in a single NICU. This organism is extremely heat resistant, can survive processing, and may flourish in the growth media of powdered formula.

Weir E. Powdered infant formula and fatal infection with *Enterobacter sakazakii*. *JMAC* 2002; 166(12):1570.

### June–July 1998: Brussels, Begium

Twelve neonates in the neonatal intensive care unit developed necrotizing entercolitis from ingestion of *Enterobacter sakazakii*. Ten of the 12 babies consumed the same brand of powdered milk formula, which was contaminated with *E. sakazakii*. Two of the infants died.

van Acker J, de Smet F, Muyldermans G, et al. Outbreak of necrotizing enterocolitis associated with *Enterobacter sakazakii* in powdered milk formula. *J Clin Microbiol* 2001; 39(1):293–297.

# Ergot Alkaloids

### 1951: Pont-Saint-Esprit, France

Ergot fungus contaminated the rye crop of a small French village, which caused mass hallucination. In the ensuing confusion and terror, seven people died.

John Grant Fuller. *The Day of St. Anthony's Fire.* New York: Hutchinson; 1969.

### 1692: Salem, Massachusetts

Ergot alkaloids were thought to be the cause of bizarre behavior, which at the time, was attributed to witchcraft and possession.

Caporael LR. Ergotism: the Satan loosed in Salem. *Science* 1976; 192:21.

### AD 994: Aquitaine, France

Ergot alkaloids were thought to cause the deaths of 40,000 people after they consumed contaminated bread.

Burgen A. St. Anthony's gift. *Eur Rev* 2003; 11:27–35.

## Escherichia coli O157:H7

### February 2004: Okinawa, Japan

Three cases of *E. coli* infection in a Japanese family were linked to eating contaminated ground beef. This resulted in the voluntary recall of about 90,000 pounds of frozen ground beef in the United States and at U.S. military bases in Asia. The first laboratory-confirmed case was in a child who was hospitalized with bloody diarrhea. All family members had eaten hamburgers made from the same ground beef. Tests confirmed *E. coli* in two other family members.

Centers for Disease Control and Prevention (CDC). *Escherichia coli* O157:H7 infections associated with ground beef from a U.S. military installation—Okinawa, Japan, February 2004. *MMWR Morbid Mortal Wkly Rep* 2004; 54(2):40–42.

### June–July 2002: USA

Beef contaminated with *E. coli* caused 28 people to become ill, seven people to be hospitalized, and five cases of hemolytic uremic syndrome (HUS). These cases were traced back to products sold by the ConAgra Beef Company. Identical isolates between patients and beef resulted in a nationwide recall of 18.6 million lbs. of fresh and frozen ground beef.

Centers for Disease Control and Prevention (CDC). Multistate outbreak of *Escherichia coli* O157:H7 infections associated with eating ground beef—United States June–July 2002. *MMWR Morbid Mortal Wkly Rep* 2002; 51(29):637–639.

### 2000: Barcelona, Spain

Two hundred five children were infected with *E. coli*; six developed hemolytic uremic syndrome (HUS) after being served contaminated sausages in the school lunch program. The same catering company supplied food to six schools in the Catalonian region.

Bosch X. Spain's *E. coli* outbreak highlights mistakes. *Lancet* 2000; 356:1665.

### 2000: Walkerton, Ontario, Canada
An outbreak of this *E. coli* was traced to the municipal water supply resulting in 1,460 illnesses and 198 laboratory-confirmed cases. Hemolytic uremic syndrome (HUS) was reported in 26 of these cases.

Canada Infectious Disease News Brief; September 22, 2000.

Public Safety and Emergency Preparedness Canada. *Canadian Disaster Database.* Available at: http://psepc-sppcc.gc.ca/res/em/cdd/search=en.asp. Accessed September 21, 2005.

### August 1999: Clark County, Washington
An outbreak of *E. coli* infection was found to be associated with swimming in Battle Ground Lake. The outbreak included 28 swimmers and eight people who had contact with swimmers.

Samadpour M, Stewart J, Steingart K, et al. Laboratory investigation of an *E. coli* O157: H7 outbreak associated with swimming in Battle Ground Lake, Vancouver, Washington. *J Environ Health* 2002; 64(10):16–20.

### 1999: Southwestern Ontario, Canada
One hundred fifty-nine cases of *E. coli* were contracted from a petting zoo at a county fair. One child developed hemolytic uremic syndrome (HUS).

Helwig D. *E. coli* outbreak linked to fall fair. *CMAJ* 2000; 162(2):245–250.

### Albany, New York
*E. coli* was found in shallow wells used by vendors at a public fair. One hundred sixteen people fell ill, 11 developed hemolytic uremic syndrome (HUS), and two died.

Helwig D. *E. coli* outbreak linked to fall fair. *CMAJ* 2000; 162(2):245–250.

### 1996–1997: Japan
In 1997, 126 people were infected and one person died from an unknown source. The source was suspected to be radishes; however, this was never confirmed. In 1996, in Sokai City, contaminated radish sprouts were believed to be the cause of 9,451 *E. coli* infections and 12 deaths.

Gutierrez E. Japan prepares as 0157 strikes again. *Lancet* 1997; 349:1156.

### 1995: Bavaria, Germany
An estimated 1,000 people were infected with *E. coli*, including 47 known cases of hemolytic uremic syndrome (HUS). All but one of the patients who developed HUS were children. Seven children died. The source was never determined.

Karcher HL. Germany fears more deaths from *E. coli* outbreak. *BMJ* 1996; 312:1500.

### 1993: Washington

Contaminated frozen hamburger patties sold by a fast-food chain made 450 people sick. Twenty-one developed hemolytic uremic syndrome (HUS), and 3 infants died.

McCarthy M. U.S. seeks to rid beef of *E. coli. Lancet* 1993; 341(8846):687.

### 1989–1990: Missouri

Sewage contamination of a rural town's drinking water affected 243 people and killed 4 others.

Swerdlow DL, Woodruff BA, et al. A waterborne outbreak in Missouri of *Escherichia coli* O157:H7 associated with bloody diarrhea and death. *Ann Intern Med* 1992; 117(10):812–819.

### 1985: London, England, United Kingdom

Nineteen nursing home residents died after being served sandwiches containing uncooked meat and poultry products.

Helwig D. *E. coli* outbreak linked to fall fair. *CMAJ* 2000; 162(2):245–250.

## Food Poisoning

### February 2004: Philadelphia, Pennsylvania

Sixty attendees of a mortgage conference fell ill and had to be hospitalized due to food poisoning. The group had eaten several meals together, but it was unclear whether the food poisoning stemmed from any particular food.

Fallik D. *Food poisoning sickens 60 at hotel.* The Philadelphia Inquirer. February 9, 2004.

## Francisella tularensis

### 2000: Sweden

A widespread outbreak of tularemia, caused by *F. tularensis*, was reported in areas of Sweden where tularemia had previously been rare. Analysis showed mosquito bites to be the main risk factor.

Eliasson H, Lindback J, Nuorti JP, et al. The 2000 tularemia outbreak: a case-control study of risk factors in disease-endemic and emergent areas, Sweden. *Emerg Infect Dis* 2002; 8(9):956–960.

## Grass-Pea Plant (*Lathyrus sativus*)

### India

A neurodegenerative disease similar to the disease state manifested by the people of Guam who consume cycads is called lathyrism. It has been conclusively linked to consumption of the grass-pea (*L. sativus, L. cicera, L. clymenum*), which contains the neurotoxin beta-N-oxalylamino-L-alanine (BOAA). Lathyrism causes fatal motor-neuron wasting.

Spencer PS, Schaumburg HH. Lathyrism: A neurotoxic disease. *Neurobehav Toxicol Teratol* 1983; 5(6):625–629.

(*Also see Cycad*)

## Grayanotoxins (Andromedotoxin)

### 1983–1988: Turkey

Eleven cases of toxic-honey intoxication were reported to Turkish health officials. The honey was produced from the *Rhododendron* species *R. luteum* and *R. ponticum,* two species that grow in northern Turkey. The compounds responsible for the human poisoning are the grayanotoxins, mainly grayanotoxin I, that occur only in the *Ericaceae* plants. Patients in another study (19 individuals) that presented with "mad" honey poisoning had symptoms of nausea, vomiting, sweating, dizziness, and weakness.

Sutlupinar N, Mat A, Satganoglu Y. Poisoning by toxic honey in Turkey. *Arch Toxicol* 1993; 67(2):148–150.

Ozhan H, Akdemir R, Yazici M, et al. Cardiac emergencies caused by honey ingestion: a single centre experience. *Emerg Med J* 2004; 21(6):742–744.

## Hantavirus

### 1999–2000: Los Santos, Panama

Eleven cases of hantavirus pulmonary syndrome were identified, and nine of the 11 were confirmed serologically. Three of the cases were fatal. This was the first reported outbreak of human hantavirus infection in Central America.

Bayard V, Kitsutani PT, Barria EO, et al. Outbreak of hantavirus pulmonary syndrome, Los Santos, Panama, 1999–2000. *Emerg Infect Dis* 2004; 10(9):1635–1642.

### 1993: New Mexico and Arizona

Ten people died from a severe flulike illness during an 8-week period and a total of 24 were infected. Initial mortality was 70% prior to infectious-agent identification, but quickly dropped to 40% once the disease entity was identified. There have been fewer than 15 cases per year since these index cases.

Yates TL, Mills JN, et al. The ecology and evolutionary history of an emergent disease: hantavirus pulmonary syndrome. *BioScience* 2002; 52(11):989–998.

### 1950–1953: Korea

Approximately 3,000 U.S. and United Nations (UN) troops became infected with hantavirus. They developed hemorrhagic fever with renal syndrome.

Hoff B, Smith C III. *Mapping Epidemics: A Historical Atlas of Disease.* C. H. Calisher, ed. New York: Franklin Watts; 2000.

## Haff Disease

### 1997: California and Missouri

Six cases of Haff disease were reported in the United States, four in California, and two in Missouri. The patients ate buffalo fish, *Ictiobus cyprinellus,* a bottom-feeder found mostly in the Mississippi River and its tributaries. Haff disease is a syndrome of unexplained rhabdomyolysis caused by an unknown toxin.

Centers for Disease Control and Prevention (CDC). Haff disease associated with eating buffalo fish—United States, 1997. *MMWR Morbid Mortal Wkly Rep* 1998; 47(50):1091–1093.

### 1960s: Russia

Haff disease was reported in Russia.

Strusevich AV. Alimentary-toxic paroxysmol myoglobinuria (Haff-luksov-Sartlan disease) [Russian]. *Arkh Patol* 1966; 28:56–60.

### 1920s: Koenigsberg Haff

Approximately 1,000 people living along this brackish inlet of the Baltic Sea experienced severe muscle pain and stiffness. It is now known that this is a syndrome of idiopathic rhabdomyolysis caused by an unidentified toxin after consuming certain fish.

Zu Jeddeloh B: Haffkrankheit (Haff disease) [German]. *Erg Inn Med* 1939; 57:138–182.

# Hemorrhagic Fever, Acute

### January 2005: Timor-Leste (East Timor)
The World Health Organization (WHO) received reports of 67 patients
hospitalized with acute hemorrhagic fever, as well as reports of eight
patient deaths. The cases occurred in Dili, Liquica, and Maliana.

World Health Organization. Epidemic and Pandemic Alert and Response (EPR): Disease Outbreak News. *Acute Haemorrhagic Fever Syndrome in Timor-Leste.* Available at: http://www.who.int/csr/don/2005_01_31/en/.

### May 18, 2004: South Sudan
Cases of acute hemorrhagic fever were reported in Hai-Cuba, Yambio, the
Western Equatoria Region of south Sudan.

World Health Organization. Epidemic and Pandemic Alert and Response (EPR): Disease Outbreak News. *Suspected cases of acute haemorrhagic fever syndrome in south Sudan.* Available at: http://www.who.int/csr/don/2004_05_18/en/.

*(Also see Rift Valley Fever)*

### May–June 2001: Kosovo
The World Health Organization (WHO) office located in Kosovo reported
27 illnesses and four deaths attributed to acute hemorrhagic fever. The
cases occurred in the southwestern area of Kosovo.

World Health Organization. Epidemic and Pandemic Alert and Response (EPR): Disease Outbreak News. *2001—Acute Haemorrhagic Fever Syndrome in Kosovo.* Available at: http://www.who.int/csr/don/2001_06_08e/en/.

### September 2000: Wadi Mawr, Yemen
As of September 2000, 134 cases of an acute hemorrhagic fever that included
31 deaths were reported. The hemorrhagic fever was suspected to be Rift
Valley Fever.

World Health Organization. Epidemic and Pandemic Alert and Response (EPR): Disease Outbreak News. *2000—Rift Valley fever in Saudi Arabia—Update/Acute Haemorrhagic Fever Syndrome in Yemen—Update.* Available at: http://www.who.int/csr/don/2000_09_29/en/.

### July 2000: Gulran, Herat Province, Afghanistan
The World Health Organization (WHO) received reports of 27 suspected
cases, including 16 deaths, of an acute hemorrhagic fever.

World Health Organization. Epidemic and Pandemic Alert and Response (EPR): Epidemic and Pandemic Alert and Response (EPR): Disease Outbreak News. *2000—Acute Haemorrhagic Fever Syndrome in Afghanistan—Update.* Available at: http://www.who.int/csr/don/2000_07_11/en/.

# Hemorrhagic Fever, Bolivian

### 1994: Magdelena, Bolivia

Bolivian hemorrhagic fever killed 6 people. The cause is the Machupo arenavirus carried by the mouse *Calomys callosus.*

Hoff B, Smith C III. *Mapping Epidemics: A Historical Atlas of Disease.* C. H. Calisher, ed. New York: Franklin Watts; 2000.

# Hepatitis A

### November 2003: Monaca, Pennsylvania

A large outbreak of hepatitis A occurred among people who ate at a single restaurant. Of the 601 patients identified, 124 were hospitalized and three died. The source was found to be green onions grown in Mexico that were apparently contaminated before they arrived at the restaurant. The onions were used in the large batches of mild salsa that were given to all the restaurant patrons. This was an unusually large outbreak of restaurant-associated hepatitis A. In 2003, the FDA issued an import ban on green onions from four Mexican farms, as well as a consumer alert.

Wheeler C, Vogt TM, Armstrong GL, et al. An outbreak of hepatitis A associated with green onions. *New Engl J Med* 2005; 353(9):890–897.

Centers for Disease Control and Prevention (CDC). Hepatitis A outbreak associated with green onions at a restaurant–Monaca, Pennsylvania, 2003. *MMWR Weekly* 2003; 52(47):1155–1157.

### June 2003: Central Australia

An outbreak of hepatitis A occurred at a 5-day youth camp, with 21 cases matching the outbreak case definition. Food was significantly related to illness, which demonstrated the importance of food safety and hygiene in large-group catering.

Munnoch SA, Ashbolt RH, Coleman DJ, et al. A multi-jurisdictional outbreak of hepatitis A related to a youth camp—implications for catering operations and mass gatherings. *Commun Dis Intell* 2004; 28(4):521–527.

### April–October 2002: Selangor State, Malaysia

An outbreak of hepatitis A occurred among students and local indigenous populations in and around Mukim Hulu Langat, Hulu Langat district. A total of 51 cases were reported. Investigations suggested that the local river water was fecally contaminated from the upstream Orang Asli community, due to a lack of toilet facilities. The outbreak was controlled by October after education and hygiene-control measures were instituted.

Venugopalan B, Nik Rubiah NA, Meftahuddin T, et al. Hepatitis A outbreak in Hulu Lagat District, Selangor State, Malaysia during April–October 2002. *Med J Malaysia* 2004; 59(5):670–673.

### 2002: Florence, Italy

Two hepatitis A outbreaks occurred on opposite sides of Florence. Both originated from immigrant children. The outbreaks occurred in a maternal school (37 cases) and a day-care center (3 cases). Federally guided vaccination began at the maternal school after the occurrence of a secondary case.

Bonanni P, Franzin A, Staderini C, et al. Vaccination against hepatitis A during outbreaks starting in schools: what can we learn from experiences in central Italy? *Vaccine* 2005; 23(17–18):2176–2180.

### 1988: Shanghai, China

A reported 290,000 cases of hepatitis A were contracted from eating infected clams.

Tang YW, Wang JX, et al. A serologically confirmed, case-control study of a large outbreak of hepatitis A in China, associated with the consumption of clams. *Epidemiol Infect* 1991; 107:651–657.

## Histoplasma capsulatum

### January 2004: Nebraska

An outbreak of histoplasmosis occurred among 25 workers in an agricultural processing plant. It was believed that the outbreak was caused by the disruption of the soil pile that was known to be contaminated with *H. capsulatum*. Histoplasmosis is generally an acute, self-limited respiratory illness. The incubation period is 1 to 2 weeks after inhalation of *H. capsulatum* spores.

Safranek T, Beecham B, et al. Outbreak of histoplasmosis among industrial plant workers—Nebraska, 2004. *MMWR Morbid Mortal Wkly Rep* 2004; 53(43):1020–1022.

## Human Immunodeficiency Virus (HIV)

### 1970s–1980s: USA

Approximately 90% of hemophilia-A patients developed HIV seroconversion after receiving contaminated concentrated cryoprecipitate preparations.

Wax PM. Toxicologic Plagues and Disasters in History. In: *Goldfrank's Toxicologic Emergencies,* 7th ed. L.R. Goldfrank, ed. New York: McGraw-Hill; 2002; pp. 23–34.

### 1980: USA

The first cases of human immunodeficiency virus were reported in San Francisco, Los Angeles, and New York.

Hoff B, Smith C III. *Mapping Epidemics: A Historical Atlas of Disease.* C.H. Calisher, ed. New York: Franklin Watts; 2000.

## Influenza, Asian

### 1957: China

A pandemic termed the "Asian Flu" spread globally from China. It was estimated that the virus affected approximately 35% of the world's population.

Hoff B, Smith C III. *Mapping Epidemics: A Historical Atlas of Disease.* C.H. Calisher, ed. New York: Franklin Watts; 2000.

## Influenza, Spanish

### March–November 1918: USA and Worldwide

A widespread outbreak of Spanish influenza killed more than 500,000 people. This was the worst epidemic in U.S. history. The strain also caused a pandemic, killing an estimated 20–50 million people world-wide.

Tompey TM, et al. Characterization of the reconstructed 1918 Spanish influenza pandemic virus. *Science* 2005; 310(5745): 77–80.

## Legionnaires' Disease (*Legionella*)

### October 2003: Ocean City, Maryland

Seven confirmed cases and one suspected case of Legionnaires' disease were identified among hotel guests from October 2003 to February 2004. The guests had all stayed at the same hotel for one to four nights. Seven of the patients were hospitalized.

Goeller D, Blythe D, Davenport M, et al. Legionnaires disease associated with potable water in a hotel—Ocean City, Maryland, October 2003—February 2004. *MMWR Morbid Mortal Wkly Rep* 2005; 54(7):165–168.

### 2002: Northwestern England, United Kingdom

One hundred thirty-one confirmed cases of Legionnaires' disease were reported. Thirteen patients required intensive care and four patients died. The source was found to be an air conditioning system at a local community center.

*Legionnaires' Disease: British Officials Believe Outbreak Slowing Down.* TB & Outbreaks Weekly; September 10, 2002; p. 13.

### Waterbury, Vermont

Sixteen patients were infected, but no deaths were reported. The source was found to be a contaminated air conditioning cooling tower in the state women's prison complex. This report indicated that eight to 18,000 cases of Legionnaires' disease are reported annually in the United States.

*Legionnaires' Disease; British Officials Believe Outbreak Slowing Down.* TB & Outbreaks Weekly; September 10, 2002, p. 13.

### Alcoy, Spain
Three hundred fifty-seven confirmed cases of Legionnaires' disease were linked to cooling towers.

Fernandez JA, Lopez P, et al. Clinical study of an outbreak of Legionnaire's disease in Alcoy, Southeastern Spain. *Eur J Clin Microbiol Infect Dis* 2002; 21(10):729–735.

### 1976: Philadelphia, Pennsylvania
Two hundred twenty-one attendees at the American Legion convention in the summer of 1976 became sick with a pneumonia-like respiratory disease that ultimately killed 34 Legionnaires. These index cases led to the realization that members of the bacterial family *Legionellaceae* had been isolated as early as 1943.

Winn WC Jr. Legionnaires disease: historical perspective. *Clin Microbiol Rev* 1988; 1(1):60–81.

*Legionnaires' Disease: British Officials Believe Outbreak Slowing Down.* TB & Outbreaks Weekly; September 10, 2002; p. 13.

## Leprosy (*Mycobacterium leprae*)
### 1179: Europe
Pope Alexander III decreed that lepers were to wear tunics embroidered with the letter *L* and to carry bells or clappers to warn others of their approach. The Pope also banned lepers from touching or looking at nonlepers.

Hoff B, Smith C III. *Mapping Epidemics: A Historical Atlas of Disease.* C.H. Calisher, ed. New York: Franklin Watts; 2000.

## Leptospirosis
### September 2000: Malaysian Borneo
The Centers for Disease Control and Prevention (CDC) investigated cases of leptospirosis reported among participants of the EcoChallange Sabah 2000 Expedition Race. Several of the 155 U.S. athletes and four Canadian athletes developed fever and muscle aches. Leptospirosis is caused by a bacterium that is transmitted to humans via water contaminated with urine from infected animals.

Centers for Disease Control and Prevention (CDC). Press Release. September 13, 2000.

Canada Infectious Diseases News Brief. Population and Public Health Branch (PPHB). September 22, 2000.

## Listeriosis

### 2002: Northeastern USA

Forty-six culture-confirmed cases with seven deaths and three fetal deaths were traced to *Listeria monocytogenes* from sliced deli turkey meat. This led to the recall of 27.4 million lbs. of fresh and frozen turkey and chicken products. The contamination was traced to a poultry processing plant in Franconia, Pennsylvania.

Centers for Disease Control (CDC). Outbreak of listeriosis—northeastern United States, 2002. *MMWR Morbid Mortal Wkly Rep* 2002; 51(42):950–951.

### May 2000: New York, Georgia, Connecticut, Ohio, Michigan, California, Pennsylvania, Tennessee, Utah, and Wisconsin

Twenty-nine cases of illness that occurred across 10 states were reported to the Centers for Disease Control (CDC). The cases of listeriosis, caused by a strain of *Listeria monocytogenes*, were linked to eating deli meat. The investigation prompted deli-meat producers to recall their product, including ready-to-eat foods and processed turkey and chicken deli meat.

Centers for Disease Control and Prevention (CDC). Multistate outbreak of listeriosis—United States, 2000. *MMWR Morbid Mortal Wkly Rep* 2000; 49(50):1129–1130.

## Lyme Disease

### 1975: Old Lyme, Connecticut

The first cases of the inflammatory disease now known as Lyme disease were described after a mysterious outbreak of arthritis in the town of Old Lyme. The source was identified as the spirochete *Borrelia burgdorferi*, transmitted via the bite of a deer tick.

Hoff B, Smith C III. *Mapping Epidemics: A Historical Atlas of Disease.* C.H. Calisher, ed. New York: Franklin Watts; 2000.

## Malaria

### 2002: Kenya

Within a one-month period, 318 people died of malaria and 200,000 were infected.

Siringi S. Failure to tackle malaria in East Africa. *Lancet* 2002; 360:317.

### 323 BC

Alexander the Great of Macedonia developed a high fever and died from an illness that was likely malaria. Alexander conquered Asia Minor, Egypt, Mesopotamia, and Persia during his reign.

Hoff B, Smith C III. *Mapping Epidemics: A Historical Atlas of Disease.* C.H. Calisher, ed. New York: Franklin Watts; 2000.

## Marburg Virus

### March 23, 2005: Uige Province, Angola, Africa

The World Health Organization (WHO) confirmed Marburg virus as the agent responsible for an outbreak of viral hemorrhagic fever. A total of 140 cases were identified from October 1, 2004 to April 1, 2005 with 132 deaths. Symptoms included fever, hemorrhage, vomiting, cough, diarrhea, and jaundice. The Marburg virus is in the family *Filoviridae*, which includes the Ebola virus.

Centers for Disease Control and Prevention (CDC). Outbreak Notice. *Update: Marburg Virus Hemorrhagic Fever, Angola, Central Africa. Interim Guidance for Travelers.* Last updated March 29, 2005. Available at: http://www.cdc.gov/travel/other/marburg_vhf_angola_2005.htm.

## Measles (*Rubivirus*)

### January 1997: Guadeloupe

An outbreak of measles in Guadeloupe was reported, mostly in the city of St. Francois. Laboratory tests confirmed 12 cases.

World Health Organization. Epidemic and Pandemic Alert and Response (EPR). Disease Outbreak News. *Measles in Guadeloupe.* Available at: http://www.who.int/csr/don/1997_01_17a/en/.

## Measles (*Rubivirus*) and/or Smallpox (*Variola major*)

### 1520: North and Central America

The Spanish brought smallpox and measles with them as they explored the Americas.

Hoff B, Smith C III. *Mapping Epidemics: A Historical Atlas of Disease.* C.H. Calisher, ed. New York: Franklin Watts; 2000.

### 165–180: Middle East

Either measles or smallpox was brought to the Middle East from Rome, in what was referred to as the Plague of Galen. Emperors Lucius Verus and Marcus Aurelius Antoninus were both afflicted with it and later died from the disease.

Hoff B, Smith C III. *Mapping Epidemics: A Historical Atlas of Disease.* C.H. Calisher, ed. New York: Franklin Watts; 2000.

## Meningitis, Bacterial (*Neisseria meningitidis*)

### 1996: Africa

Bacterial meningitis killed more than 17,000 people in Africa during 1996.

Hoff B, Smith C III. *Mapping Epidemics: A Historical Atlas of Disease.* C.H. Calisher, ed. New York: Franklin Watts; 2000.

### 1936–1937: Chad

More than 3,000 people died from bacterial meningitis caused by *Neisseria meningitidis.*

Hoff B, Smith C III. *Mapping Epidemics: A Historical Atlas of Disease.* C.H. Calisher, ed. New York: Franklin Watts; 2000.

## Meningitis, Meningococcal

### February 1997: Togo

An outbreak of meningitis began in Togo in November 1997 with approximately 1,235 cases. There were 151 deaths.

World Health Organization. Epidemic and Pandemic Alert and Response (EPR): Disease Outbreak News. *Meningitis outbreak in Togo.* Available at: http://www.who.int/csr/don/1997_02_07c/en/index.html.

### January 1997: Burkina Faso

A total of 461 cases with 64 deaths were reported in an outbreak of meningococcal meningitis.

World Health Organization. Epidemic and Pandemic Alert and Response (EPR): Disease Outbreak News. *Meningitis in West Africa.* Available at: http://www.who.int/csr/don/1997_01_31a/en/.

### January 1997: Ghana and Mali

Meningitis was reported in Ghana (181 cases, 17 deaths) and Mali (180 cases, 26 deaths) in West Africa.

World Health Organization. Epidemic and Pandemic Alert and Response (EPR): Disease Outbreak News. *Meningitis in West Africa.* Available at: http://www.who.int/csr/don/1997_01_31a/en/.

### January 1997: Togo

A total of 961 cases with 143 deaths were reported in an outbreak of meningitis.

World Health Organization. Epidemic and Pandemic Alert and Response (EPR): Disease Outbreak News. *Meningitis in West Africa.* Available at: http://www.who.int/csr/don/1997_01_31a/en/.

## Microcystins

### 1996: Caruaru, Brazil

Eighty-nine percent of dialysis patients had visual disturbances, nausea, and vomiting associated with hemodialysis. Microcystins produced by cyanobacteria were detected in water samples from the dialysis center. One hundred one patients out of 124 had acute liver failure as a result, and 52 died of what is now known as Caruaru syndrome.

Jochimsen EM, Carmichael WW, et al. Liver failure and death after exposure to microcystins at a hemodialysis center in Brazil. *N Engl J Med* 1998; 338(13):873–878.

Carmichael WW, Azevedo SM, An JS, Molica RJ, et al. Human fatalities from cyanobacteria: chemical and evidence for cyanotoxins. *Environ Health Perspect* 2001; 109(7): 663–668.

## *Mycobacterium chelonae*

### 1996–1997

Thirty-four of 82 patients who had tumescent liposuction performed by the same surgeon developed cutaneous abscesses within a six-month period. The source was the tap water in the surgeon's office, which was used to wash and reuse the suction tubing. The surgeon had also been washing the "sterile" towels himself.

Meyers H, Brown-Elliot BA, et al. An outbreak of *Mycobacterium chelonae* infection following liposuction. *Clin Infect Dis* 2002; 34:1500–1507.

## Niacin Deficiency

### 1902: USA

Epidemics of pellagra, a systemic disease resulting from niacin deficiency, occurred in the American south. The most frequently observed risk factors were poverty and corn consumption as a dietary staple. Diets based on unfortified maize were found to be pellagragenic because they are low in tryptophan, the amino-acid precursor of niacin.

Rajakumar K. Pellagra in the United States: a historical perspective. *South Med J* 2000; 93(3):272–277.

## 3-Nitropropionic Acid

### 1972–1989: China
This fungal metabolite causes coma followed by spasticity. Fungi that was growing on sugarcane caused 885 poisonings and 88 deaths in northern China during this time period. The sugarcane was stored over the winter months to be used for New Years celebrations.

World Health Organization. *Neurotoxicity Risk Assessment for Human Health: Principles and Approaches. Environmental Health Criteria 223.* Geneva, Switzerland, 2001. Available at: http://www.inchem.org/documents/ehc/ehc/ehc223.htm#223230000.

He F, Zhang S, Zhang C. Mycotoxin induced encephalopathy and dystonia in children. Volans GN, Sims J, Sullivan FM, Turner P, eds. In: *Basic Science in Toxicology.* London, England, UK: Taylor & Francis; 1990; p. 596.

## Norovirus (formerly Norwalk-like virus)

### September 2005: Mississippi and Texas
As a result of Hurricane Katrina, the Centers for Disease Control and Prevention (CDC) received reports of approximately 1,000 cases of acute gastroenteritis among hurricane evacuees. Tests confirmed norovirus in stool specimens of patients located in Texas.

Centers for Disease Control and Prevention (CDC). Infectious disease and dermatologic conditions in evacuees and rescue workers after Hurricane Katrina—multiple states, August–September, 2005. *MMWR Dispatch* 2005; 54(Dispatch):1–4.

### January–December 2002
Twenty-one outbreaks of acute gastroenteritis aboard 17 cruise ships were reported to the CDC's vessel sanitation program in one calendar year. Of the outbreaks, nine were laboratory confirmed to be associated with norovirus infection. In the previous year (2001), there were four confirmed outbreaks. Noroviruses (i.e., Norwalk-like viruses) are part of a group of common microorganisms that cause gastrointestinal symptoms for 24–48 hours. Many reports of cruise-ship outbreaks and resulting disinfection have surfaced over the last several years, including the *Amsterdam* and Disney's *Magic.*

Centers for Disease Control and Prevention (CDC). Outbreaks of gastroenteritis associated with noroviruses on cruise ships–United States, 2002. *MMWR Morbid Mortal Wkly Rep* 2002; 51(49):1112–1115.

### July 2001: Virginia
An outbreak of gastroenteritis associated with a Norwalk-like virus at a large youth encampment was reported.

Centers for Disease Control and Prevention (CDC). Norwalk-like virus-associated gastroenteritis in a large, high density encampment—Virginia, July 2001. *MMWR Morbid Mortal Wkly Rep* 2002; 51(3):661–663.

### 2001: England, United Kingdom
Forty-nine people who developed gastroenteritis were determined to have eaten at the same restaurant the same weekend prior to symptom onset. Six people showed evidence of norovirus infection. Eating prepared salad was strongly correlated with illness, and one of the chefs who had previously been ill with gastrointestinal symptoms had been present in the food preparation area.

Holtby I, Tebbutt GM. Outbreak of Norwalk-like virus infection associated with salad provided in a restaurant. *Commun Dis Public Health* 2001; 4(4):305–310.

### 2001: Northern Wisconsin
An outbreak of gastroenteritis at two summer recreational camps in Wisconsin was reported. The transmission was attributed to person-to-person dissemination of a norovirus.

Centers for Disease Control and Prevention (CDC). Norwalk-like virus outbreaks at two summer camps—Wisconsin, June 2001. *MMWR Morbid Mortal Wkly Rep* 2001; 50(30):642–643.

### New Delhi, India
After a farewell party, an outbreak of acute gastroenteritis in the nurses' hostel of a hospital was reported. All affected patients had eaten salad sandwiches at the party. Specimens tested positive for genogroup II norovirus.

Girish R, Broob S, et al. Foodborne outbreak caused by a Norwalk-like virus in India. *J Med Virol* 2002; 67(4):603–607.

### January 2001: United Kingdom
Thirty-eight staff as well as 20 patients of an acute elderly care ward became ill with an outbreak of a gastrointestinal infection. The causative agent was found to be a norovirus.

McCall J, Smithson R. Rapid response and strict control measures can contain a hospital outbreak of Norwalk-like virus. *Commun Dis Public Health* 2002; 5(3):243–246.

### 1999: Sweden
An outbreak of gastroenteritis was attributed to a Norwalk-like virus at 30 day-care centers in Sweden.

Gotz H, Ekdahl K, et al. Clinical spectrum and transmission characteristics of infection with Norwalk-like virus: findings from a large community outbreak in Sweden. *Clin Infect Dis* 2001; 33(5):622–628.

### 1999: Toledo, Ohio

Ninety-three people who attended the same Christmas dinner developed
gastroenteritis. All of the patients had eaten tossed salad prepared by a
local caterer; eight received medical attention, and one was hospitalized.
Eight of 12 stool specimens tested positive for a Norwalk-like virus.

Kassa H. An outbreak of Norwalk-like viral gastroenteritis in a frequently penalized
food service operation: a case for mandatory training of food handlers in safety and
hygiene. *J Environ Health* 2001; 64(5):9–12.

### September 1998: Florida

Diarrhea and vomiting was reported by many of the members of the North
Carolina football team during a game in Florida. Stool samples tested positive for a genogroup 1 Norwalk-like virus. This case demonstrated close-
contact, person-to-person transmission of the virus.

Becker KM, Moe CL, et al. Transmission of Norwalk virus during football game.
*N Engl J Med* 2000; 343(17):1223–1227.

### 1997–1999: Japan

Approximately 265 gastroenteritis cases were reported to be associated with a
small, round-structured virus, or Norwalk-like virus.

Inouye S, Yamashita K, et al. Surveillance of viral gastroenteritis in Japan: pediatric
cases and outbreak incidents. *J Infect Dis* 2000; 181(Suppl 2):S270–S274.

### January 1982: Tate, Georgia

Twenty-seven patients presented to local physicians during an outbreak of
Norwalk-virus gastroenteritis. Illness was characterized by the abrupt onset
of nausea, abdominal cramps, diarrhea and/or vomiting, headache, and
low-grade fever. After a municipal survey, it was found that as many as 500
people may have been ill during this outbreak. An investigation found that
the Tate water system was the source for norovirus infection.

Community outbreak of Norwalk gastroenteritis—Georgia. *MMWR Morbid Mortal
Wkly Rep* 1982; 31(30):405–407.

## Palytoxin Poisoning

### October–November 2000: Kochi Prefecture, Japan

A total of 11 people experienced symptoms of severe muscle pain, low-back
pain, and black urine after ingestion of a serranid fish. Testing revealed the
agent responsible to be palytoxin (PTX).

Taniyama S, Mahmud Y, Terada M, Takatani T, Arakawa O, Noguchi T. Occurrence of a food poisoning incident by palytoxin from a serranid *Epinephelus sp.* in Japan. *J Nat Toxins* 2002; 11(4):277–282.

## Paralytic Shellfish Poisoning (PSP; Saxitoxin)

### June 5, 1990: Georges Bank, Massachusetts
Food-borne illness occurred in six fishermen aboard a fishing boat off the Nantucket coast. The fishermen had eaten blue mussels (*Mytilus edulis*) and developed vomiting, periorbital edema, and numbness of the mouth, throat, and tongue approximately one to two hours after shellfish inges- tion. The uneaten mussels contained saxitoxin levels significantly higher than the maximum safe level (80 μg/100 mg). The harvesting area had been identified as having high levels of shellfish saxitoxin.

Centers for Disease Control and Prevention (CDC). Epidemiologic notes and reports paralytic shellfish poisoning—Massachusetts and Alaska, 1990. *MMWR Morbid Mortal Wkly Rep* 1991; 40(10):157–161.

### June 1990: Alaska
An Alaskan Native American man died after consuming butter clams from the Alaska Peninsula. Within an hour of ingestion, the man had tingling and numbness of the mouth, face, and fingers; two hours later he suffered cardiopulmonary arrest. Two other crew members from the same boat, and four members from another crew also ingested the shellfish and experienced numbness and tingling. Other episodes in the area resulted in a PSP outbreak with 13 cases among 21 persons.

Centers for Disease Control and Prevention (CDC). Epidemiologic notes and reports paralytic shellfish poisoning—Massachusetts and Alaska, 1990. *MMWR Morbid Mortal Wkly Rep* 1991; 40(10):157–161.

### July–August 1987 City: Champerico, Guatemala
An outbreak of PSP occurred on the Pacific coast of Guatemala and included the typical neurologic symptoms (paresthesis of mouth and extremities, ataxia, muscle paralysis). One hundred eighty-seven people were affected; 26 died. The vehicle for saxitoxin poisoning was found to be the clam *Amphichaena kindernami.*

Rodriguez DC, Etzel RA, de Porras E, et al. Lethal paralytic shellfish poisoning in Guatemala. *Am J Trop Med Hyg* 1990; 42(3):267–271.

Centers for Disease Control and Prevention (CDC). Epidemiologic notes and reports paralytic shellfish poisoning—Massachusetts and Alaska, 1990. *MMWR Morbid Mortal Wkly Rep* 1991; 40(10):157–161.

### *1987*
Two mass human poisonings were reported, with symptoms including dizziness, diarrhea, vomiting, disorientation, respiratory distress, and eye irritation. The source was found to be saxitoxin, produced by algae, and concentrated in shellfish that consumed the algae. A single 0.2 mg dose of saxitoxin could be fatal.

Edwards N. Saxitoxin: from food poisoning to chemical warfare. The Chemical Laboratories, School of Chemistry, Physics, & Environmental Science. University of Sussex at Brighton. Available at: http://www.bris.ac.uk/Depts/Chemistry/MOTM/stx/saxi1.htm.

### *1950s: USA*
The CIA covertly experimented with saxitoxin as a possible chemical-warfare agent, reportedly using it in suicide capsules provided to their agents.

Edwards N. *Saxitoxin: from food poisoning to chemical warfare.* The Chemical Laboratories, School of Chemistry, Physics, & Environmental Science. University of Sussex at Brighton. Available at: http://www.bris.ac.uk/Depts/Chemistry/MOTM/stx/saxi1.htm.

### *June 15, 1793: British Columbia, Canada*
The explorer Captain George Vancouver described the deaths of two crewmen from paralytic shellfish poisoning during his expedition into what is now Vancouver in British Columbia, Canada.

Northwest Fisheries Science Center. Harmful Algal Blooms. *Paralytic Shellfish Poisoning.* Available at: http://www.nwfsc.noaa.gov/hab/HABs_Toxins/Marine_Biotoxins/PSP/.

## Poliomyelitis (Polio)

### *2000: Dominican Republic and Haiti*
From July through November 2000, 19 people in the Dominican Republic were stricken with an acute flaccid paralysis. Six of these patients were determined via laboratory testing to have been infected by poliovirus type 1. All patients were either unvaccinated or inadequately vaccinated. In Haiti, one laboratory-confirmed poliovirus type 1 case was identified in a child who was inadequately vaccinated.

Centers for Disease Control and Prevention (CDC). Public Health Dispatch: Outbreak of Poliomyelitis—Dominican Republic and Haiti, 2000. *MMWR Morbid Mortal Wkly Rep* 2000; 49(48):1094, 1103.

### *May 1999: Kunduz Province, Afghanistan*
Twenty-six cases of acute flaccid paralysis were reported. Wild poliovirus type 1 was isolated from five of the patients. The cause of the outbreak is not

known, but the 1997 discontinuation of polio vaccination due to civil unrest may have contributed to the outbreak.

Centers for Disease Control and Prevention (CDC). Public Health Dispatch: Outbreak of Poliomyelitis—Kunduz, Afghanistan, 1999. *MMWR Morbid Mortal Wkly Rep* 1999; 48(34):761–762.

### 1952: USA

In the worst epidemic of polio since 1916, there were 57,628 cases of polio reported, with 3,300 deaths occurring from the poliovirus.

Centers for Disease Control and Prevention (CDC): National Immunization Program. *Polio Vaccine Timeline,* 2005. Available at: http://www.cdc.gov/nip/events/polio-vacc-50th/timeline.htm. Accessed October 24, 2005.

### 1949: USA and Worldwide

Polio caused 2,720 deaths in the United States. There were 42,173 cases reported worldwide.

Cook EM Jr, Anton T, Sherwood ES. The 1949 poliomyelitis epidemic. *J Maine Med Assoc* 1950; 41(8):337–339.

### 1916: USA

During America's worst polio epidemic, there were 27,363 cases of polio (infantile paralysis) with more than 7,000 deaths.

Hoff B, Smith C III. *Mapping Epidemics: A Historical Atlas of Disease.* C.H. Calisher, ed. New York: Franklin Watts; 2000.

## Pontiac Fever (*Legionella pneumophila*)

### 1990s: Japan

In a Japanese outbreak of Pontiac fever, all the occupants of a building reported similar symptoms, including fever, arthralgias, headache, and general fatigue.

Mori M, Hoshino K, et al. An outbreak of Pontiac fever due to *Legionella* serogroup 7. I. Clinical aspects. *Kansenshogaka Zasshi* [Japanese] 1995; 69:646–653.

### 1987: New York City, New York

An outbreak of Pontiac fever occurred in an office building, with a clustering of cases in an office that was air-conditioned by a dedicated, separate cooling tower. A high concentration of *Legionella pneumophila* cells were quantified in the cooling tower, and it was difficult to eliminate the organism from the tower.

Friedman S, Spitalny K, et al. Pontiac fever outbreak associated with a cooling tower. *Am J Public Health* 1987; 77(5):568–572.

### 1982: Michigan

After using a whirlpool, 14 female church-group members reported symptoms of chills, fever, chest pain, cough, and nausea. These symptoms were consistent with Pontiac fever, and the whirlpool likely served as a reservoir for the *Legionella pneumophila* organisms.

Mangione EJ, Remis RS, et al. An outbreak of Pontiac fever related to whirlpool use, Michigan, 1982. *JAMA* 1985; 253(4):535–539.

### 1981

Three hundred and seventeen automobile assembly-plant workers were affected by Pontiac fever. Molecular analysis showed that the etiologic agent was a new *Legionella* species.

Herwaldt LA, Gorman GW, et al. A new *Legionella* species, *L. feeleii* species nova, causes Pontiac fever in an automobile plant. *Ann Intern Med* 1984; 100(3):333–338.

### 1968: Pontiac, Michigan

An epidemic of acute febrile illness occurred at a county health department, characterized by fever, headache, myalgia, and malaise. This affected 144 people, including 95 of 100 people working at the health department. A defective air conditioning system was implicated, but the etiology remained unknown. The bacterial agent was thought to resemble that which causes Legionnaires' disease.

Glick TH, Gregg MB, et al. Pontiac fever. An epidemic of unknown etiology in a health department: I. Clinical and epidemiologic aspects. *Am J Epidemiol* 1978; 107(2):149–160.

## Prion Disease Epizootics ("Mad Cow Disease")

### 1986–1996: United Kingdom

There is a probable connection between the bovine spongiform encephalopathy (BSE) epidemic observed in the United Kingdom since 1986 and an outbreak of a new form of Creutzfeldt-Jakob disease (CJD) first reported in 1996. As of June 1997, 17 cases of the new variant CJD have been reported in the United Kingdom, possibly caused by the spread of BSE to humans.

Bosque PJ. Bovine spongiform encephalopathy, chronic wasting disease, scrapie, and the threat to humans from prion disease epizootics. *Curr Neurol Neurosci Rep* 2002; 2(6):488–495.

Calza L, et al. Prion diseases. [Italian]. *Ann Ital Med Int* 1998; 13(4):209–216.

Schonberger LB. New variant Creutzfeldt-Jakob disease and bovine spongiform encephalopathy. *Infect Dis Clin North Am* 1998; 12(1):111–121.

## Propofol Contamination

### 1990s

The Centers for Disease Control and Prevention (CDC) conducted investigations at 7 hospitals after reports of postoperative infections. These infections were traced to contamination of propofol, a lipid-based anesthetic agent, by strains of *Staphylococcus aureus, Candida albicans, Moraxella osloensis, Enterobacter agglomerans,* or *Serratia marcescens.*

Bennett SN, McNeil MM, et al. Postoperative infections traced to contamination of an intravenous anesthetic, propofol. *N Engl J Med* 1995; 333(3):147–154.

## Pseudomonas fluorescens

### December 2004–February 2005: Missouri, New York, Texas, and Michigan

At least 36 cases of *Pseudomonas* infection were reported across four states in patients who had received a heparin/saline flush in their indwelling central venous catheters. The flushes were prepared by IV Flush, which was determined to be the source of the *P. fluorescens.* A CDC investigation concluded that the heparin/saline flush, preloaded in syringes by IV Flush, was contaminated with *P. fluorescens* during commercial preparation. The product was recalled, and most of the patients required surgical removal of their catheters due to bloodstream infection.

Centers for Disease Control and Prevention (CDC). *Pseudomonas* bloodstream infections associated with a heparin/saline flush—Missouri, New York, Texas, and Michigan, 2004–2005. *MMWR Morbid Mortal Wkly Rep* 2005; 54(11):269–272.

## Q Fever

### 1983: Bagnes, Switzerland

More than 300 people presented with an acute illness that included high fever, chills, malaise, headache, and arthralgias. Of those patients, 191 clinical cases of Q fever were serologically confirmed. Twelve patients were hospitalized with severe bronchopneumonia. Q fever is a zoonosis caused by *Coxiella burnetii*; the movement of sheep flocks was implicated in infection dissemination. During the investigation, it was suggested that unusually dry summer and autumn seasons may have encouraged the propagation of infectious aerosols and dusts.

Centers for Disease Control and Prevention (CDC). Q fever outbreak—Switzerland. *MMWR Morbid Mortal Wkly Rep* 1984; 33(25):335–356, 361.

## *Rickettsia typhi*

### 2002: Hawaii
Murine typhus, caused by *Rickettsia typhi*, is uncommon in the United States. However, 47 cases were reported in Hawaii in 2002, the largest number recorded since 1947. Patients experienced symptoms of fever, headache, chills, myalgias, and abdominal pain.

Hoskinson S, Lipetz M, et al. Murine typhus—Hawaii, 2002. *MMWR Morbid Mortal Wkly Rep* 2003; 52(50):1224–1226.

### 1998: Kauai, Hawaii
Five cases of murine typhus, caused by *Rickettsia typhi*, occurred on southwestern Kauai. Two of the patients had concurrent leptospirosis.

Manea SJ, Sasaki DM, Ikeda JK, Bruno PP. Clinical and epidemiological observations regarding the 1998 Kauai murine typhus outbreak. *Hawaii Med J* 2001; 60(1):7–11.

### 1552: France
At the Battle of Metz, 10,000 men fighting for the Holy Roman Emperor Charles V died of typhus.

Hoff B, Smith C III. *Mapping Epidemics: A Historical Atlas of Disease.* C.H. Calisher, ed. New York: Franklin Watts; 2000.

### 1528: Naples, Italy
Typhus decimated the French military ranks as they attempted to forcibly take Naples.

Hoff B, Smith C III. *Mapping Epidemics: A Historical Atlas of Disease.* C.H. Calisher, ed. New York: Franklin Watts; 2000.

## Rift Valley Fever

### September 2000: Jizan Province, Saudi Arabia
As of September 2000, 160 suspected cases of Rift Valley Fever were reported, including 33 deaths.

World Health Organization. Epidemic and Pandemic Alert and Response (EPR): Disease Outbreak News. *2000—Rift Valley fever in Saudi Arabia—Update/Acute Haemorrhagic Fever Syndrome in Yemen—Update.* Available at: http://www.who.int/csr/don/2000_09_29/en/.

### 1977: Egypt
The first human epidemic of Rift Valley Fever occurred.

Hoff B, Smith C III. *Mapping Epidemics: A Historical Atlas of Disease.* C.H. Calisher, ed. New York: Franklin Watts; 2000.

## Rotavirus

### 1990: Worldwide

Rotaviruses are responsible for more than 600,000 pediatric deaths per year from diarrhea-associated dehydration.

Centers for Disease Control and Prevention (CDC). National Center for Infectious Diseases, Respiratory and Enteric Viruses Branch. *Disease Information: Rotavirus.* Last Updated January 20, 2005. Available at: http://www.cdc.gov/ncidod/dvrd/revb/gastro/rotavirus.htm.

## Rotavirus, Group A

### March–April 2000: Washington, DC

An outbreak of acute gastroenteritis among students, some of whom reported eating tuna or chicken salad sandwiches from one of the dining halls on campus, was reported. The DC health department's investigation indicated that group A rotavirus transmitted by food was the cause of the outbreak.

Centers for Disease Control and Prevention (CDC). Foodborne outbreak of group A rotavirus gastroenteritis among college students—District of Columbia, March–April 2000. *MMWR Morbid Mortal Wkly Rep* 2000; 49(50):1131–1133.

*Rubivirus (See Measles)*

## Salmonella enterica

### September 24, 2003: Oregon

Eighteen cases of infection with *Salmonella enterica*, serotype *typhimurium*, were linked to kits for making egg salad distributed by a vendor to a local supermarket chain. The patients all sought care in an Oregon hospital.

Keene WE, Hedberg K, Cieslak P, et al. *Salmonella* serotype *typhimurium* outbreak associated with commercially processed egg salad—Oregon, 2003. *MMWR Morbid Mortal Wkly Rep* 2003; 53(48):1132–1134.

## Salmonella enteritidis

### June 2, 2004: USA

A cluster of *Salmonella enteritidis* cases were identified and traced to consumption of natural raw almonds from Paramount Farms, California. The almonds were sold internationally. The Food and Drug Administration (FDA) recalled the product.

World Health Organization. Epidemic and Pandemic Alert and Response (EPR): Disease Outbreak News. *Salmonella Enteritidis in the United States of America.* Available at: http://www.who.int/csr/don/2004_06_02a/en/.

## Salmonella kottbus

### March 2001: California

After a multistate outbreak of food-borne disease, the California Department of
Health Services detected an increased number of *Salmonella* serotype *kottbus*
isolates in raw sprouts. Their case-control study found sickness to be associated with alfalfa-sprout consumption and, when traced back, a single sprouter
was identified. *Salmonella kottbus* was found in ungerminated seeds and floor
drains within the facility. The implicated sprouts had undergone heat treatment and soaking with a 2,000-ppm sodium hypochlorite solution rather
than the FDA-recommended 20,000-ppm calcium hypochlorite soak.

Winthrop KL, Palumbo MS, Farrar JA, et al. Alfalfa sprouts and *Salmonella kottbus*
infection: a multistate outbreak following inadequate seed disinfection with heat
and chlorine. *J Food Prot* 2003; 66(1):13–17.

## Salmonella mbandaka

### 1999: Multistate, USA

An outbreak of salmonellosis associated with consumption of *Salmonella*
*mbandaka*-contaminated alfalfa sprouts was reported in multiple states.
The contamination was thought to be a result of inadequate or faulty treatment processes. It was determined that aqueous heat treatments alone do
not appear to be a viable alternative to hyperchlorination techniques as an
effective way to eradicate *Salmonella*.

Suslow TV, Wu J, Fett WF, Harris LJ. Detection and elimination of *Salmonella*
*mbandaka* from naturally contaminated alfalfa seed by treatment with heat or
calcium hypochlorite. *J Food Prot* 2002; 65(3):452–458.

## Typhoid Fever (Salmonella typhimurium DT 104)

### August 2000: West Midlands, England, United Kingdom

The Public Health Laboratory Service (PHLS) reported that it positively identified 372 cases of *S. typhimurium*, with 7 infected patients being admitted
to the hospital, 2 people developing septicemia, and 1 patient dying. The
likely source was lettuce, tomatoes, or cucumbers found in food purchased
at take-away shops 3 days prior to symptom onset.

Public Health Laboratory Service. Press Release; September 13, 2000.

Population and Public Health Branch (PPHB). Canada Infectious Diseases News Brief;
September 22, 2000.

### 1999: Colorado

An outbreak of enteric infections associated with *Salmonella typhimurium*
occurred, with 52% of the affected people recalling consumption of raw

alfalfa-style sprouts. The investigators implicated clover sprouts grown by two sprouters. Only one of the two producers presoaked the sprouts as recommended (presoaking seeds in 20,000-ppm calcium hypochlorite solution), and it was noted that fewer infections were attributed to this particular sprouter. Once the implicated sprouts were recalled, *S. typhimurium* illness declined.

Brooks JT, Rowe SY, Shillam P, et al. *Salmonella typhimurium* infections transmitted by chlorine-pretreated clover sprout seeds. *Am J Epidemiol* 2001; 154(11):1020–1028.

### 1998-1999: Florida
Sixteen cases of typhoid fever were linked to the consumption of mamey, a fruit imported from Guatemala and Honduras.

Katz DJ, Cruz MA, et al. An outbreak of typhoid fever in Florida associated with an imported frozen fruit. *J Infec Dis* 2002; 186:234–239.

### 1984: Prince Edward Island and Ontario, Canada
Several hundred cases of salmonellosis were reported. The outbreak was caused by *Salmonella typhimurium* phage type 10 contaminating cheeses produced by Amalgamated Dairies, Ltd. The cheeses, sold under different labels, were recalled in Canada.

Centers for Disease Control and Prevention (CDC). Salmonellosis associated with cheese consumption—Canada. *MMWR Morbid Mortal Wkly* 1984; 33(27):387.

### September–October 1984: The Dalles, Oregon
A community outbreak of *Salmonella* gastroenteritis was reported, with a total of 751 afflicted persons identified as eating or working at area restaurants. The outbreak of salmonellosis was found to have been caused by the intentional contamination of restaurant salad bars by members of a religious cohort.

Torok TJ, Tauxe RV, Wise RP, et al. A large community outbreak of salmonellosis caused by intentional contamination of restaurant salad bars. *JAMA* 1997; 278(5):389–395.

### October–November 1981: Jackson, Michigan
Eighteen cases of typhoid fever were identified among 310 United Way volunteers. The volunteers had eaten a lunch served at a community banquet hall, and although no specific food source could be identified, one of the food handlers who prepared the lunch was probably a chronic carrier of *Salmonella typhi*. All 18 patients reported fever, fatigue, and headache. There were four relapses, but there were no gastrointestinal hemorrhages, perforations, or deaths.

Centers for Disease Control and Prevention (CDC). Epidemiologic notes and reports typhoid fever—Michigan. *MMWR Morbid Mortal Wkly Rep* 1982; 31(40):544, 549–550.

### 1905: New York

Mary Mallon, a cook hired by several affluent families, became known as "Typhoid Mary"—the first known healthy carrier of typhoid fever. She was forcibly detained after she was linked to several outbreaks of typhoid among the families for whom she had worked.

Hoff B, Smith C III. *Mapping Epidemics: A Historical Atlas of Disease.* C.H. Calisher, ed. New York: Franklin Watts; 2000.

### 1898: North America

Typhoid fever killed more than 1,500 American soldiers during the Spanish-American War.

Hoff B, Smith C III. *Mapping Epidemics: A Historical Atlas of Disease.* C.H. Calisher, ed. New York: Franklin Watts; 2000.

## Scarlet Fever (Group A *Streptococcus*), Bubonic Plague (*Yersinia pestis*), Smallpox (*Variola major*), or Typhus (*Rickettsia*)

### 430 BC: Athens, Greece

The historian Thucydides, when describing the "Great Plague of Athens," was most likely referring to an outbreak of one of these diseases. Illness spread through the Athenian Army, debilitating the troops and prolonging the Peloponnesian War.

Hoff B, Smith C III. *Mapping Epidemics: A Historical Atlas of Disease.* C.H. Calisher, ed. New York: Franklin Watts; 2000.

## Scombotoxin

### 2003: Canberra, Australia

Six people reported symptoms consistent with scombroid poisoning after all ate fish at the same restaurant. Symptoms included tingling of the lips, flushing, dizziness, nausea, and diarrhea. One patient presented with significant hypotension. Scombroid poisoning is also known as "histamine fish poisoning."

Hall M. Something fishy: Six patients with an unusual cause of food poisoning! *Emerg Med* 2003; 15:293–295.

### 1992: Australia

Seven cases of scombroid poisoning were reported from the ingestion of juvenile western Australian salmon (*Arripis truttaceus*). Symptoms included tingling of the lips, flushing, dizziness, nausea, and diarrhea. Scombroid poisoning is also known as "histamine fish poisoning."

Hall M. Something fishy: Six patients with an unusual cause of food poisoning! *Emerg Med* 2003; 15:293–295.

Smart DR. Scombroid poisoning. A report of seven cases involving the Western Australian salmon, *Arripis truttaceus*. *Med J Aust* 1992; 157:748–751.

### 1973: Japan
The largest recorded outbreak of scombroid poisoning involved 2,656 cases of poisoning from the ingestion of dried horse mackerel (*Trachurus japonicus*). Symptoms included tingling of the lips, flushing, dizziness, nausea, and diarrhea. Scombroid poisoning is also known as "histamine fish poisoning."

Hall M. Something fishy: Six patients with an unusual cause of food poisoning! *Emerg Med* 2003; 15:293–295.

### 1830: Scotland, United Kingdom
Five crew members of the ship *Triton of Leith* fell ill after eating bonito, a fish commonly associated with scombroid poisoning. Scombroid poisoning may include symptoms of tingling of the lips, flushing, dizziness, nausea, and diarrhea. Scombroid poisoning is also known as "histamine fish poisoning."

Hall M. Something fishy: Six patients with an unusual cause of food poisoning! *Emerg Med* 2003; 15:293–295.

Henderson PB. Case of poisoning from the bonito (*Scomber pelamis*). *Edinburgh Med J* 1830; 34:317–318.

## Serratia marcescans
### 2002: United Arab Emirates
Thirty-six infants in a special-care baby unit were colonized with this bacterium, which caused four cases of bacteremia, two cases of meningitis, two cases of sepsis, and five deaths. The source of the bacteria was the air-conditioning system.

Uduman SA, Farrukh AS, et al. An outbreak of *Serratia marcescans* infection in a special care baby unit of a community hospital in United Arab Emirates: the importance of the air conditioner duct as a nosocomial reservoir. *J Hosp Infect* 2002; 52(3):175–180.

### 1998: United Arab Emirates

Eight cases of *Serratia marcescans* bacteremia in a single cardiac intensive care unit were traced to a respiratory therapist believed to be tampering with the fentanyl supply, as well as using it himself (confirmed by hair analysis). The therapist was not charged, and there were no further cases after his dismissal.

Ostrowsky BE, Whitener C, et al. *Serratia marcescans* bacteremia traced to an infused narcotic. *N Engl J Med* 2002; 346(20):1529–1537.

### 1950–1951: San Francisco, California

An outbreak of urinary tract infections was reported in the Stanford University hospital, caused by nosocomial *S. marcescens*, and followed covert experiments that utilized *S. marcescens* as a stimulant.

Christopher GW, Cieslak TJ, Pavlin JA, Eitzen EM Jr. Biological warfare: a historical perspective. *JAMA* 1997; 278(5):412–418.

## Severe Acute Respiratory Syndrome (SARS)

### 2002–2003: China, Hong Kong, Singapore, Toronto, and Hanoi

SARS was first reported in southern China in late 2002 as a new human disease, and then was transported to Hong Kong in 2003 by an infected traveler. Ten secondary cases spread SARS to other cities. The novel coronavirus (SARS-CoV) was identified as the causative agent; the disease spread to 27 countries and probably infected a total of 8,096 patients.

Cherry JD. The chronology of the 2002–2003 SARS mini pandemic. *Paediatr Respir Rev* 2004; 5(4):262–269.

## Severe Acute Respiratory Syndrome-(SARS) like Pneumonia

### August 2003: Surrey, Vancouver, Canada

Almost 150 residents and staff of the Kinsmen Place Lodge reported symptoms that resembled a much milder version of SARS. Most recovered, but six people died of pneumonia-related illness. Laboratory testing showed a coronavirus similar to that which causes SARS. Presently, the World Health Organization (WHO) remains unconvinced that this was a new SARS outbreak.

Ho A. *SARS may be here again.* Singapore Government SARS Web site. Available at: http://www.sars.gov.sg/archive/Sars%20May%20Be%20Here%20Again%20(ST).html. Accessed August 20, 2003.

## Shigellosis

### *May 2004: Sudan*

An outbreak of shigellosis was detected in North Darfur in the Abu Shoak Internally Displaced Persons camp. As of June 30, 2004, 1,340 cases of bloody diarrhea with 11 deaths had been documented. Of the 13 stool samples taken, three were positive for *Shigella dysenteriae* type 1.

World Health Organization. Epidemic and Pandemic Alert and Response (EPR): Disease Outbreak News. *Shigellosis in Sudan.* Available at: http://www.who.int/csr/don/2004_07_14/en/.

## Smallpox (*Variola major*)

### *1763: North America*

Sir Jeffrey Amherst, commander of the British forces in North America, first suggested that smallpox deliberately be used to reduce the Native American population. After an outbreak of smallpox at Fort Pitt, the contaminated blankets were given to the Native Americans. This was followed by a smallpox epidemic among tribes of the Ohio River valley. This is an early example of using a bioweapon against a targeted population.

Christopher GW, Cieslak TJ, Pavlin JA, Eitzen EM Jr. Biological warfare: a historical perspective. *JAMA* 1997; 278(5):412–418.

### *1721: Boston, Massachusetts*

An epidemic of smallpox around the Boston area prompted Dr. Zabdiel Boylston to administer inoculations to 287 Bostonians. This is one of the first documented inoculation programs.

Hoff B, Smith C III. *Mapping Epidemics: A Historical Atlas of Disease.* C.H. Calisher, ed. New York: Franklin Watts; 2000.

Best M, Neuhauser D, Slavin L. "Cotton Mather, you dog, dam you! I'l [sic] inoculate you with this; with a pox to you": smallpox inoculation, Boston, 1721. *Qual Saf Health Care* 2004; 13:82–83.

### *1617–1619: Massachusetts*

Smallpox killed approximately 90% of the Native American population in and around Massachusetts Bay.

Hoff B, Smith C III. *Mapping Epidemics: A Historical Atlas of Disease.* C.H. Calisher, ed. New York: Franklin Watts; 2000.

### *1525–1527: Central America*

Smallpox killed 200,000 Incas.

Hoff B, Smith C III. *Mapping Epidemics: A Historical Atlas of Disease.* C.H. Calisher, ed. New York: Franklin Watts; 2000.

***735: Japan***
Smallpox afflicted members of the ruling Fujiwara family.

Hoff B, Smith C III. *Mapping Epidemics: A Historical Atlas of Disease.* C.H. Calisher ed.
New York: Franklin Watts; 2000.


## Sporothrix schenckii

### June–September, 1983

Twelve cases of cutaneous sporotrichosis among workers who had been
part of three different hay-mulching crews were reported. Each of the
three crews had used hay produced from the same fields in south-central
Oklahoma; the crop had been left in the field for five to six weeks because
of rainfall before being baled. *S. schenckii* is a fungus found in soil, plants,
and decaying vegetation. Sporotrichosis occurs after inoculation of spores
into human skin.

Cook W, Sexton DJ, Gildon B, et al. Sporotrichosis among hay-mulching workers—
Oklahoma, New Mexico. *MMWR Morbid Mortal Wkly* 1984; 33(48):682–683.


## Staphylococcus aureus

### September 2005: Dallas, Texas

As a result of Hurricane Katrina, the Centers for Disease Control and
Prevention (CDC) received reports of a cluster of infections with
methicillin-resistant *Staphylococcus aureus* (MRSA) in approximately
30 evacuees from the New Orleans area. The patients were both children
and adults. Three of these MRSA cases were culture-confirmed.

Centers for Disease Control and Prevention (CDC). Infectious disease and dermatologic conditions in evacuees and rescue workers after Hurricane Katrina—multiple
states, August–September, 2005. *MMWR Dispatch* 2005; 54(Dispatch):1–4.


## Tetrodotoxin

### 1975: Japan

The famous kabuki actor, Mitsugoro Bando, died eight hours after eating fugu
(*Takifugu rubripes*, puffer fish) liver. The fish is a delicacy; Bando enjoyed
the tingling the liver created on his lips and tongue. Bando experienced
paralysis of the arms and legs, difficulty breathing, and finally death.
Tetrodotoxin is a potent neurotoxin that blocks sodium ions and stops
nerve impulses. Fugu chefs have to be licensed in Japan.

Newman C. Twelve toxic tales. *National Geographic*; May 2005.

## *Tinea corporis*

### September 2005: Mississippi

As a result of Hurricane Katrina, the Centers for Disease Control and Prevention (CDC) received reports of 17 cases of tinea corporis infections among hurricane rescue workers. The cases occurred in 2 locations among the rescuers who were working in the wet environment of the initial evacuation plan.

Centers for Disease Control and Prevention (CDC). Infectious disease and dermatologic conditions in evacuees and rescue workers after Hurricane Katrina—multiple states, August–September, 2005. *MMWR Dispatch* 2005; 54(Dispatch):1–4.

## Tricothecene Mycotoxins

### February 13, 1982: Tuol Chrey, Kampuchea

Three artillery shells exploded near a camp of Khmer Rouge guerillas, who reportedly smelled a sweet, perfume-like odor and were quickly incapacitated. There were at least 100 casualties.

Stahl CJ, Green CC, Farnum JB. The incident at Tuol Chey: pathologic and toxicologic examinations of a casualty after chemical attack. *J Forensic Sci* 1985; 30(2):317–337.

## African Sleeping Sickness (*Trypanosoma brucei*)

### 1992: Congo

Rwandan refugee camps are stricken with African sleeping sickness in the Democratic Republic of Congo. African sleeping sickness is caused by the protozoan parasite *Trypanosoma brucei.*

Hoff B, Smith C III. *Mapping Epidemics: A Historical Atlas of Disease.* C.H. Calisher, ed. New York: Franklin Watts; 2000.

## West African Sleeping Sickness (*Trypanosoma brucei gambiensis*)

### 2001: Tanzania

Nine cases of trypanosomiasis with one death were reported after patients visited the Tarangire and Serengeti National Parks.

Jelinek T, Bisoffi A, et al. Cluster of African trypanosomiasis in travelers to Tanzanian national parks. *Emerg Infect Dis* 2002; 8(6):634–635.

## Tuberculosis (*Mycobacterium tuberculosis*)

### September 2005: Philadelphia, Pennsylvania

As a result of Hurricane Katrina, the Centers for Disease Control and Prevention (CDC) initiated a search for all known tuberculosis patients that were originally located in the affected Gulf region in order to assure their therapy continued. Through early screening, a new case of tuberculosis was identified. The diagnosed patient was a homeless individual who was evacuated from New Orleans. The patient was isolated and promptly administered treatment; culture confirmed the diagnosis of tuberculosis.

Centers for Disease Control and Prevention (CDC). Infectious disease and dermatologic conditions in evacuees and rescue workers after Hurricane Katrina—multiple states, August–September, 2005. *MMWR Dispatch* 2005; 54(Dispatch):1–4.

### 1989–1992: Maine

An outbreak of tuberculosis in a small town in Maine included 21 active cases of tuberculosis among shipyard workers and local residents.

Allos BM, Genshelmer KF, et al. Management of an outbreak of tuberculosis in a small community. *Ann Intern Med* 1996; 125(2):114–117.

### 1930: Lubeck, Germany

Two hundred seven of 251 newborn babies who were given oral bacillus Calmette-Guerin (BCG) vaccination to prevent tuberculosis ended up developing tuberculosis as a result of the vaccination. Seventy-two babies died. The occurrence was due to the preparation containing nonattenuated human tubercle bacilli being replaced with the nonvirulent BCG vaccine.

Wax PM. Toxicologic plagues and disasters in history. L.R. Goldfrank, ed. In: *Goldfrank's Toxicologic Emergencies*, 7th ed. New York: McGraw-Hill; 2002; pp. 23–34.

Lambert ED. *Modern Medical Mistakes*. Bloomington, IN: University Press; 1978.

## Typhoid Fever (*Salmonella typhimurium*), Dysentery (*Shigella dysenteriae*), or Malaria

### 1081: Rome, Italy

The army of Holy Roman Emperor Henry IV was afflicted with an outbreak of typhoid fever, dysentery, or malaria during the army's attack on Rome.

Hoff B, Smith C III. *Mapping Epidemics: A Historical Atlas of Disease*. C. H. Calisher, ed. New York: Franklin Watts; 2000.

## Typhus (see *Rickettsia typhi*)

## Venom, Scorpion

### AD *199: Hatra, Iraq*

Romans attacked the city of Hatra, in what is now Iraq. In retaliation, the citizens of Hatra lobbed scorpion-filled clay pots over the walls of the city. This is an early example of biological warfare.

Newman C. Twelve toxic tales. *National Geographic;* May 2005.

## *Vibrio cholerae*

### *January 1997: Zaire*

Fifty-six cases of cholera with two deaths were reported in the Tingi Tingi Rwandan refugee camp.

World Health Organization. Epidemic and Pandemic Alert and Response (EPR): Disease Outbreak News, *Health situation in Rwandan refugee camp in Zaire.* Available at: http://www.who.int/csr/don/1997_01_20/en/.

### *Yacuiba, Bolivia*

An outbreak of cholera was reported in Yacuiba, Tarija Province, on the border of Argentina. Approximately 492 cases were reported, with another 231 cases, including six deaths, occurring in other Bolivian provinces. Fifty percent of these cases were confirmed with laboratory tests.

World Health Organization. Epidemic and Pandemic Alert and Response (EPR): Disease Outbreak News. *Cholera in Bolivia.* Available at: http://www.who.int/csr/don/1997_01_22/en/.

### *Rumonge, Burundi*

An outbreak of cholera was reported with approximately 482 cases and 21 deaths. The affected village was the target of an armed group, and there was a breakdown of water supplies. That lack of water, in conjunction with poor hygiene practices and an increase in displaced persons, contributed to the outbreak.

World Health Organization. Epidemic and Pandemic Alert and Response (EPR): Disease Outbreak News. *Cholera in Burundi—Update.* Available at: http://www.who.int/csr/don/1997_01_17b/en/.

### *November 1995: Suleimaniyah, Iraq*

UNICEF indicated that the local water was not being chlorinated. The lack of chlorine resulted in a cholera outbreak culminating in 340 confirmed cases and three deaths. Cholera was confirmed in Arbil and Dohuk.

United Nations Commission of Human Rights: Report on the situation of human rights in Iraq. Submitted by the Special Rapportuer, Mr. Max van der Stoel, in accordance with Commission resolution 1995/76. March 4, 1996. E/CN.4/1996/61.

### 1982: Truk, Federated States of Micronesia, Trust Territories of the Pacific Islands

Approximately 892 cases of diarrhea and 11 deaths due to diarrhea were reported. The outbreak began in the outer islands of Pulap, Pulusuk, Puluwat, and Tamatan. *Vibrio cholerae* O1 was isolated from stool cultures in 109 patients.

Centers for Disease Contol and Prevention (CDC). Vibrio cholerae—Truk, Federated States of Micronesia. *MMWR Morbid Mortal Wkly Rep* 1982; 31(39):539.

### 1881–1896: India

After previous cholera outbreaks, a fifth cholera pandemic spread from India to both the East and West. However, many of the major European and American cities were spared from this outbreak due to improved urban sanitation.

Hoff B, Smith C III. *Mapping Epidemics: A Historical Atlas of Disease.* C.H. Calisher, ed. New York: Franklin Watts; 2000.

### 1863: India

An 1863 cholera epidemic in India spread to Europe and the United States by the year 1866.

Hoff B, Smith C III. *Mapping Epidemics: A Historical Atlas of Disease.* C.H. Calisher, ed. New York: Franklin Watts; 2000.

### 1826–1837: Europe and Americas

After a cholera pandemic subsided in 1826, a second pandemic began in India and spread from Asia to Russia; Ottoman, Turkey; and then to Europe and the Americas.

Hoff B, Smith C III. *Mapping Epidemics: A Historical Atlas of Disease.* C.H. Calisher, ed. New York: Franklin Watts; 2000.

### 1817–1823: Asia, Middle East

A pandemic of cholera that originated in India moved to Asia, the Middle East, and then Russia.

Hoff B, Smith C III. *Mapping Epidemics: A Historical Atlas of Disease.* C.H. Calisher, ed. New York: Franklin Watts; 2000.

## *Vibrio cholerae* O1 El Tor

### *June 15, 2004: Cameroon*

Reports from the Ministry of Health note that a total number of 2,924 cases and 46 deaths from January–June 2004 have been linked to *Vibrio cholerae* O1 El Tor.

World Health Organization. Epidemic and Pandemic Alert and Response (EPR): Disease Outbreak News. *Cholera in Cameroon.* Available at: http://www.who.int/csr/don/2004_06_15/en/.

## *Vibrio parahemolyticus*

### *September 2005: Arkansas, Arizona, Georgia, Louisiana, Mississippi, Oklahoma, and Texas*

As a result of Hurricane Katrina, the Centers for Disease Control and Prevention (CDC) received reports of 24 cases of *Vibrio vulnificus* and *V. parahaemolyticus* wound infections among hurricane evacuees. There were 6 deaths.

Centers for Disease Control and Prevention (CDC). Infectious disease and dermatologic conditions in evacuees and rescue workers after Hurricane Katrina–multiple states, August–September, 2005. *MMWR Dispatch* 2005; 54(Dispatch):1–4.

### *1998: Galveston Bay, Texas*

Four hundred sixteen cases of gastroenteritis were associated with eating oysters harvested from the bay.

Shapiro RL, Alterkruse S, et al. The role of Gulf Coast oysters harvested in winter months in *vibrio vulnificus* infections in the United States, 1998–1996. Vibrio Working Group. *J Infect Dis* 1998; 178:752–759.

### *1974–1975: Caribbean*

Outbreaks of gastrointestinal illness associated with *V. parahaemolyticus* occurred on 2 cruise ships; a total of 697 passengers and 27 crew members were affected. Seafood was implicated as the vehicle of transmission after it was cooked in seawater from the ships' internal seawater distribution systems. There were no more outbreaks once seawater was no longer used in the ships' food-handling areas.

Lawrence DN, Blake PA, Yashuk JC, et al. *Vibrio parahaemolyticus* gastroenteritis outbreaks aboard two cruise ships. *Am J Epidemiol* 1979; 109(1):71–80.

## Vibrio vulnificus

### September 2005: Arkansas, Arizona, Georgia, Louisiana, Mississippi, Oklahoma, and Texas

As a result of Hurricane Katrina, the Centers for Disease Control and Prevention (CDC) received reports of 24 cases of *Vibrio vulnificus* and *V. parahaemolyticus* wound infections among hurricane evacuees. There were six deaths.

Centers for Disease Control and Prevention (CDC). Infectious disease and dermatologic conditions in evacuees and rescue workers after Hurricane Katrina—multiple states, August–September, 2005. *MMWR Dispatch* 2005; 54(Dispatch):1–4.

## Vitamin B$_6$

### 1983–1984: USA

Excessive intake of vitamin B$_6$ led to sensory neuropathy.

World Health Organization. *Neurotoxicity Risk Assessment for Human Health: Principles and Approaches. Environmental Health Criteria 223.* Geneva, Switzerland, 2001. Available at: http://www.inchem.org/documents/ehc/ehc/ehc223.htm#223230000.

Spencer PS, Schaumburg HH, Ludolph AC. *Experimental and Clinical Neurotoxicology,* 6th ed. New York: Oxford University Press; 2000.

## West Nile Virus

### 2000: Zerifin, Israel

Thirty-five patients were admitted to a local hospital; nearly two thirds had a neurological finding on presentation. Two patients died as a result of meningoencephalopathy.

Klein C, Pollack L, et al. Neurological features of West Nile infection during the 2000 outbreak in a regional hospital in Israel. *J Neuro Sci* 2002; 200:63–66.

### 1999: New York City, New York

Seven deaths were associated with the West Nile virus. This may have been the first appearance of the West Nile virus in North America.

West Nile Virus; International Cases Provide Blueprint for Understanding U.S. Outbreak. *TB & Outbreaks Weekly,* September 10, 2002; p. 6.

Hoff B, Smith C III. *Mapping Epidemics: A Historical Atlas of Disease.* C.H. Calisher, ed. New York: Franklin Watts; 2000.

### July 1999: Russia

Five hundred illnesses were reported to be associated with the West Nile virus, resulting in 40 deaths. Of the patients who died, 76% had meningococcal meningitis and were over 60 years of age.

West Nile Virus; International Cases Provide Blueprint for Understanding U.S. Outbreak. *TB & Outbreaks Weekly*; September 10, 2002; p. 6.

### 1996: Southeastern Romania

Three hundred ninety-three people were infected with West Nile virus, and 17 people died. Many of the patients were located in and around Bucharest or other urban settings.

West Nile Virus; International Cases Provide Blueprint for Understanding U.S. Outbreak. *TB & Outbreaks Weekly*; September 10, 2002; p. 6.

## Yellow Fever

### May–June 2004: Burkina Faso

As of May 10, 2004, the Ministry of Health Burkina Faso had reported 25 suspected cases of yellow fever occurring in the districts of Bobo-Dioulasso and Gaoua. Four of the cases were laboratory confirmed and are believed to have originated in Bobo-Dioulasso. Both the commencement of the rainy season and presence of *Aedes aegypti*, the vector for yellow fever transmission, prompted the World Health Organization (WHO) to recommend a mass vaccination campaign.

World Health Organization. Epidemic and Pandemic Alert and Response (EPR): Disease Outbreak News. *Yellow fever in Burkina Faso*. Available at: http://www.who.int/csr/don/2004_05_11/en/.

World Health Organization. Epidemic and Pandemic Alert and Response (EPR): Disease Outbreak News. *Yellow Fever in Burkina Faso—update*. Available at: http://www.who.int/csr/don/2004_06_01/en/.

### 1878: Memphis, Tennessee

An outbreak of yellow fever in the lower Mississippi Valley killed more than 13,000 people.

Hoff B, Smith C III. *Mapping Epidemics: A Historical Atlas of Disease*. C. H. Calisher, ed. New York: Franklin Watts; 2000.

### 1853: New Orleans, Louisiana

Yellow fever caused the deaths of more than 7,000 people.

Hoff B, Smith C III. *Mapping Epidemics: A Historical Atlas of Disease*. C.H. Calisher, ed. New York: Franklin Watts; 2000.

### 1803: Haiti

French troops fell ill with yellow fever on the island of Hispaniola. This outbreak forced France to cede control of what is present-day Haiti to African slaves who had rebelled against French authority.

Hoff B, Smith C III. *Mapping Epidemics: A Historical Atlas of Disease.* C.H. Calisher, ed. New York: Franklin Watts; 2000.

### 1668: New York

An epidemic of yellow fever struck New York, and was probably the earliest recorded episode in nontropical America.

Hoff B, Smith C III. *Mapping Epidemics: A Historical Atlas of Disease.* C.H. Calisher, ed. New York: Franklin Watts; 2000.

### 1647: Barbados

More than 5,000 people died from yellow fever.

Hoff B, Smith C III. *Mapping Epidemics: A Historical Atlas of Disease.* C.H. Calisher, ed. New York: Franklin Watts; 2000.

## Yersinia enterocolitica

### December 2002–January 2003: Chicago, Illinois

A cluster of *Y. enterocolitica* infections was reported during a 10-week period among nine infants under the age of one year. Caretakers of six of the nine infants purchased chitterlings from the same grocery store chain, but from three different locations. Chitterlings are pig intestines, stewed and then frequently battered and fried. Chitterlings are a known source of *Y. enterocolitica* gastroenteritis. All of the infants recovered.

Jones RC, Fernandez JR, Gerber SI, et al. *Yersinia enterocolitica* gastroenteritis among infants exposed to chitterlings—Chicago, Illinois, 2002. *MMWR Morbid Mortal Wkly Rep* 2003; 52(40):956–958.

### June–July 1982: Southern USA

An interstate outbreak of *Y. enterocolitica* infections occurred in Arkansas, Tennessee, and Mississippi. A total of 172 culture-positive cases were identified; most of the patients required hospitalization and 148 patients had enteric infections. An epidemiologic investigation found that the source of infection was milk pasteurized at a plant in Memphis, Tennessee.

Centers for Disease Control and Prevention (CDC). Epidemiologic notes and reports multi-state outbreak of Yersiniosis. *MMWR Morbid Mortal Wkly Rep* 1982; 31(37):505–506.

## Bubonic Plague (*Yersinia pestis*)

### January 1997: Namwala, Zambia

Ninety cases of plague with 22 deaths were reported in the Southern Province of Zambia. The outbreak was thought to be linked to heavy rain and flooding, causing rats to invade inhabited areas. Fleas were also reported to be abundant.

World Health Organization. Epidemic and Pandemic Alert and Response (EPR): Disease Outbreak News. *Bubonic plague in Zambia.* Available at: http://www.who.int/csr/don/1997_01_31b/en/.

### 1720: Marseilles, France

An epidemic of plague killed one third of the local population.

Hoff B, Smith C III. *Mapping Epidemics: A Historical Atlas of Disease.* C.H. Calisher, ed. New York: Franklin Watts; 2000.

### October–November 1630: Venice, Italy

The Venetian plague of 1630 was extensively documented. Records show that over 1,000 people died, a large number of whom were women. A smallpox epidemic was raging simultaneously with the plague epidemic.

Ell SR. Three days in October of 1630: detailed examination of mortality during an early modern plague epidemic in Venice. *Rev Infect Dis* 1989; 11(1):128–141.

### 1300s: Caffa

The Tatar soldiers of the 14th century purportedly threw contaminated corpses into a Christian stronghold in Caffa, which sparked an epidemic of the plague throughout Crimea. The plague, or "Black Death," is thought to have been caused by the gram-negative zoonotic bacterium *Y. pestis*, and some believe this was the source of the bacteria that swept through Europe. If true, this would be one of the first incidents of bioterrorism.

Wheelis M. Biological warfare at the 1346 Siege of Caffa. *Emerg Infect Dis* 2002; 8(9):971–975.

Sabbatani S. Observations of the 1348 pest epidemic. Measures taken to combat its tragic effects and avoid epidemic recrudescence. *Infect Med* 2003; 11(1):49–61.

### 542: Mediterranean

A pandemic of bubonic plague, termed the "Plague of Justinian," swept through the Mediterranean countries.

Hoff B, Smith C III. *Mapping Epidemics: A Historical Atlas of Disease.* C.H. Calisher, ed. New York; Franklin Watts; 2000.

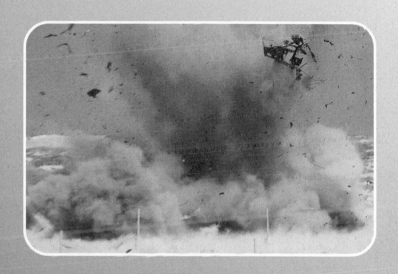

# RADIOLOGICAL EVENTS

# Chapter 3

# RADIOLOGICAL EVENTS

## Cesium 137

### November 1994: Tammiku, Estonia

Three brothers stole a small quantity of cesium 137 from a radioactive waste facility. The source was transported in a jacket pocket and then hung in a hallway of the thief's home. Four days later, he was hospitalized and died from kidney failure. Two weeks later, the son of the deceased found the source and moved it to the kitchen. He received burns to his hand that hospital staff identified as radiation-related burns. Four people in total were injured and one died. A dog also died from radiation exposure.

International Atomic Energy Agency (IAEA). *The Radiological Accident in Tammiku.* Vienna, Austria: IAEA; 1998. Available at: http://www-pub.iaea.org/MTCD/publications/PDF/Pub1053_web.pdf.

### September 13, 1987: Goiânia, Brazil

Scavengers found an abandoned radiotherapy unit in a demolished clinic and sold it to a junkyard owner who noticed a blue glow coming from the container at night. He opened the shielded container and distributed the unusual material to many of his neighbors, some of whom spread it on their skin. Several people became ill after contacting the material. Eventually, the wife of the junkyard owner transported a sample of the material by public bus to a hospital, stating it was the cause of her family's illness. Despite this claim, tropical disease was suspected by all but one physician, who fortunately contacted a medical physicist to evaluate the material. The medical physicist confirmed the material to be radioactive. More than 100,000 people were screened for radiation exposure; 129 were found to be contaminated and 20 were hospitalized. A total of five people died and 23 were injured. Eighty-five homes were demolished in the clean-up process.

da Cruz AD, Volpe JP, Saddi V, et al. Radiation risk estimation in human populations: Lessons from the radiological accident in Brazil. *Mutat Res* 1997; 373(2):207–214.

International Atomic Energy Agency (IAEA). *Dosimetric and Medical Aspects of the Radiological Accident in Goiânia in 1987.* IAEA-TECDOC-1009.Vienna, Austria: IAEA; 1998. Available at: http://www-pub.iaea.org/MTCD/publications/PDF/te_1009_prn.pdf.

Valverde NJ, Oliveira AR. The Early Medical Response to the Goiânia Accident. In: *Restoration of Environments Affected by Residues from Radiological Accidents: Approaches to Decision Making. Proceedings of an International Workshop held in Rio de Janeiro and Goiânia, Brazil, 29 August–2 September 1994.* IAEA-TECDOC-1131. Vienna, Austria: IAEA; 2000; pp. 138–141. Available at: http://www-pub.iaea.org/MTCD/publications/PDF/te_1131_prn.pdf.

Agency for Toxic Substances and Disease Registry (ATSDR). *Toxicological Profile for Ionizing Radiation.* Atlanta: ATDSR, U.S. Department of Health and Human Services; 1999; pp. 195–197. Available at: http://www.atsdr.cdc.gov/toxprofiles/tp149.html.

## Cesium 137 and Cobalt 60

### August 2000–March 2001: Panama City, Panama
Errors in radiotherapy dosage calculations at the Instituto Oncológico Nacional resulted in 28 patients developing symptoms of radiation overexposure. Seventeen deaths were attributed to radiation exposure, 13 of which were associated with rectal complications. Many of the nonlethal exposures resulted in bowel-related radiation injury.

Borras C, Bares JP, Rudder D, et al. Clinical effects in a cohort of cancer patients overexposed during external beam pelvic radiotherapy. *Int J Radiat Oncol Biol Phys* 2004; 59(2):538–550.

International Atomic Energy Agency (IAEA). *Investigation of an Accidental Exposure of Radiotherapy Patients in Panama: Report of a Team of Experts, 26 May–1 June 2001.* Vienna, Austria: IAEA; 2001. Available at: http://www-pub.iaea.org/MTCD/publications/PDF/Pub1114_scr.pdf.

## Cobalt 60

### January 20, 2000–February 24, 2000: Samut Prakarn, Thailand
Radioactive material contained in its protective housing was purchased by a Thai man as scrap metal on January 24, 2000. The source of this material was unknown. After successfully dismantling the housing, multiple people were exposed to the material and became ill. Local physicians identified radiation exposure as the likely cause. The material was not secured until

February 20, 2000, and the total number of persons exposed is unknown. Three individuals died and seven were injured due to exposure. Injuries were primarily radiation burns.

International Atomic Energy Agency (IAEA). *The Radiological Accident in Samut Prakarn.* Vienna, Austria: IAEA; 2002. Available at: http://www.pub.iaea.org/MTCD/publications/PDF/Pub1124_scr.pdf.

### August 22, 1996–September 27, 1996: San José, Costa Rica

A radiotherapy unit in Costa Rica was miscalibrated, which resulted in a 60% overexposure to a source of cobalt 60. Estimates of total morbidity and mortality vary widely, but are significant. Between seven and 17 deaths were attributed to radiation overdose. Of the surviving patients, it is estimated that 81 received varying degrees of injury. Twenty-two patients had no discernable injury.

International Atomic Energy Agency (IAEA). *Accidental Overexposure of Radiotherapy Patients in San José, Costa Rica.* Vienna, Austria: IAEA; 1998. Available at: http://www-pub.iaea.org/MTCD/publications/PDF/P027_scr.pdf.

Ortiz P, Oresegun M, Wheatley J. *Lessons from Major Radiation Accidents.* International Radiation Protection Association (IRPA) International Congress Proceedings: IRPA 10—Scientific Topics; Radiologic & Nuclear Accidents. Ref. P-11-230. Available at: http://www.irpa.net/irpa10/cdrom/00140.pdf.

### November 19, 1992: Jilin, Xinzhou Province, China

A cobalt 60 source was stolen by a construction worker during decommissioning of an industrial irradiation facility. The source was transported to the worker's home, and eight individuals were exposed to high levels of radiation. The construction worker, his brother, and his father all died from radiation exposure. Local medical personnel did not recognize the radiation injuries and were themselves exposed when the source was brought to the hospital. The source was neither recognized nor secured for more than 70 days. Five additional individuals, including medical staff, received significant radiation-related injury.

Nenot JC. Radiation accidents: lessons learnt for future radiological protection. *Int J Radiat Biol* 1998; 73(4):435–442.

United Nations Scientific Committee on the Effects of Atomic Radiation (UNSCEAR). Annex E: Occupational radiation exposures. In: *Sources and Effects of Ionizing Radiation.* United Nations Scientific Committee on the Effects of Atomic Radiation. UNSCEAR 2000 Report to the General Assembly, with Scientific Annexes, Volume I: Sources. Vienna, Austria: UNSCEAR; 2000. Available at: http://www.unscear.org/pdffiles/annexe.pdf.

### February 5, 1989: San Salvador, El Salvador

During repair of a medical sterilizing facility, a cobalt 60 source fell into an unshielded area. Radiation monitors were disabled at the time, and several employees received radiation exposure. One person died and two sustained radiation injury.

International Atomic Energy Association (IAEA). *The Radiological Accident in San Salvador.* Vienna, Austria: IAEA; 1990. Available at: http://www-pub.iaea.org/MTCD/publications/PDF/Pub847_web.pdf.

### December 1983–February 1984: Ciudad Juarez, Mexico

A medical radiotherapy source containing several thousand 1-mm pellets of cobalt 60 was illegally purchased from a Texas hospital by the Centro Médico in Ciudad Juarez, Mexico. A local handyman stole the source from a warehouse and in turn sold it to a recycling plant. There it was dismantled and unknowingly recycled into a variety of radioactive consumer products. Products included table bases, construction rebar, and various forms of industrial steel. This steel was sold throughout Mexico, Canada, and the United States. Radioactive steel was eventually discovered at the Los Alamos National Laboratory in New Mexico, when radiation detectors sounded as a truck driver hauling radioactive rebar stopped to ask for directions. The source was eventually traced to the recycling plant in Ciudad Juarez. An estimated 600 tons of radioactive steel were shipped into 23 U.S. states. One hundred nine houses in Sinaloa, Mexico were constructed with radioactive rebar and subsequently demolished. U.S. reconnaissance helicopters have found 22 radioactive sites between Chihuahua and Juarez. The U.S. Federal Nuclear Regulatory Commission has initiated radiation monitoring at all border crossings. One fatality and four radiation injuries are attributed to this accident. Clean-up costs are in excess of a million dollars.

Texas Department of State Health Services, Bureau of Radiation Control. Incident Investigation Program. *Significant Events.* Available at: http://www.tdh.state.tx.us/radiation/complaints.htm.

Lister BAJ. Contaminated Mexican steel incident. *J Soc Radiol Protect* 1985; 5:145–147.

### 1975: Brescia, Italy

Poor safety control at a food irradiation facility resulted in significant radiation exposure at a conveyor entrance. One person died 13 days after exposure.

United Nations Scientific Committee on the Effects of Atomic Radiation (UNSCEAR). Annex E: Occupational radiation exposures. In: *Sources and Effects of Ionizing Radiation: United Nations Scientific Committee on the Effects of Atomic Radiation.* UNSCEAR 2000 Report to the General Assembly, with Scientific Annexes, Volume 1. Vienna, Austria: UNSCEAR; 2000. Available at: http://www.unscear.org/pdffiles/annexe.pdf.

### January 1963: Sanlian Province, China

A cobalt 60 source was unearthed from an underground waste site and taken to a private residence where six people received radiation exposure. Two of them died and four were injured. One person suffered a leg amputation.

Ortiz P, Oresegun M, Wheatley J. Lessons for Major Radiation Accidents, International Radiation Protection Association (IRPA) International Congress Proceedings: IRPA 10 Scientific Topics; Radiologic and Nuclear Accidents. Ref. P-11-230. Available at: http://www.irpa.net/irpa10/cdrom/00140.pdf.

### 1962: Mexico City, Mexico

A cobalt 60 source was lost from an industrial radiographic site. Four people unwittingly received lethal doses of radiation.

Ortiz P, Oresegun M, Wheatley J. Lessons for Radiation Accidents, International Radiation Protection Association (IRPA) International Congress Proceedings: IRPA 10 Scientific Topics; Radiologic and Nuclear Accidents. Ref. P-11-230. Available at: http://www.irpa.net/irpa10/cdrom/00140.pdf.

## Ionizing Radiation

### 1954: Marshall Islands

Fallout from the nuclear testing program led to the development of thyroid cancer in local inhabitants.

United Nations Scientific Committee on the Effects of Atomic Radiation (UNSCEAR). *Sources, Effects and Risks of Ionizing Radiation.* United Nations Scientific Committee on the Effects of Atomic Radiation. UNSCEAR 1988 Report to the General Assembly, with Annexes. Vienna, Austria: UNSCEAR; 1988.

## Iridium 192

### June 22, 2002: Cochabamba, Bolivia

An industrial radiographic source used to inspect welding seams malfunctioned in the field. The field radiographer elected to return the source to the capital, La Paz, about 400 km by passenger bus, believing it to be properly housed. However, the source was not fully within its shielding and the bus commuters were exposed during the eight-hour ride to La Paz. Once in La Paz, the source was transported by taxi, and only after its return was it discovered to be emitting dangerous levels of radiation. No employees were injured and although few passengers were located, none reported signs of injury.

International Atomic Energy Agency (IAEA). *The Radiological Accident in Cochabamba.* Vienna, Austria: IAEA; 2004. Available at: http://www-pub.iaea.org/MTCD/publications/PDF/Pub1199_web.pdf.

### March 1984: Casablanca, Morocco
A radiography source was misplaced and taken home by an employee. The employee kept the source on a bedroom table for approximately two weeks. Eight family members died and three received radiation injury.

International Atomic Energy Agency (IAEA). *The Radiological Accident in Goiânia.* Vienna, Austria: IAEA; 1988. Available at: http://www-pub.iaea.org/MTCD/publications/PDF/Pub815_web.pdf.

### July 29, 1981: Tulsa, Oklahoma
Douglas Crofut, an unemployed industrial radiographer, stole a source of iridium 192 and sustained self-inflicted radiation injuries. He later died from radiation exposure.

Mize K. *Classical Radiological Dispersal Devices (RDD).* Office of Emergency Response, National Nuclear Security Administration. Available at: http://www.nlectc.org/training/nij2004/mize.pdf.

### May 1978: Sétif, Algeria
An industrial radiographic source was found by two children. After playing with the source, the children's grandmother stored it in her kitchen. Six persons received radiation injury. Both children required finger amputation and one miscarriage was attributed to radiation exposure. The grandmother later died from radiation injury.

Cosset JM. ESTRO Breur Gold Medal Award Lecture 2001: irradiation accidents– lessons for oncology? *Radiother Oncol* 2002; 63(1):1–10.

## Nitric Acid and Plutonium Explosion
### December 30, 1958: Los Alamos, New Mexico
A mixture of nitric acid and plutonium-bearing solids was combined with emulsion in a tank, and shortly after initiating a nonnuclear reaction, the operator and a nearby employee observed a "blue flash." The employee died 35 hours later from the effects of radiation, and two other employees received radiation exposure.

*Operational Accidents and Radiation Exposure Experience Within the United States Atomic Energy Commission, 1943–1970.* WASH 1192. Washington, DC: U.S. Government Printing Office; 1971.

McLaughlin TP, Monahan SP, Pruvost NL. *A Review of Criticality Accidents, 2000 Revision.* Tech Report No. LA-13638. Los Alamos: Los Alamos National Laboratories; 2000.

## Plutonium 239

### January 16, 1966: Palomares, Spain

During a mid-air refueling operation, a U.S. Air Force (USAF) B-52 bomber
carrying four nuclear weapons collided with a USAF KC-135 tanker over
the southern Spanish coast. Two weapons landed near Palomares, resulting
in various amounts of radioactive contamination over 558 acres. The
USAF removed the surface soil layer, and of the 714 people examined
through 1988, 124 had urine plutonium concentrations greater than the
minimum detection limits.

Agency for Toxic Substances and Disease Registry (ATSDR). *Toxicological Profile for
Ionizing Radiation.* Atlanta: ATDSR, U.S. Department of Health and Human Services;
1999; pp. 195–197. Available at: http://www.atsdr.cdc.gov/toxprofiles/tp149.html.

## Plutonium 240, 238

### January 1968: Thule, Greenland

A U.S. Air Force plane experienced an onboard fire and crashed during emergency landing procedures. The force of the crash and onboard explosions
caused the dispersion of plutonium debris over a 100 m × 700 m area. The
radionuclides settled into the bottom sediments of local water basins, and
the bivalve and crustacean levels of plutonium increased by a factor of 10
to 1,000.

Agency for Toxic Substances and Disease Registry (ATSDR). *Toxicological Profile for
Ionizing Radiation.* Atlanta: ATDSR, U.S. Department of Health and Human Services;
1999; pp. 195–197. Available at: http://www.atsdr.cdc.gov/toxprofiles/tp149.html.

## Plutonium-Contaminated Materials

### 1957, 1969: Rocky Flats, Colorado

There have been several incidents at the Rocky Flats Nuclear Weapons Plant,
including two fires in 1957 and leakage of plutonium-containing cutting
oils from storage drums. These incidents led to the disturbance of filtration
and storage, allowing plutonium contamination of soil and local water
sources. However, subsequent epidemiologic investigations did not find
significant increases in cancer rates for the region.

Agency for Toxic Substances and Disease Registry (ATSDR). *Toxicological Profile for
Ionizing Radiation.* Atlanta: ATDSR, U.S. Department of Health and Human Services;
1999; pp. 195–197. Available at: http://www.atsdr.cdc.gov/toxprofiles/tp149.html.

## Plutonium Criticality

### August 21, 1945: Los Alamos, New Mexico

An employee accidentally dropped a brick of tungsten carbide onto a plutonium assembly, which provided the necessary neutron reflection to reach
a supercritical power excursion. Although the worker quickly removed the
brick and dismantled the plutonium metal assembly, he received a dose of
510 rem radiation and died about a month later. A nearby Army guard
sustained a dose of 50 rem radiation.

McLaughlin TP, Monahan SP, Pruvost NL. *A Review of Criticality Accidents, 2000
Revision*. Tech Report No. LA-13638. Los Alamos: Los Alamos National Laboratories;
2000.

## Radiation Exposure

### 1999: Kingisepp, Russia

The radioactive core of a radiothermal generator was discovered at a bus stop
in Kingisepp, Russia. The source was stolen from a lighthouse in the vicinity and intended for scrap metal. The three men who stole the source died
of radiation-related injuries and an unknown number of people were
exposed.

Bodrov O. *Thieves Steal Radioactive Object in Russia*. Pravda; April 17, 2003.

Rashid A. *Radioisotope Thermoelectric Generators*. Bellona Foundation; April 2, 2005.
Available at: http://www.bellona.no/en/international/russia/navy/northern_fleet/
incidents/37598.htm.

### September 13, 1999: Grozny, Chechnya

Six individuals attempted to steal radioactive material from the Radon Special
Combine chemical plant in Grozny. Within 30 minutes of taking the material, one suspect died and another collapsed. All of the suspects were ap-
prehended and eventually hospitalized. Three of the suspects died and
three sustained radiation injuries.

Krock L, Deusser R. *Dirty Bomb: Chronology of Events*. NOVA; February 2003. Public
Broadcasting System (PBS). Available at: http://www.pbs.org/wgbh/nova/dirtybomb/
chrono.html.

Parrish S, ed. *Criminal dies stealing radioactive material*. Washington, DC: Center for
Nonproliferation Studies, Nuclear Threat Initiative (NTI; 21 October 1999). Available
at: http://www.nti.org/db/nistraff/1999/19990810.htm.

## Radioactive Leak

### November 1996: Sosnovy-Bor, Russia

The Finnish Center for Radiation and Nuclear Safety, which monitors the activity of the Leningrad Nuclear Power Plant, discovered leaks in the reactor-cooling turbine condensers. The center believes these leaks to be the result of the corrosive salt water used to lower reactor temperatures.

Badkhen A. *Nuclear Plant Whistleblower 'Silenced'*. St. Petersburg Times; September 7, 1999.

## Radioactive Steam

### 1961: North Atlantic Ocean

A Russian K-19 submarine developed a leak in the cooling circuit of its nuclear reactor. The leak was inaccessible to maintenance, forcing the crew to release radioactive steam and gases into the reactor compartment. Eight crew members later died from radiation exposure and 31 others received radiation injuries.

Huchthausen P. *K-19: The Widowmaker*. Washington, DC: National Geographic Books; 2002.

Nilsen T, Kudrik I, Nikitin A. Nuclear submarine accidents. In: *Report 2, 1996: The Russian Northern Fleet*. Bellona Foundation; 1996 Available at: http://www.bellona.no/imaker?sub=1&id=11084.

## Radioactive Water

### January 1990: Ontario, Canada

Computer software error caused 12 metric tons of heavy water coolant to spill into the reactor vault after the brakes on the fueling machine bridge were released. This occurred at the Bruce A nuclear station's Unit 4 reactor.

*Nucleonics Week*; May 31, 1990.

### 1920s: USA

"Radithor," or radioactive water, was sold as radium-containing patent medication. It was sold all over the world as "harmless in every respect" and was promoted as a sexual stimulant. More than 400,000 bottles were sold. The 1932 death of a prominent Radithor connoisseur from chronic radiation exposure helped reform the era of radioactive patent medications.

Wax PM. Toxicologic plagues and disasters in history. In: LR Goldfrank, ed. *Goldfrank's Toxicologic Emergencies*, 7th ed. New York: McGraw-Hill; 2002; pp. 23–34.

Macklis RM. Radithor and the era of mild radium therapy. *JAMA* 1990; 264(5): 614–618.

# Radium

### 1994: Bear Lake, Michigan

It was discovered that a house located in Bear Lake was significantly contaminated with radium. The family was relocated by the Environmental Protection Agency (EPA), and the home was demolished. The debris, soil, and the family's contaminated possessions were disposed of as radioactive waste.

U.S. Environmental Protection Agency (EPA). Radiation Protection Program: Radiological Emergency Response. *Radioactively Contaminated Sites.* Available at: http://www.epa.gov/radiation/rert/rad_cont_sites.html.

### 1910s–1920s: Orange, New Jersey and Worldwide

One of the first mass exposures to radiation occurred among thousands of teenaged girls and young women who worked in the dial-painting industry. The compound used to paint luminous numbers on watch and instrument dials contained radium. Exposure occurred by licking the brushes and inhaling the radium-containing dust. It was not until 1923 that systemic and oropharyngeal injuries were recognized. Morbidity and mortality incidence is difficult to ascertain, but nine persons are known to have died. Hundreds of others are estimated to have been injured.

Rentetzi M. The women radium dial painters as experimental subjects (1920–1990) or what counts as human experimentation. *NTM* 2004; 12(4):233–248.

Wax PM. Toxicologic plagues and disasters in history. In: LR Goldfrank, ed. *Goldfrank's Toxicologic Emergencies*, 7th ed. New York: McGraw-Hill; 2002; pp. 23–34.

Polednak AP, Stehney AF, Rowland RE. Mortality among women first employed before 1930 in the U.S. radium dial-painting industry. A group ascertained from employment lists. *Am J Epidemiol* 1978; 107(3):179–195.

Martland HS. Occupational poisoning in manufacture of luminous watch dials. *JAMA* 1929; 92:466–473, 552–559.

# Radium 226, Cesium 132, and Cobalt 60

### June 1996–October 1997: Tbilsi, Georgia

Soldiers at the Lilo Training Center developed mysterious burns on their skin and reported gastrointestinal distress. A Moscow hematologist and dosimetrist confirmed the diagnosis of radiation burns. Sixteen locations with more than 200 lost or poorly stored radioactive sources were found on the base. Locations included a jacket pocket, soccer field, smoking area, and junkyard. Eleven people incurred radiation injury.

Gottlober P, Bezold G, Weber L, et al. The radiation accident in Georgia: clinical appearance and diagnosis of cutaneous radiation syndrome. *J Am Acad Dermatol* 2000; 42(3):453–458.

International Atomic Energy Agency (IAEA). *The Radiological Accident in Lilo.* Vienna, Austria: IAEA; 2000. Available at: http://www-pub.iaea.org/MTCD/publications/PDF/Pub1097_web.pdf.

## Thorium 232

### 1920s–1950s: USA

Patients who had been injected with Thorotrast (a medium used to enhance radiographic imaging) received chronic internal exposure to thorium 232, which is a naturally occurring $\alpha$-emitter. This resulted in an elevated risk of death from hepatic and hematologic cancers, as well as chromosomal damage.

Platz EA, Wiencke JK, Kelsey KT, et al. Chromosomal aberrations and hprt mutant frequencies in long-term American thorotrast survivors. *Int J Radiol Biol* 2000; 76(7):955–961.

## Thorium, Radioactive

### April 1997: Pargny sur Saulx, France

The former industrial site of Orflam-Plast milled monazite, which contains elevated levels of natural radioactivity. Sixteen drums of radioactive thorium waste were found, prompting investigators to study cancer mortality in the surrounding populations. There was an excess lung- and bladder-cancer mortality in the surrounding communities between 1968 and 1994.

de Vathaire F, de Vathaire CC, Ropers J, Mollie A. Cancer mortality in the commune of Pargny sur Saulx in France. *J Radiol Prot* 1998; 18(1):23–27.

## Uranium 235

### September 30, 1999: Tokaimura, Japan

Employees at a fuel fabrication plant incorrectly placed uranium 235 in improper precipitation tanks for dispensing. A blue flash was observed while adding a seventh batch of uranium solution to the tank. Gamma radiation detectors sounded throughout the building and all employees were evacuated. The two individuals pouring the uranium died of radiation exposure despite stem-cell transplant. One employee sitting at a desk close to the accident was hospitalized for radiation injury, but later recovered. Local residents were exposed to high levels of radiation.

Fujimoto K. Nuclear accident in Tokai, Japan. *J Radiol Protect* 1999; 19:377–380.

McLaughlin TP, Monahan SP, Pruvost NL. *A Review of Criticality Accidents, 2000 Revision.* Tech Report No. LA-13638. Los Alamos: Los Alamos National Laboratories; 2000; pp. 53–63.

United Nations Scientific Committee on the Effects of Atomic Radiation (UNSCEAR).
Annex E: Occupational radiation exposures. In: *Sources and Effects of Ionizing Radiation.* United Nations Scientific Committee on the Effects of Atomic Radiation. UNSCEAR 2000 Report to the General Assembly, with Scientific Annexes, Volume I: Sources. Vienna, Austria: UNSCEAR; 2000. Available at: http://www.unscear.org/pdffiles/annexe.pdf.

Watts J. Radiation leak in Japan threatens thousands. *Lancet* 1999; 354:1271.

## Uranium Alloy

### August–September 1999: Razdolnoye, Russia

Six people were arrested for allegedly trying to sell radioactive uranium alloy, which was stolen from military facilities. The alloy was a mix of uranium 238 and nickel.

Medetsky A. *Uranium Sellers Arrested.* Vladivostok News; September 3, 1999.

## Uranium Criticality

### July 24, 1964: Wood River Junction, Rhode Island

Highly concentrated uranium solution was combined with a carbonate reagent that resulted in a criticality excursion of 1.0 to $1.1 \times 10^{17}$. As a result, there was a flash of light and the operator in the room was splashed with radioactive solution. Two additional supervisors received doses of radiation from a second excursion that occurred an hour and half later. The operator who was in the room for the initial excursion received a radiation dose of approximately 10,000 rad and died two days later.

McLaughlin TP, Monahan SP, Pruvost NL. *A Review of Criticality Accidents, 2000 Revision.* Tech Report No. LA-13638. Los Alamos: Los Alamos National Laboratories; 2000.

### January 2, 1958: Mayak Enterprise, Russia

Operators of a test apparatus circumvented the standard draining procedure by unbolting a 400-liter tank, lifting it, and draining fissile solution directly into receiving containers. By doing this, the operators' presence provided the neutron reflection necessary to cause a criticality excursion. A flash of light was reported, and solution was blown five meters up in the air. The three operators who physically lifted the tank received radiation doses of approximately 6,000 rad. They died five to six days after the accident. A fourth operator suffered acute radiation sickness.

McLaughlin TP, Monahan SP, Pruvost NL. *A Review of Criticality Accidents, 2000 Revision.* Tech Report No. LA-13638. Los Alamos: Los Alamos National Laboratories; 2000.

### April 21, 1957: Mayak Enterprise, Russia

A large amount of uranium precipitate collected in a filter vessel and then it began to expel gas, solution, and precipitate. Operators did not realize that a criticality excursion had happened until 20 minutes later. During this interim, an operator who had handled precipitate began to feel ill. She received a whole-body radiation dose of 3,000 rad and died 12 days later. Five other operators received doses over 300 rad and experienced radiation sickness.

McLaughlin TP, Monahan SP, Pruvost NL. *A Review of Criticality Accidents, 2000 Revision*. Tech Report No. LA-13638. Los Alamos: Los Alamos National Laboratories; 2000.

## Uranium Hexafluoride ("Hex") Explosion

### September 2, 1944: Philadelphia, Pennsylvania

Two chemists for the Manhattan Project at the Naval Research Laboratory were killed when a cylinder of uranium hexafluoride feed stock exploded. The explosion ruptured adjacent steam pipes, resulting in hydrogen fluoride release. The accident also injured four civilians and four soldiers.

Ahern JJ. International Journal of Naval History. *The United States Navy's Early Atomic Energy Research, 1939–1946*. Available at: http://www.ijnhonline.org/volume1_number1_Apr02/article_ahern_atomic_nrl.doc.htm.

## Yttrium 90

### 1980: Houston, Texas

A radiotherapy accident resulted in seven patient deaths.

Ricks RC, Berger ME, Holloway EC, Goans RE. *2000, REAC/TS Radiation Accident Registry: Update of Accidents in the United States*. International Radiation Protection Association (IRPA) International Congress Proceedings: IRPA 10—Scientific Topics; Radiologic & Nuclear Accidents. Ref. P-11-238. Available at: http://www.irpa.net/irpa10/cdrom/00325.pdf.

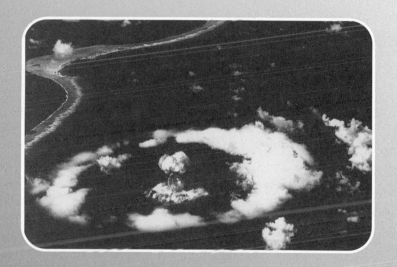

# NUCLEAR EVENTS

Chapter **4**

# NUCLEAR EVENTS

## Nuclear Contamination

### 1948–1956: Southern Urals, Russia
Fission products that totaled a $\beta/\gamma$ activity of $10^{17}$ Bq (2.75 Mci) were released into the Techa river system, which was the only water source for 24 local villages. The contamination was continuously released over several years, and a total of 124,000 people received exposure to radionuclides that included cesium 137, ruthenium 106, and zirconium 95. The villagers also ingested strontium 89, strontium 90, and cesium 137. It has been estimated that approximately eight percent of the local population, mainly comprised of Russian and Tartar-Bashkir ethnic groups, received radiation doses higher than 1.0 Gy.

Testa A, Padovani L, Mauro F, et al. Cytogenetic study on children living in Southern Urals contaminated areas (nuclear incidents 1948–1967). *Mutat Res* 1998; 401(1-2): 193–197.

## Nuclear Explosions

### 1945: Hiroshima and Nagasaki, Japan
The first atomic bombs were dropped on Japan at the end of World War II. The clinical effects of the radiation exposure are still evident today. Long-term follow-up studies show increased leukemia, other cancers, radiation cataracts, hyperparathyroidism, and chromosomal abnormalities 60 years after the bombings.

Wax PM. Toxicologic Plagues and Disasters in History. In: Goldfrank LR, ed. *Goldfrank's Toxicologic Emergencies*, 7th ed. New York: McGraw-Hill; 2002; pp. 23–34.

Kodama K, Mabuchi K, Shigematsu I. A long-term cohort study of the atomic-bomb survivors. *J Epidemiol* 1996; 6(3 Suppl):S95–S105.

## Nuclear Irradiation

### 1967: Lake Karachay, Southern Urals, Russia

Wind redistribution spread radioactive wastes over an area of 1,800 km$^2$, irradiating approximately a half million people with $2.2 \times 10^{13}$ Bq (600 Ci). The radioactive material contained four Ebq of strontium 90 and cesium 137. The material was deposited in the dry lake bed.

Testa A, Padovani L, Mauro F, et al. Cytogenetic study on children living in Southern Urals contaminated areas (nuclear incidents 1948–1967). *Mutat Res* 1998; 401(1-2): 193–197.

## Nuclear Submarine Accident

### August 2000: Barents Sea

The *Kursk*, a Russian nuclear submarine, suffered multiple explosions and sank in the Barents Sea. All 118 crew members died. The submarine was recovered and defueled without complication in February 2003.

Bellona Foundation. *The Kursk Accident.* All about the *Kursk* accident in the Barents Sea; August 12, 2000. Available at: http://www.bellona.no/en/international/russia/navy/northern_fleet/incidents/kursk/index.html.

## Radioactive Explosion

### May 14, 1997: Hanford, Washington

Evaporation caused chemicals to react and explode inside a plutonium tank at the Hanford Plutonium Reclamation Facility. Although the surrounding area did not show evidence of a radioactive release, several employees were sent to the local hospital.

U.S. Department of Energy. Memorandum: Chemical Safety Concerns. *Significant Occurrences May, 1997.* Available at: http://www.dne.bnl.gov/etd/csc/1997/may97.html.

Washington State Department of Health. Division of Environmental Health: Office of Radiation Protection. *Report on the Response to the Accident on May 14, 1997 on the Hanford Site.* Available at: http://www.doh.wa.gov/ehp/rp/air/prf-rpt.pdf.

### August 10, 1985: Vladivostok, Russia

A major accident occurred aboard a Soviet nuclear submarine during refueling. Vital control rods were pulled out of the nuclear reactor, sparking an explosion. This incident killed 10 sailors and spread radioactive materials into both the air and sea.

Bellona Foundation. *Nuclear submarine accidents.* The Russian Northern Fleet Nuclear Submarine Accidents. Report 2: 1996; the Russian Northern Fleet. Bellona Foundation: 1996. Available at: bellona.no/en/international/russia/navy/northern_fleet.report_2–1996/11084.html.

## Reactor Core Incident

### December 1995: France
Salt was placed into a cooling contour at one of the Blayais reactors by saboteurs.

Bukharin O. Problems of Nuclear Terrorism. In: Bertsch G, ed., for Center for International Trade and Security at the University of Georgia. *The Monitor: Nonproliferation, Demilitarization and Arms Control. Terrorism and Weapons of Mass Destruction.* Athens, GA: Center for International Trade and Security at the University of Georgia; 1997; 3(2):8–10. Available at: http://www.uga.edu/cits/documents/pdf/monitor/monitor_sp_1997.pdf.

### April 1986: Chernobyl, Ukraine
While performing an unauthorized engineering test on a generator, power instabilities occurred in the reactor system. Within three seconds, the internal fission rate increased and the resulting steam explosion lifted the 90-ton reactor cover and ejected debris from the facility. Thirty-one people died and 135,000 residents were evacuated after the explosion released a cloud containing 40 million Ci of iodine 131, 3 million Ci of cesium 137, and 50 million Ci of xenon isotopes.

Bonte FJ. Chernobyl retrospective. *Semin Nucl Med* 1988; 18(1):16–24.

Agency for Toxic Substances and Disease Registry (ATSDR). *Toxicological Profile for Ionizing Radiation.* Atlanta: ATDSR, U.S. Department of Health and Human Services; 1999; pp. 195–197. Available at: http://www.atsdr.cdc.gov/toxprofiles/tp149.html.

### March 28, 1979: Three Mile Island, Pennsylvania
An accident occurred at the Unit 2 civilian nuclear power reactor when feed water pumps malfunctioned, interrupting the steam-generator water supply. This resulted in a loss of reactor core cooling, and radioactive material (xenon 133 and iodine 131) flowed onto the containment room floor. Little radioactivity was released into the environment, and no radiation effects were reported by the surrounding population, despite the psychological effects of the accident.

Agency for Toxic Substances and Disease Registry (ATSDR). *Toxicological Profile for Ionizing Radiation.* Atlanta: ATDSR, U.S. Department of Health and Human Services; 1999; pp. 195–197. Available at: http://www.atsdr.cdc.gov/toxprofiles/tp149.html.

Talbott EO, Youk AO, et al. Mortality among the residents of the Three Mile Island accident area: 1979–1992. *Environ Health Perspect* 2000; 108(6):545–552.

### March 22, 1975: Brown's Ferry, Alabama

Two electricians, trying to seal air leaks, were working below the Brown's Ferry nuclear power station's control room for Units 1 and 2. The electricians were using candles to determine if the leaks had been sealed by observing the movements of the flame, as caused by escaping air. The electrical engineer placed the candle too close to foam rubber, causing it to burst into flame. A fire ensued, disabling many of the electrical safety systems at the plant. A meltdown accident almost occurred since the entire emergency cooling system was shut down for Unit 1, but workers averted crisis by controlling Unit 1 with a makeshift system.

Comey DD. Institution of Chemical Engineers. Safety and Loss Prevention Subject Group. *The Fire at Brown's Ferry Nuclear Power Station.* Available at: http://www.ccnr. org/browns_ferry.html.

### 1961: Idaho Falls, Idaho

Three deaths and 22 radiation injuries were reported when a maintenance crew removed a central control rod from a nuclear reactor core beyond the proper limit. The resulting explosion flooded the reactor room with 500–1000 rem/hour.

*Operational Accidents and Radiation Exposure Experience Within the United States Atomic Energy Commission, 1943–1970.* WASH 1192. Washington, DC: U.S. Government Printing Office; 1971.

### October 1957: Windscale, England, United Kingdom

Radioactive material was released in a nuclear reactor accident due to operator error. There was a subsequent graphite fire that lasted three days, releasing iodine 131, cesium 137, polonium 210, ruthenium 106, and xenon 133. The contamination of surrounding pastureland was extensive, and the greatest threat came from the ingestion of cow's milk contaminated with iodine 131.

Agency for Toxic Substances and Disease Registry (ATSDR). *Toxicological Profile for Ionizing Radiation.* Atlanta, GA: ATSDR, U.S. Department of Health and Human Services; 1999; pp. 195–197. Available at: http://www.atsdr.cdc.gov/toxprofiles/tp149.html.

## Reactor Waste Explosion

### September 1957: Kyshtym, Russia

Underground steel storage tanks overheated when the cooling system failed, resulting in an explosion that released a cloud of cerium 144 , zirconium 95, niobium 95, and strontium 90. Approximately 10,000 people were evacuated from the high-contamination area, and there were 1,118 deaths.

Agency for Toxic Substances and Disease Registry (ATSDR). *Toxicological Profile for Ionizing Radiation.* Atlanta: ATSDR, U.S. Department of Health and Human Services; 1999; pp. 195–197. Available at: http://www.atsdr.cdc.gov/toxprofiles/tp149.html.

**, 1947: Texas City, Texas**

 nitrate exploded on the cargo ship *Grandchamp* that was deliver-
lizer. The blast was estimated to be on the kiloton level and resulted
al wave that hit Texas City. The explosion left 576 dead and more
,000 injured. An additional 175 people were never located.

State Historical Association (TSHA). *The Handbook of Texas Online. 1997–*
ilable at: http://www.tsha.utexas.edu/handbook/online/articles/TT/lyt1.html

t *100 Years, Looking Back: Freighter Explosion Rocked Texas City Region.* Hous-
ronicle Archives. April 15, 2001.

**mber 21, 1921: Oppau, Germany**

xplosion at the Bradishe Aniline chemical works plant, which manufac-
ured nitrates, destroyed the plant as well as a nearby village. More than
,500 people were injured and 561 people died.

shington University and Washington State Department of Labor & Industries.
ISHA Training Module: Process Safety Management (PSM) Part 1: Review of Indus-
al Catastrophes Related to PSM. Available at: wisha-training.lni.wa.gov/ training/
esentations/PSMoverview1.ppt.

Rosenthal I, Kleindorfer P, Kunreuther H, et al. *OECD Workshop on Lessons Learned
from Chemical Accidents and Incidents.* Available at: http://grace.wharton.upenn.edu/
risk/downloads/Final%20%20Fnl%20DD%20Sweden%20WS%20August%206%
202004.pdf.

UNEP-APELL. *Ammonium nitrate explosion in Toulouse, France. Other Accidents
Involving Ammonium Nitrate.* Available at: http://www.uneptie.org/pc/apell/disasters/
toulouse/other_accidents.htm

## Beer Flood

**October 16, 1814: London, England, United Kingdom**

The Meux and Co. Brewery on Tottenham Court Road had one of the largest
beer vats in the city, held together by metal hoops. Smaller vats were also
housed in the same building. The vat was showing signs of age: the metal
hoops snapped and beer exploded into the building, causing the other be
vats to rupture. Approximately 8,500 barrels of beer smashed through th
brick wall and rushed into the surrounding streets of St. Giles. Eight peo
died.

Page W, ed. Industries: Brewing. In: *A History of the County of Middlesex: Volume 2*
Boydeil & Brewer; 1911; p. 168–178.

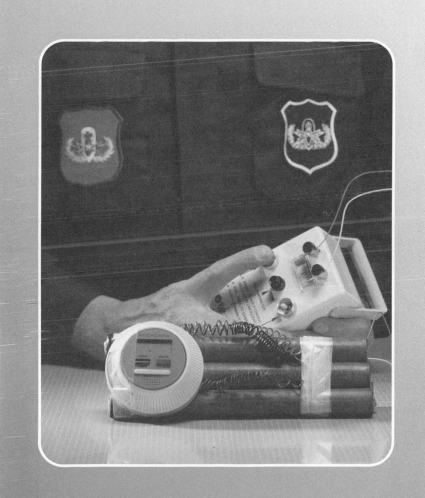

## EXPLOSIVE AND FIRE EVENTS

# EXPLOSIVE AND FIRE H

The Texas
2000. Av

Our Fir
ton Ch

**Septe**
An e
t

Wa
W
tr
p

## Aluminum Dust Explosion

### October 29, 2003: Huntington, Indiana

An accumulation of aluminum dust, a flammable by
production process, caused a series of explosions at
manufacturing plant. The plant manufactured cast-a
wheels. Two workers were severely burned and a third
sult of the explosions. One of the burned workers subs
his injuries.

U.S. Chemical Safety and Hazard Investigation Board. CSB investig
page. *Hayes Lemmerz Dust Explosions and Fire: Huntington, IN, Octo
able at: http://www.csb.gov/index.cfm?folder=completed_investigation
info&INV_ID=44

## Ammonium Nitrate Explosions

### September 21, 2001: Toulouse, France

Two hundred to 300 tons of ammonium nitrate granules produced at
izer factory exploded, leaving 31 dead and 2,442 injured. The blast w
to be the equivalent of a 3.4-Richter-scale-grade earthquake.

UNEP-APELL. *Ammonium Nitrate Explosion in Toulouse-France 21 September 2001.
Available at: http://www.unep.fr/pc/apell/disasters/toulouse/home.html

# Benzoyl Peroxide Explosion

### January 2, 2003: Gnadenhutten, Ohio

A vacuum dryer at the Catalyst Systems Inc. production plant exploded, injuring one employee and damaging the facility. The vacuum dryer was holding nearly 200 pounds of benzyl peroxide, which is unstable at high concentrations. At the time of the explosion, employees were in the process of drying granular benzoyl peroxide.

U.S. Chemical Safety and Hazard Investigation Board. CSB investigation information page. *Catalyst Systems Inc. Reactive Chemical Explosion: Gnadenhutten, OH, January 2, 2003.* Available at: http://www.csb.gov/index.cfm?folder=completed_investigations& page=info&INV_ID=40

# Butane Explosion

### November 19, 1984: Mexico City, Mexico

An explosion of liquefied butane at a storage facility near Mexico City resulted in more than 400 deaths.

Arturson G. The tragedy of San Juanico—the most severe LPG disaster in history. *Burns Incl Therm Inj* 1987; 13(2):87–102.

# Chemical Explosions

### August 10, 2005: Romulus, Michigan

An explosion and fire at a chemical plant in Romulus, Michigan caused the evacuation of residents within a half-mile of the plant. The cause of the explosion was not immediately determined, but further explosions were reported as the fire spread to additional chemical tanks. At least 16 people were treated for minor respiratory problems.

Brand-Williams O, Hunter G, Donnelly FX. *Plant explosion rocks Romulus.* The Detroit News; August 10, 2005.

### December 3, 2004: Houston, Texas

A storage tank at the Marcus Oil and Chemical polyethylene wax facility failed catastrophically, leading to a blast that was felt up to 20 miles away. Large fires were ignited, and two firefighters were injured during emergency response.

U.S. Chemical Safety and Hazard Investigation Board. CSB investigation information page. *Marcus Oil and Chemical Tank Explosion: Houston, TX, December 3, 2004.* Available at: http://www.csb.gov/index.cfm?folder=current_investigations&page= info&INV_ID=50

### April 22, 2004: Ryongchon, North Korea (Near the Chinese Border)

Two trains carrying oil and liquefied petroleum gas collided and exploded in a North Korea train station. At least 3,000 people were killed or injured.

CBS News World. *Train Disaster Shakes N. Korea.* Available at: http://www.cbsnews.com/stories/2004/04/23/world/main613302.shtml

### February 18, 2004: Neyshabur, Iran

A train carrying fuel, fertilizer, and industrial chemicals rolled out of a switch-yard and derailed at a speed of 90 mph. After derailing, the 51-car train caught fire and exploded, destroying five villages and killing at least 200 people.

CNN.com. *Major Train Disasters since 1900.* Available at: http://www.cnn.com/2004/WORLD/meast/02/18/iran.train.disaster.ap/

### July 29, 2003: Beijing, China

An explosion at a Chinese fireworks factory killed at least 29 and injured more than 140 people.

CBS News. *China Fireworks Blast Kills Dozens.* July 29, 2003. http://www.cbsnews.com/stories/2003/07/29/world/main565603.shtml.

### February 7, 2003: Cranston, Rhode Island

An explosion at Technic Inc. seriously injured one worker when maintenance on a ventilation system that connected multiple chemical reactors led to an accumulation of hazardous materials. Eighteen other employees were taken to the hospital and local residents were evacuated. The plant produced precious-metal-processing chemicals. Authorities believed that an employee tapped on the ventilation duct with a hammer because he believed it to be clogged. The blow of the hammer likely caused a chemical reaction inside the duct that resulted in the explosion.

U.S. Chemical Safety and Hazard Investigation Board. *Investigation Report: Vent Collection System Explosion.* Report No. 2003-08-I-RI. Washington, DC: CSB Investigation Board; 2003. Available at: http://www.csb.gov/completed_investigations/docs/CSB_Technic_Report.pdf

### October 13, 2002: Pascagoula, Mississippi

A violent explosion occurred in a chemical distillation tower at the First Chemical Corporation, scattered major debris over a wide area in the plant. Three control-room workers were injured by shattered glass. The explosion debris also punctured one nitrotoluene storage tank, which ignited a fire that burned for several hours.

U.S. Chemical Safety and Hazard Investigation Board. CSB investigation information page. *First Chemical Corp. Reactive Chemical Explosion: Pascagoula, MS, October 13, 2002.* Available at: http://www.csb.gov/index.cfm?folder=completed_investigations &page=info&INV_ID=24

### June 21, 2002: Kingsville, Ontario, Canada

An industrial fire incinerated four million pounds of styrene and forced the evacuation of 2,500 people.

Public Safety and Emergency Preparedness Canada. *Canadian Disaster Database.* Available at: http://www.psepc-sppcc.gc.ca/red/em/cdd/search-em.asp. Accessed September 21, 2005.

### April 25, 2002: New York City, New York

An explosion at Kaltech Industries, a Chelsea sign manufacturer in New York City, hospitalized 36 people, including 14 members of the public. The explosion was caused by a reaction between waste chemicals and began in the basement of a mixed-use commercial building. Damage was reported up to the fifth floor.

U.S. Chemical Safety and Hazard Investigation Board. *Investigation Report: Chemical Waste-Mixing Incident.* Report No. 2002-02-I-NY. Washington, DC: CSB Investigation Board; 2003. Available at: http://www.csb.gov/completed_investigations/docs/KaltechFinalReport.pdf

### November 5, 2000: Nigeria

An oil tanker crashed into a stand of parked vehicles at a police checkpoint between the areas of Ife and Ibadan. The incident killed 96 people.

CNN.com Africa. *At Least 96 Killed in Nigerian Petrol Tanker Explosion.* Available at: http://archives.cnn.com/2000/WORLD/africa/11/06/crash.nigeria.03.ap/index.html

### April 8, 1998: Paterson, New Jersey

During the production of Automate Yellow 96 dye, an explosion and fire occurred from a runaway reaction. This reaction overpressurized a 2,000-gallon vessel, releasing and igniting flammable material. Nine employees were injured.

U.S. Chemical Safety and Hazard Investigation Board. CSB investigation information page. *Morton International Inc. Runaway Chemical Reaction: Paterson, NJ, April 8, 1998.* Available at: http://www.csb.gov/index.cfm?folder=completed_investigations&page=info&INV_ID=18

### January 7, 1998: Mustang, Nevada

Two explosions that occurred in rapid succession destroyed Sierra Chemical
Company's Kean Canyon plant, four workers were killed and six others
injured.

U.S. Chemical Safety and Hazard Investigation Board. CSB investigation information
page. *Sierra Chemical Co. High Explosives Accident: Mustang, NV, January 7, 1998.*
Available at: http://www.csb.gov/index.cfm?folder=completed_investigations&page=
info&INV_ID=4

### May 25, 1994: Sydney, Nova Scotia, Canada

A PCB-transformer explosion and fire at a steel factory threatened a major
toxic discharge; 500 residents downwind of Witney Pier were evacuated.
Although soil analysis did not reveal any contamination by PCB, dioxin, or
furan, the clean-up process generated 15 barrels of hazardous waste.

Public Safety and Emergency Preparedness Canada. *Canadian Disaster Database.* Available at: http://www.psepc-sppcc.gc.ca/red/em/cdd/search-em.asp. Accessed September
21, 2005.

### August 13, 1920: Pounding Mills, Virginia

Detonation of explosive materials at the Pounding Mills rock quarry killed
nine people.

CDC and NIOSH Safety and Health Research. *Historical Mining Disasters.* Available at:
http://www.cdc.gov/niosh/mining/statistics/discoal.htm. Accessed September 21, 2005.

## Chemical Fires

### July 10, 1997: Hamilton, Ontario, Canada

A fire broke out at a plastics recycling plant without a suppressant system,
causing severe air pollution. Approximately 4,000 people were evacuated.
The plant mainly recycled plastics and polyvinyl chloride from the automotive industry.

Public Safety and Emergency Preparedness Canada. *Canadian Disaster Database.* Available at: http://www.psepc-sppcc.gc.ca/red/em/cdd/search-em.asp. Accessed September
21, 2005.

### October 21, 1994: Montreal, Québec, Canada

A building of a bankrupt petrochemical industry was being cleaned and prepared when an unused reservoir of 700 m$^3$ of fuel oil and light hydrocarbons exploded and burned. One nearby worker was killed instantly and
another sustained severe burns. The burned worker died shortly thereafter.

Public Safety and Emergency Preparedness Canada. *Canadian Disaster Database.* Available at: http://www.psepc-sppcc.gc.ca/red/em/cdd/search-em.asp. Accessed September 21, 2005.

## Chlorine Gas Explosion

### 1945: Baci, Italy

An American ship carrying chlorine gas exploded. Three hundred sixty people died in the ensuing disaster, mainly from gas inhalation.

Eckert WG. Mass deaths by gas or chemical poisoning: a historical perspective. *Am J Forens Med Pathol* 1991; 12(2):119–125.

## Coal Mine Explosions

### 2006–2000

### January 2, 2006: Upshur County, West Virginia

An explosion at the Sago mine trapped 13 miners underground for an extended amount of time. Despite substantial rescue efforts, 12 of the miners died. The surviving miner sustained severe injury. The Mine Safety and Health Administration launched an extensive investigation into the accident to determine what caused the explosion, the manner in which emergency information was disseminated, and if any safety standards were violated. The families of the trapped miners were initially led to believe that the miners survived the explosion due to false communication.

U.S. Department of Labor, Mine Safety and Health Administration. *Sago Mine Information Single Source Page.* Available at http://www.msha.gov/sagomine/sagomine.asp

### April 2002: Southwestern China

Twenty-three people died in an explosion at the Huashan coal mine. China pledged to cut mining-related deaths by closing 8,000 small coal mines.

Workplace Disasters. Mine blast kills 23. *Hazards and Workers' Health International Newsletter.* Available at: http://www.hazards.org/disasters/

### September 23, 2001: Brookwood, Alabama

An explosion at the Jim Walter Resources, Inc. coal mine number five killed 13 people.

CDC and NIOSH Safety and Health Research. *Coal Mining Disasters.* Available at: http://www.cdc.gov/niosh/mining/statistics/discoal.htm. Accessed September 21, 2005.

### December 7, 1992: Norton, Virginia
An explosion at the Southmountain coal mine number three killed eight people.

CDC and NIOSH Safety and Health Research. *Coal Mining Disasters.* Available at: http://www.cdc.gov/niosh/mining/statistics/discoal.htm. Accessed September 21, 2005.

### 1989–1980
### September 13, 1989: Sullivan, Kentucky
An explosion at the number nine slope of the Pyro Mining Company, killed ten people.

CDC and NIOSH Safety and Health Research. *Coal Mining Disasters.* Available at: http://www.cdc.gov/niosh/mining/statistics/discoal.htm. Accessed September 21, 2005.

### June 21, 1983: McClure, Virginia
An explosion in the Clinchfield Coal McClure number one coal mine killed seven people.

CDC and NIOSH Safety and Health Research. *Coal Mining Disasters.* Available at: http://www.cdc.gov/niosh/mining/statistics/discoal.htm. Accessed September 21, 2005.

### January 20, 1982: Craynor, Kentucky
An explosion in the number one shaft of a local coal mine killed seven people.

CDC and NIOSH Safety and Health Research. *Coal Mining Disasters.* Available at: http://www.cdc.gov/niosh/mining/statistics/discoal.htm. Accessed September 21, 2005.

### December 8, 1981: Whitewell, Tennessee
An explosion at the Grundy Mining Co. Mine #21 killed 13 people.

CDC and NIOSH Safety and Health Research. *Coal Mining Disasters.* Available at: http://www.cdc.gov/niosh/mining/statistics/discoal.htm. Accessed September 21, 2005.

### December 7, 1981: Kite, Kentucky
An explosion in the Adkins Coal Mine Explosion #11 facility killed eight people.

CDC and NIOSH Safety and Health Research. *Coal Mining Disasters.* Available at: http://www.cdc.gov/niosh/mining/statistics/discoal.htm. Accessed September 21, 2005.

### April 15, 1981: Redstone, Colorado
An explosion in the Mid-Continent Resources Dutch Creek number one coal facility killed 15 people.

CDC and NIOSH Safety and Health Research. *Coal Mining Disasters.* Available at: http://www.cdc.gov/niosh/mining/statistics/discoal.htm. Accessed September 21, 2005.

### November 7, 1980: Uneeda, West Virginia
An explosion in the #17 shaft of the Ferrell coal mine killed five people.

CDC and NIOSH Safety and Health Research. *Coal Mining Disasters*. Available at:
http://www.cdc.gov/niosh/mining/statistics/discoal.htm. Accessed September 21, 2005.

### 1979–1970
### March 11, 1976: Whitesburg, Kentucky
An explosion at the Scotia coal mine killed 11 people, including federal
  inspectors.

CDC and NIOSH Safety and Health Research. *Coal Mining Disasters*. Available at:
http://www.cdc.gov/niosh/mining/statistics/discoal.htm. Accessed September 21, 2005.

### March 9, 1976: Whitesburg, Kentucky
An explosion at the Scotia coal mine killed 15 people.

CDC and NIOSH Safety and Health Research. *Coal Mining Disasters*. Available at:
http://www.cdc.gov/niosh/mining/statistics/discoal.htm. Accessed September 21, 2005.

### December 16, 1972: Itmann, West Virginia
An explosion in the number three shaft of the Itmann coal mine killed five
  people.

CDC and NIOSH Safety and Health Research. *Coal Mining Disasters*. Available at:
http://www.cdc.gov/niosh/mining/statistics/discoal.htm. Accessed September 21, 2005.

### July 22, 1972: Blacksville, West Virginia
An explosion in the number one shaft of the Blacksville coal mine killed nine
  people.

CDC and NIOSH Safety and Health Research. *Coal Mining Disasters*. Available at:
http://www.cdc.gov/niosh/mining/statistics/discoal.htm. Accessed September 21, 2005.

### December 30, 1970: Hyden, Kentucky
Explosions in shafts numbers 15 and 16 of the Finley coal mine killed 38
  people.

CDC and NIOSH Safety and Health Research. *Coal Mining Disasters*. Available at:
http://www.cdc.gov/niosh/mining/statistics/discoal.htm. Accessed September 21, 2005.

### 1969–1960
### November 20, 1968: Farmington, West Virginia
An explosion in the number nine shaft of the Consol coal mine killed 78 people.

CDC and NIOSH Safety and Health Research. *Coal Mining Disasters*. Available at:
http://www.cdc.gov/niosh/mining/statistics/discoal.htm. Accessed September 21, 2005.

### August 7, 1968: Greenville, Kentucky

An explosion at the River Queen coal mine killed nine people.

CDC and NIOSH Safety and Health Research. *Coal Mining Disasters.* Available at: http://www.cdc.gov/niosh/mining/statistics/discoal.htm. Accessed September 21, 2005.

### July 23, 1966: Mount Hope, West Virginia

An explosion at the Siltex Mine killed seven people.

CDC and NIOSH Safety and Health Research. *Coal Mining Disasters.* Available at: http://www.cdc.gov/niosh/mining/statistics/discoal.htm. Accessed September 21, 2005.

### December 28, 1965: Redstone, Colorado

An explosion at the Dutch Creek Mine killed nine people.

CDC and NIOSH Safety and Health Research. *Coal Mining Disasters.* Available at: http://www.cdc.gov/niosh/mining/statistics/discoal.htm. Accessed September 21, 2005.

### October 16, 1965: Wilsonburg, West Virginia

An explosion in the number two shaft of the Mars coal mine killed seven people.

CDC and NIOSH Safety and Health Research. *Coal Mining Disasters.* Available at: http://www.cdc.gov/niosh/mining/statistics/discoal.htm. Accessed September 21, 2005.

### May 24, 1965: Robbins, Tennessee

An explosion in the number two shaft of the C.L. Cline coal mine killed five people.

CDC and NIOSH Safety and Health Research. *Coal Mining Disasters.* Available at: http://www.cdc.gov/niosh/mining/statistics/discoal.htm. Accessed September 21, 2005.

### December 16, 1963: Helper, Utah

An explosion in the number two shaft of the Carbon Fuel coal mine killed nine people.

CDC and NIOSH Safety and Health Research. *Coal Mining Disasters.* Available at: http://www.cdc.gov/niosh/mining/statistics/discoal.htm. Accessed September 21, 2005.

### April 25, 1963: Dola, West Virginia

An explosion in the number two shaft of the Compass coal mine killed 22 people.

CDC and NIOSH Safety and Health Research. *Coal Mining Disasters.* Available at: http://www.cdc.gov/niosh/mining/statistics/discoal.htm. Accessed September 21, 2005.

### December 6, 1962: Carmichaels, Pennsylvania

An explosion in the number three shaft of the Robena coal mine killed 37 people.

CDC and NIOSH Safety and Health Research. *Coal Mining Disasters.* Available at: http://www.cdc.gov/niosh/mining/statistics/discoal.htm. Accessed September 21, 2005.

### January 10, 1962: Herrin, Illinois

An explosion in the number two shaft of the Blue Blaze coal mine killed 11 people.

CDC and NIOSH Safety and Health Research. *Coal Mining Disasters.* Available at: http://www.cdc.gov/niosh/mining/statistics/discoal.htm. Accessed September 21, 2005.

### March 2, 1961: Terre Haute, Indiana

An explosion at the Viking Mine coal mine killed 22 people.

CDC and NIOSH Safety and Health Research. *Coal Mining Disasters.* Available at: http://www.cdc.gov/niosh/mining/statistics/discoal.htm. Accessed September 21, 2005.

### 1959–1950
### March 23, 1959: Robbins, Tennessee

An explosion at the Phillips & West coal mine killed nine people.

CDC and NIOSH Safety and Health Research. *Coal Mining Disasters.* Available at: http://www.cdc.gov/niosh/mining/statistics/discoal.htm. Accessed September 21, 2005.

### October 28, 1958: Craigsville, West Virginia

An explosion at the Burton coal mine killed 14 people.

CDC and NIOSH Safety and Health Research. *Coal Mining Disasters.* Available at: http://www.cdc.gov/niosh/mining/statistics/discoal.htm. Accessed September 21, 2005.

### October 27, 1958: McDowell County, West Virginia

An explosion in the # 34 shaft of the Bishop coal mine killed 22 people.

CDC and NIOSH Safety and Health Research. *Coal Mining Disasters.* Available at: http://www.cdc.gov/niosh/mining/statistics/discoal.htm. Accessed September 21, 2005.

### December 27, 1957: McDowell County, West Virginia

An explosion in the # 31 shaft of the Amonate coal mine killed 11 people.

CDC and NIOSH Safety and Health Research. *Coal Mining Disasters.* Available at: http://www.cdc.gov/niosh/mining/statistics/discoal.htm. Accessed September 21, 2005.

### *September 23, 1957: Marianna, Pennsylvania*
An explosion in the # 58 shaft of the Marianna coal mine killed six
   people.

CDC and NIOSH Safety and Health Research. *Coal Mining Disasters.* Available at:
http://www.cdc.gov/niosh/mining/statistics/discoal.htm. Accessed September 21, 2005.

### *February 4, 1957: McDowell County, West Virginia*
An explosion in the # 34 shaft of the Bishop coal mine killed 37 people.

CDC and NIOSH Safety and Health Research. *Coal Mining Disasters.* Available at:
http://www.cdc.gov/niosh/mining/statistics/discoal.htm. Accessed September 21, 2005.

### *January 18, 1957: Jonesville, Alaska*
An explosion at the Evan Jones coal mine killed five people.

CDC and NIOSH Safety and Health Research. *Coal Mining Disasters.* Available at:
http://www.cdc.gov/niosh/mining/statistics/discoal.htm. Accessed September 21, 2005.

### *November 13, 1954: Farmington, West Virginia*
An explosion in the number nine shaft of the Jamison coal mine killed 16
   people.

CDC and NIOSH Safety and Health Research. *Coal Mining Disasters.* Available at:
http://www.cdc.gov/niosh/mining/statistics/discoal.htm. Accessed September 21, 2005.

### *March 30, 1953: Lovilia, Iowa*
An explosion at the O'Brien coal mine killed five people.

CDC and NIOSH Safety and Health Research. *Coal Mining Disasters.* Available at:
http://www.cdc.gov/niosh/mining/statistics/discoal.htm. Accessed September 21, 2005.

### *February 2, 1952: Carpentertown, Pennsylvania*
An explosion at the Carpentertown coal mine killed six people.

CDC and NIOSH Safety and Health Research. *Coal Mining Disasters.* Available at:
http://www.cdc.gov/niosh/mining/statistics/discoal.htm. Accessed September 21, 2005.

### *December 21, 1951: West Frankfort, Illinois*
An explosion in the number two shaft of the Orient coal mine killed 119
   people.

CDC and NIOSH Safety and Health Research. *Coal Mining Disasters.* Available at:
http://www.cdc.gov/niosh/mining/statistics/discoal.htm. Accessed September 21, 2005.

### *October 31, 1951: United, West Virginia*
An explosion in the number one shaft of the United Gas coal plant killed 12
   people.

CDC and NIOSH Safety and Health Research. *Coal Mining Disasters*. Available at: http://www.cdc.gov/niosh/mining/statistics/discoal.htm. Accessed September 21, 2005.

### October 15, 1951: Cassville, West Virginia

An explosion at the Bunker coal mine killed ten people.

CDC and NIOSH Safety and Health Research. *Coal Mining Disasters*. Available at: http://www.cdc.gov/niosh/mining/statistics/dlscoal.htm. Accessed September 21, 2005.

### March 29, 1951: Wilkes-Barre, Pennsylvania

An explosion at the Buttonwood coal mine killed five people.

CDC and NIOSH Safety and Health Research. *Coal Mining Disasters*. Available at: http://www.cdc.gov/niosh/mining/statistics/discoal.htm. Accessed September 21, 2005.

### January 8, 1951: Kermit, West Virginia

An explosion at the Burning Springs coal mine killed 11 people.

CDC and NIOSH Safety and Health Research. *Coal Mining Disasters*. Available at: http://www.cdc.gov/niosh/mining/statistics/discoal.htm. Accessed September 21, 2005.

### 1949–1940
### July 30, 1948: Birmingham, Alabama

An explosion at the Edgewater coal mine killed 11 people.

CDC and NIOSH Safety and Health Research. *Coal Mining Disasters*. Available at: http://www.cdc.gov/niosh/mining/statistics/discoal.htm. Accessed September 21, 2005.

### July 27, 1948: Princeton, Indiana

An explosion at the King coal mine killed 13 people.

CDC and NIOSH Safety and Health Research. *Coal Mining Disasters*. Available at: http://www.cdc.gov/niosh/mining/statistics/discoal.htm. Accessed September 21, 2005.

### February 28, 1948: Excelsior, Arkansas

An explosion at the Sun Excelsior coal mine killed eight people.

CDC and NIOSH Safety and Health Research. *Coal Mining Disasters*. Available at: http://www.cdc.gov/niosh/mining/statistics/discoal.htm. Accessed September 21, 2005.

### December 11, 1947: Wilkes-Barre, Pennsylvania

An explosion at the Franklin coal mine killed eight people.

CDC and NIOSH Safety and Health Research. *Coal Mining Disasters*. Available at: http://www.cdc.gov/niosh/mining/statistics/discoal.htm. Accessed September 21, 2005.

**July 24, 1947: West Frankfort, Illinois**
An explosion in the number eight shaft of the Old Ben coal mine killed 27
  people.

CDC and NIOSH Safety and Health Research. *Coal Mining Disasters.* Available at:
http://www.cdc.gov/niosh/mining/statistics/discoal.htm. Accessed September 21, 2005.

**April 30, 1947: Terre Haute, Indiana**
An explosion at the Spring Hill coal mine killed eight people.

CDC and NIOSH Safety and Health Research. *Coal Mining Disasters.* Available at:
http://www.cdc.gov/niosh/mining/statistics/discoal.htm. Accessed September 21, 2005.

**April 10, 1947: Exeter, Pennsylvania**
An explosion at the Schooley coal mine killed ten people.

CDC and NIOSH Safety and Health Research. *Coal Mining Disasters.* Available at:
http://www.cdc.gov/niosh/mining/statistics/discoal.htm. Accessed September 21, 2005.

**March 25, 1947: Centralia, Illinois**
An explosion in the number five shaft of a local coal mine killed 111 people.

CDC and NIOSH Safety and Health Research. *Coal Mining Disasters.* Available at:
http://www.cdc.gov/niosh/mining/statistics/discoal.htm. Accessed September 21, 2005.

**January 15, 1947: Plymouth, Pennsylvania**
An explosion at the Nottingham coal mine killed 15 people.

CDC and NIOSH Safety and Health Research. *Coal Mining Disasters.* Available at:
http://www.cdc.gov/niosh/mining/statistics/discoal.htm. Accessed September 21, 2005.

**April 18, 1946: McCoy, Virginia**
An explosion at the Great Valley coal mine killed 12 people.

CDC and NIOSH Safety and Health Research. *Coal Mining Disasters.* Available at:
http://www.cdc.gov/niosh/mining/statistics/discoal.htm. Accessed September 21, 2005.

**January 15, 1946: Havaco, West Virginia**
An explosion in the number nine shaft of the Havaco coal mine killed 15
  people.

CDC and NIOSH Safety and Health Research. *Coal Mining Disasters.* Available at:
http://www.cdc.gov/niosh/mining/statistics/discoal.htm. Accessed September 21, 2005.

**December 26, 1945: Fourmile, Kentucky**
An explosion in the number one shaft of the Belva coal mine killed 25 people.

CDC and NIOSH Safety and Health Research. *Coal Mining Disasters*. Available at: http://www.cdc.gov/niosh/mining/statistics/discoal.htm. Accessed September 21, 2005.

### May 9, 1945: Sunnyside, Utah

An explosion in the number one shaft of a local coal mine killed 23 people.

CDC and NIOSH Safety and Health Research. *Coal Mining Disasters*. Available at: http://www.cdc.gov/niosh/mining/statistics/discoal.htm. Accessed September 21, 2005.

### March 14, 1945: Kenilworth, Utah

An explosion at the Kenilworth coal mine killed seven people.

CDC and NIOSH Safety and Health Research. *Coal Mining Disasters*. Available at: http://www.cdc.gov/niosh/mining/statistics/discoal.htm. Accessed September 21, 2005.

### January 17, 1945: Haileyville, Oklahoma

An explosion at the Bond Valley coal mine killed nine people.

CDC and NIOSH Safety and Health Research. *Coal Mining Disasters*. Available at: http://www.cdc.gov/niosh/mining/statistics/discoal.htm. Accessed September 21, 2005.

### July 28, 1944: Brilliant, New Mexico

An explosion in the number two shaft of the Brilliant coal mine killed six people.

CDC and NIOSH Safety and Health Research. *Coal Mining Disasters*. Available at: http://www.cdc.gov/niosh/mining/statistics/discoal.htm. Accessed September 21, 2005.

### March 24, 1944: Lumberport, West Virginia

An explosion in the number four shaft of the Katherine coal mine killed 16 people.

CDC and NIOSH Safety and Health Research. *Coal Mining Disasters*. Available at: http://www.cdc.gov/niosh/mining/statistics/discoal.htm. Accessed September 21, 2005.

### November 6, 1943: Madison, West Virginia

An explosion in the number three shaft of the Nellis coal mine killed 11 people.

CDC and NIOSH Safety and Health Research. *Coal Mining Disasters*. Available at: http://www.cdc.gov/niosh/mining/statistics/discoal.htm. Accessed September 21, 2005.

### September 24, 1943: Minersville, Pennsylvania

An explosion at the Primrose Colliery killed 14 people.

CDC and NIOSH Safety and Health Research. *Coal Mining Disasters*. Available at: http://www.cdc.gov/niosh/mining/statistics/discoal.htm. Accessed September 21, 2005.

### September 16, 1943: Three Point, Kentucky

An explosion at the Three Point coal mine killed 12 people.

CDC and NIOSH Safety and Health Research. *Coal Mining Disasters.* Available at:
http://www.cdc.gov/niosh/mining/statistics/discoal.htm. Accessed September 21, 2005.

### August 28, 1943: Sayreton, Alabama

An explosion in the number two shaft of the Sayreton coal mine killed 28
    people.

CDC and NIOSH Safety and Health Research. *Coal Mining Disasters.* Available at:
http://www.cdc.gov/niosh/mining/statistics/discoal.htm. Accessed September 21, 2005.

### May 11, 1943: Praco, Alabama

An explosion in the number ten shaft of the Praco coal mine killed 12 people.

CDC and NIOSH Safety and Health Research. *Coal Mining Disasters.* Available at:
http://www.cdc.gov/niosh/mining/statistics/discoal.htm. Accessed September 21, 2005.

### May 5, 1943: La Follette, Tennessee

An explosion at the NuRex coal mine killed ten people.

CDC and NIOSH Safety and Health Research. *Coal Mining Disasters.* Available at:
http://www.cdc.gov/niosh/mining/statistics/discoal.htm. Accessed September 21, 2005.

### February 27, 1943: Washoe, Montana

An explosion at the Smith coal mine killed 74 people.

CDC and NIOSH Safety and Health Research. *Coal Mining Disasters.* Available at:
http://www.cdc.gov/niosh/mining/statistics/discoal.htm. Accessed September 21, 2005.

### January 8, 1943: Pursglove, West Virginia

A fire in the #15 shaft of a local coal mine killed 13 people.

CDC and NIOSH Safety and Health Research. *Coal Mining Disasters.* Available at:
http://www.cdc.gov/niosh/mining/statistics/discoal.htm. Accessed September 21, 2005.

### November 30, 1942: Wheatcroft, Kentucky

An explosion in the number ten shaft of the West Kentucky coal mine killed
    six people.

CDC and NIOSH Safety and Health Research. *Coal Mining Disasters.* Available at:
http://www.cdc.gov/niosh/mining/statistics/discoal.htm. Accessed September 21, 2005.

### July 9, 1942: Pursglove, West Virginia

An explosion in the number two shaft of the Pursglove coal mine killed 20
    people.

CDC and NIOSH Safety and Health Research. *Coal Mining Disasters*. Available at: http://www.cdc.gov/niosh/mining/statistics/discoal.htm. Accessed September 21, 2005.

### May 12, 1942: Osage, West Virginia

An explosion in the number three shaft of the Christopher coal mine killed 56 people.

CDC and NIOSH Safety and Health Research. *Coal Mining Disasters*. Available at: http://www.cdc.gov/niosh/mining/statistics/discoal.htm. Accessed September 21, 2005.

### May 11, 1942: Excelsior, Arkansas

An explosion in the number two shaft of the Peerless coal mine killed six people.

CDC and NIOSH Safety and Health Research. *Coal Mining Disasters*. Available at: http://www.cdc.gov/niosh/mining/statistics/discoal.htm. Accessed September 21, 2005.

### January 27, 1942: Mount Harris, Colorado

An explosion at the Wadge coal mine killed 34 people.

CDC and NIOSH Safety and Health Research. *Coal Mining Disasters*. Available at: http://www.cdc.gov/niosh/mining/statistics/discoal.htm. Accessed September 21, 2005.

### December 28, 1941: Harco, Illinois

An explosion in the #47 shaft of a local coal mine killed eight people.

CDC and NIOSH Safety and Health Research. *Coal Mining Disasters*. Available at: http://www.cdc.gov/niosh/mining/statistics/discoal.htm. Accessed September 21, 2005.

### October 27, 1941: Daniel Boone, Kentucky

An explosion at the Daniel Boone coal mine killed 15 people.

CDC and NIOSH Safety and Health Research. *Coal Mining Disasters*. Available at: http://www.cdc.gov/niosh/mining/statistics/discoal.htm. Accessed September 21, 2005.

### July 10, 1941: Acmar, Alabama

An explosion in the number six shaft of the Acmar coal mine killed 11 people.

CDC and NIOSH Safety and Health Research. *Coal Mining Disasters*. Available at: http://www.cdc.gov/niosh/mining/statistics/discoal.htm. Accessed September 21, 2005.

### June 30, 1941: McIntyre, Pennsylvania

An explosion in the number two shaft of the Kent coal mine killed seven people.

CDC and NIOSH Safety and Health Research. *Coal Mining Disasters*. Available at: http://www.cdc.gov/niosh/mining/statistics/discoal.htm. Accessed September 21, 2005.

### June 4, 1941: Adamsville, Alabama

An explosion at the Docena coal mine killed five people.

CDC and NIOSH Safety and Health Research. *Coal Mining Disasters.* Available at: http://www.cdc.gov/niosh/mining/statistics/discoal.htm. Accessed September 21, 2005.

### May 22, 1941: Bicknell, Indiana

An explosion in the number two shaft of the Panhandle coal mine killed 14 people.

CDC and NIOSH Safety and Health Research. *Coal Mining Disasters.* Available at: http://www.cdc.gov/niosh/mining/statistics/discoal.htm. Accessed September 21, 2005.

### May 18, 1941: Benwood, West Virginia

An explosion at the Hitchman coal mine killed five people.

CDC and NIOSH Safety and Health Research. *Coal Mining Disasters.* Available at: http://www.cdc.gov/niosh/mining/statistics/discoal.htm. Accessed September 21, 2005.

### January 22, 1941: Kimball, West Virginia

An explosion at Carswell coal mine killed six people.

CDC and NIOSH Safety and Health Research. *Coal Mining Disasters.* Available at: http://www.cdc.gov/niosh/mining/statistics/discoal.htm. Accessed September 21, 2005.

### December 17, 1940: Raleigh, West Virginia

An explosion in the number four shaft of a local coal mine killed nine people.

CDC and NIOSH Safety and Health Research. *Coal Mining Disasters.* Available at: http://www.cdc.gov/niosh/mining/statistics/discoal.htm. Accessed September 21, 2005.

### November 29, 1940: Cadiz, Ohio

An explosion at the Nelms coal mine killed 31 people.

CDC and NIOSH Safety and Health Research. *Coal Mining Disasters.* Available at: http://www.cdc.gov/niosh/mining/statistics/discoal.htm. Accessed September 21, 2005.

### August 27, 1940: Bates, Arkansas

An explosion in the number two shaft of a local coal mine killed ten people.

CDC and NIOSH Safety and Health Research. *Coal Mining Disasters.* Available at: http://www.cdc.gov/niosh/mining/statistics/discoal.htm. Accessed September 21, 2005.

### July 15, 1940: Portage, Pennsylvania

An explosion at the Sonman coal mine killed 63 people.

CDC and NIOSH Safety and Health Research. *Coal Mining Disasters.* Available at: http://www.cdc.gov/niosh/mining/statistics/discoal.htm. Accessed September 21, 2005.

### March 16, 1940: St. Clairsville, Ohio
An explosion in the number ten shaft of the Willow Grove coal mine killed 72
people.

CDC and NIOSH Safety and Health Research. *Coal Mining Disasters*. Available at:
http://www.cdc.gov/niosh/mining/statistics/discoal.htm. Accessed September 21, 2005.

### January 10, 1940: Bartley, West Virginia
An explosion in the number one shaft of the Pond Creek coal mine killed 91
people.

CDC and NIOSH Safety and Health Research. *Coal Mining Disasters*. Available at:
http://www.cdc.gov/niosh/mining/statistics/discoal.htm. Accessed September 21, 2005.

### 1939–1930
### July 14, 1939: Providence, Kentucky
An explosion at the Duvin coal mine killed 28 people.

CDC and NIOSH Safety and Health Research. *Coal Mining Disasters*. Available at:
http://www.cdc.gov/niosh/mining/statistics/discoal.htm. Accessed September 21, 2005.

### June 2, 1938: Pittston, Pennsylvania
An explosion at the Butler Slope coal mine killed ten people.

CDC and NIOSH Safety and Health Research. *Coal Mining Disasters*. Available at:
http://www.cdc.gov/niosh/mining/statistics/discoal.htm. Accessed September 21, 2005.

### April 27, 1938: Pottsville, Pennsylvania
An explosion at the number one slope of a coal mine killed eight people.

CDC and NIOSH Safety and Health Research. *Coal Mining Disasters*. Available at:
http://www.cdc.gov/niosh/mining/statistics/discoal.htm. Accessed September 21, 2005.

### April 22, 1938: Hanger, Virginia
An explosion at the Keen Mountain coal mine killed 45 people.

CDC and NIOSH Safety and Health Research. *Coal Mining Disasters*. Available at:
http://www.cdc.gov/niosh/mining/statistics/discoal.htm. Accessed September 21, 2005.

### February 11, 1938: Afton, Wyoming
An explosion at the Vail (Star Valley) coal mine killed five people.

CDC and NIOSH Safety and Health Research. *Coal Mining Disasters*. Available at:
http://www.cdc.gov/niosh/mining/statistics/discoal.htm. Accessed September 21, 2005.

### *January 12, 1938: Harwick, Pennsylvania*
An explosion at the Harwick coal mine killed ten people.

CDC and NIOSH Safety and Health Research. *Coal Mining Disasters.* Available at:
http://www.cdc.gov/niosh/mining/statistics/discoal.htm. Accessed September 21, 2005.

### *October 26, 1937: Jonesville, Alaska*
An explosion at the Jonesville coal mine killed 14 people.

CDC and NIOSH Safety and Health Research. *Coal Mining Disasters.* Available at:
http://www.cdc.gov/niosh/mining/statistics/discoal.htm. Accessed September 21, 2005.

### *October 15, 1937: Mulga, Alabama*
An explosion at the Mulga coal mine killed 34 people.

CDC and NIOSH Safety and Health Research. *Coal Mining Disasters.* Available at:
http://www.cdc.gov/niosh/mining/statistics/discoal.htm. Accessed September 21, 2005.

### *July 15, 1937: Sullivan, Indiana*
An explosion at the Baker coal mine killed 20 people.

CDC and NIOSH Safety and Health Research. *Coal Mining Disasters.* Available at:
http://www.cdc.gov/niosh/mining/statistics/discoal.htm. Accessed September 21, 2005.

### *June 21, 1937: Keystone, Ohio*
Detonation of explosives at the Rupert Mine killed six people.

CDC and NIOSH Safety and Health Research. *Coal Mining Disasters.* Available at:
http://www.cdc.gov/niosh/mining/statistics/discoal.htm. Accessed September 21, 2005.

### *March 28, 1937: Du Bois, Pennsylvania*
An explosion at the Kramer coal mine killed nine people.

CDC and NIOSH Safety and Health Research. *Coal Mining Disasters.* Available at:
http://www.cdc.gov/niosh/mining/statistics/discoal.htm. Accessed September 21, 2005.

### *March 11, 1937: Macbeth, West Virginia*
An explosion in the Macbeth coal mine killed 18 people.

CDC and NIOSH Safety and Health Research. *Coal Mining Disasters.* Available at:
http://www.cdc.gov/niosh/mining/statistics/discoal.htm. Accessed September 21, 2005.

### *November 19, 1936: Bates, Arizona*
An explosion at the Bates coal mine killed five people.

CDC and NIOSH Safety and Health Research. *Coal Mining Disasters.* Available at:
http://www.cdc.gov/niosh/mining/statistics/discoal.htm. Accessed September 21, 2005.

### September 2, 1936: Macbeth, West Virginia
An explosion at the Macbeth coal mine killed ten people.

CDC and NIOSH Safety and Health Research. *Coal Mining Disasters*. Available at: http://www.cdc.gov/niosh/mining/statistics/discoal.htm. Accessed September 21, 2005.

### August 24, 1936: West Pittston, Pennsylvania
An explosion at the Clear Spring coal mine killed five people.

CDC and NIOSH Safety and Health Research. *Coal Mining Disasters*. Available at: http://www.cdc.gov/niosh/mining/statistics/discoal.htm. Accessed September 21, 2005.

### January 20, 1936: Broomfield, Colorado
An explosion in the number two shaft of the Monarch coal mine killed eight people.

CDC and NIOSH Safety and Health Research. *Coal Mining Disasters*. Available at: http://www.cdc.gov/niosh/mining/statistics/discoal.htm. Accessed September 21, 2005.

### July 17, 1935: Van Lear, Kentucky
An explosion in the #155 shaft of a local coal mine in Van Lear killed nine people.

CDC and NIOSH Safety and Health Research. *Coal Mining Disasters*. Available at: http://www.cdc.gov/niosh/mining/statistics/discoal.htm. Accessed September 21, 2005.

### January 21, 1935: Gilberton, Pennsylvania
An explosion at the Gilberton coal mine killed 13 people.

CDC and NIOSH Safety and Health Research. *Coal Mining Disasters*. Available at: http://www.cdc.gov/niosh/mining/statistics/discoal.htm. Accessed September 21, 2005.

### August 6, 1934: Big Stone Gap, Virginia
An explosion in the number three shaft of the Derby coal mine killed 17 people.

CDC and NIOSH Safety and Health Research. *Coal Mining Disasters*. Available at: http://www.cdc.gov/niosh/mining/statistics/discoal.htm. Accessed September 21, 2005.

### March 12, 1934: Wheatcroft, Kentucky
A fire in the number 10 shaft of a local coal mine killed five people.

CDC and NIOSH Safety and Health Research. *Coal Mining Disasters*. Available at: http://www.cdc.gov/niosh/mining/statistics/discoal.htm. Accessed September 21, 2005.

### September 11, 1933: Barking, Pennsylvania
An explosion at the Oakmont coal mine killed seven people.

CDC and NIOSH Safety and Health Research. *Coal Mining Disasters.* Available at: http://www.cdc.gov/niosh/mining/statistics/discoal.htm. Accessed September 21, 2005.

### December 24, 1932: Moweaqua, Illinois
An explosion at the Moweaqua coal mine killed 54 people.

CDC and NIOSH Safety and Health Research. *Coal Mining Disasters.* Available at: http://www.cdc.gov/niosh/mining/statistics/discoal.htm. Accessed September 21, 2005.

### December 9, 1932: Yancey, Kentucky
An explosion at the Zero coal mine killed 23 people.

CDC and NIOSH Safety and Health Research. *Coal Mining Disasters.* Available at: http://www.cdc.gov/niosh/mining/statistics/discoal.htm. Accessed September 21, 2005.

### December 7, 1932: Madrid, New Mexico
An explosion at the Morgan-Jones coal mine killed 14 people.

CDC and NIOSH Safety and Health Research. *Coal Mining Disasters.* Available at: http://www.cdc.gov/niosh/mining/statistics/discoal.htm. Accessed September 21, 2005.

### June 13, 1932: Splashdam, Virginia
An explosion in the number six shaft of the Splashdam coal mine killed ten people.

CDC and NIOSH Safety and Health Research. *Coal Mining Disasters.* Available at: http://www.cdc.gov/niosh/mining/statistics/discoal.htm. Accessed September 21, 2005.

### February 27, 1932: Boissevain, Virginia
An explosion at the Boissevain coal mine killed 38 people.

CDC and NIOSH Safety and Health Research. *Coal Mining Disasters.* Available at: http://www.cdc.gov/niosh/mining/statistics/discoal.htm. Accessed September 21, 2005.

### January 18, 1932: Parrott, Virginia
An explosion at the Parrott coal mine killed six people.

CDC and NIOSH Safety and Health Research. *Coal Mining Disasters.* Available at: http://www.cdc.gov/niosh/mining/statistics/discoal.htm. Accessed September 21, 2005.

### December 28, 1931: Irondale, Alabama
An explosion in the number one shaft of the Overton coal mine killed five people.

CDC and NIOSH Safety and Health Research. *Coal Mining Disasters*. Available at: http://www.cdc.gov/niosh/mining/statistics/discoal.htm. Accessed September 21, 2005.

### November 3, 1931: Holden, West Virginia
An explosion in the # 20 shaft of a coal mine in Holden killed five people.

CDC and NIOSH Safety and Health Research. *Coal Mining Disasters*. Available at: http://www.cdc.gov/niosh/mining/statistics/discoal.htm. Accessed September 21, 2005.

### May 29, 1931: Mount Carmel, Pennsylvania
An explosion at the Richard Colliery coal mine killed five people.

CDC and NIOSH Safety and Health Research. *Coal Mining Disasters*. Available at: http://www.cdc.gov/niosh/mining/statistics/discoal.htm. Accessed September 21, 2005.

### January 28, 1931: Dugger, Indiana
An explosion at the Little Betty coal mine killed 28 people.

CDC and NIOSH Safety and Health Research. *Coal Mining Disasters*. Available at: http://www.cdc.gov/niosh/mining/statistics/discoal.htm. Accessed September 21, 2005.

### January 6, 1931: Glen Rogers, West Virginia
An explosion in the number two shaft of a local coal mine in Glen Rogers killed eight people.

CDC and NIOSH Safety and Health Research. *Coal Mining Disasters*. Available at: http://www.cdc.gov/niosh/mining/statistics/discoal.htm. Accessed September 21, 2005.

### January 3, 1931: Midvale, Ohio
An explosion in the number four shaft of the Midvale coal mine killed five people.

CDC and NIOSH Safety and Health Research. *Coal Mining Disasters*. Available at: http://www.cdc.gov/niosh/mining/statistics/discoal.htm. Accessed September 21, 2005.

### December 6, 1930: Madrid, New Mexico
An explosion at the Lamb coal mine killed five people.

CDC and NIOSH Safety and Health Research. *Coal Mining Disasters*. Available at: http://www.cdc.gov/niosh/mining/statistics/discoal.htm. Accessed September 21, 2005.

### November 29, 1930: Lutie, Oklahoma
An explosion in the number five shaft of the Lutie coal mine killed 15 people.

CDC and NIOSH Safety and Health Research. *Coal Mining Disasters*. Available at: http://www.cdc.gov/niosh/mining/statistics/discoal.htm. Accessed September 21, 2005.

### November 5, 1930: Millfield, Ohio

An explosion in the number six shaft of a local coal mine in Millfield killed 82
  people.

CDC and NIOSH Safety and Health Research. *Coal Mining Disasters.* Available at:
http://www.cdc.gov/niosh/mining/statistics/discoal.htm. Accessed September 21, 2005.

### October 27, 1930: McAlester, Oklahoma

An explosion in the number four shaft of the Wheatley coal mine killed 30
  people.

CDC and NIOSH Safety and Health Research. *Coal Mining Disasters.* Available at:
http://www.cdc.gov/niosh/mining/statistics/discoal.htm. Accessed September 21, 2005.

### April 12, 1930: Carbonado, Washington

An explosion at the Carbonado coal mine killed 17 people.

CDC and NIOSH Safety and Health Research. *Coal Mining Disasters.* Available at:
http://www.cdc.gov/niosh/mining/statistics/discoal.htm. Accessed September 21, 2005.

### March 30, 1930: Kettle Island, Kentucky

An explosion at the Pioneer coal mine killed 16 people.

CDC and NIOSH Safety and Health Research. *Coal Mining Disasters.* Available at:
http://www.cdc.gov/niosh/mining/statistics/discoal.htm. Accessed September 21, 2005.

### March 26, 1930: Arnettsville, West Virginia

An explosion at the Yukon coal mine killed 12 people.

CDC and NIOSH Safety and Health Research. *Coal Mining Disasters.* Available at:
http://www.cdc.gov/niosh/mining/statistics/discoal.htm. Accessed September 21, 2005.

### March 8, 1930: Lynn, Utah

An explosion at the New Peerless coal mine killed five people.

CDC and NIOSH Safety and Health Research. *Coal Mining Disasters.* Available at:
http://www.cdc.gov/niosh/mining/statistics/discoal.htm. Accessed September 21, 2005.

### February 6, 1930: Standardville, Utah

An explosion at the Standard coal mine killed 23 people.

CDC and NIOSH Safety and Health Research. *Coal Mining Disasters.* Available at:
http://www.cdc.gov/niosh/mining/statistics/discoal.htm. Accessed September 21, 2005.

### January 19, 1930: Lillybrook, West Virginia

An explosion in the number one shaft of a local coal mine in Lillybrook killed
  eight people.

CDC and NIOSH Safety and Health Research. *Coal Mining Disasters*. Available at: http://www.cdc.gov/niosh/mining/statistics/discoal.htm. Accessed September 21, 2005.

### January 13, 1930: Straven, Alabama

An explosion at the Peerless coal mine killed seven people.

CDC and NIOSH Safety and Health Research. *Coal Mining Disasters*. Available at: http://www.cdc.gov/niosh/mining/statistics/discoal.htm. Accessed September 21, 2005.

### 1929–1920
### December 17, 1929: McAlester, Oklahoma

An explosion at the Old Town coal mine killed 61 people.

CDC and NIOSH Safety and Health Research. *Coal Mining Disasters*. Available at: http://www.cdc.gov/niosh/mining/statistics/discoal.htm. Accessed September 21, 2005.

### December 1, 1929: West Frankfort, Illinois

An explosion in the number eight shaft of the Old Ben coal mine killed seven people.

CDC and NIOSH Safety and Health Research. *Coal Mining Disasters*. Available at: http://www.cdc.gov/niosh/mining/statistics/discoal.htm. Accessed September 21, 2005.

### September 27, 1929: Tahona, Oklahoma

An explosion at the Covington coal mine killed eight people.

CDC and NIOSH Safety and Health Research. *Historical Mining Disasters*. Available at: http://www.cdc.gov/niosh/mining/statistics/discoal.htm. Accessed September 21, 2005.

### May 27, 1929: Yolande, Alabama

An explosion at the Connellsville coal mine killed ten people.

CDC and NIOSH Safety and Health Research. *Coal Mining Disasters*. Available at: http://www.cdc.gov/niosh/mining/statistics/discoal.htm. Accessed September 21, 2005.

### March 21, 1929: Parnassus, Pennsylvania

An explosion at the Kinloch coal mine killed 46 people.

CDC and NIOSH Safety and Health Research. *Coal Mining Disasters*. Available at: http://www.cdc.gov/niosh/mining/statistics/discoal.htm. Accessed September 21, 2005.

### January 26, 1929: Kingston, West Virginia

An explosion in the number five shaft of the Kingston coal mine killed 14 people.

CDC and NIOSH Safety and Health Research. *Coal Mining Disasters*. Available at: http://www.cdc.gov/niosh/mining/statistics/discoal.htm. Accessed September 21, 2005.

### December 18, 1928: Drakesboro, Kentucky

An explosion in the number two shaft of a local coal mine in Drakesboro killed six people.

CDC and NIOSH Safety and Health Research. *Coal Mining Disasters.* Available at: http://www.cdc.gov/niosh/mining/statistics/discoal.htm. Accessed September 21, 2005.

### November 30, 1928: Roderfield, West Virginia

An explosion at the Princess Poca coal mine killed six people.

CDC and NIOSH Safety and Health Research. *Coal Mining Disasters.* Available at: http://www.cdc.gov/niosh/mining/statistics/discoal.htm. Accessed September 21, 2005.

### October 22, 1928: McAlpin, West Virginia

An explosion at the McAlpin coal mine killed six people.

CDC and NIOSH Safety and Health Research. *Coal Mining Disasters.* Available at: http://www.cdc.gov/niosh/mining/statistics/discoal.htm. Accessed September 21, 2005.

### August 15, 1928: Coalport, Pennsylvania

An explosion in the number three shaft of the Irvonis coal mine killed 13 people.

CDC and NIOSH Safety and Health Research. *Coal Mining Disasters.* Available at: http://www.cdc.gov/niosh/mining/statistics/discoal.htm. Accessed September 21, 2005.

### August 9, 1928: Johnstown, Pennsylvania

An explosion at the Hillside coal mine killed five people.

CDC and NIOSH Safety and Health Research. *Coal Mining Disasters.* Available at: http://www.cdc.gov/niosh/mining/statistics/discoal.htm. Accessed September 21, 2005.

### May 25, 1928: Parsons, Pennsylvania

An explosion in the number five shaft of the Baltimore coal mine killed ten people.

CDC and NIOSH Safety and Health Research. *Coal Mining Disasters.* Available at: http://www.cdc.gov/niosh/mining/statistics/discoal.htm. Accessed September 21, 2005.

### May 22, 1928: Kenvir, Kentucky

An explosion in the #30 shaft of a local coal mine in Kenvir killed eight people.

CDC and NIOSH Safety and Health Research. *Coal Mining Disasters.* Available at: http://www.cdc.gov/niosh/mining/statistics/discoal.htm. Accessed September 21, 2005.

### May 22, 1928: Yukon, West Virginia

An explosion in the number one shaft of a local coal mine in Yukon killed 17 people.

CDC and NIOSH Safety and Health Research. *Coal Mining Disasters.* Available at: http://www.cdc.gov/niosh/mining/statistics/discoal.htm. Accessed September 21, 2005.

### May 19, 1928: Mather, Pennsylvania

An explosion in the number one shaft of the Mather coal mine killed 195 people.

CDC and NIOSH Safety and Health Research. *Coal Mining Disasters.* Available at: http://www.cdc.gov/niosh/mining/statistics/discoal.htm. Accessed September 21, 2005.

### April 2, 1928: Keystone, West Virginia

An explosion in the number two shaft of the Keystone coal mine killed eight people.

CDC and NIOSH Safety and Health Research. *Coal Mining Disasters.* Available at: http://www.cdc.gov/niosh/mining/statistics/discoal.htm. Accessed September 21, 2005.

### February 24, 1928: Jenny Lind, Arkansas

An explosion in the number three shaft of the Mama coal mine killed 13 people.

CDC and NIOSH Safety and Health Research. *Coal Mining Disasters.* Available at: http://www.cdc.gov/niosh/mining/statistics/discoal.htm. Accessed September 21, 2005.

### February 20, 1928: Parnassus, Pennsylvania

An explosion in the Kinloch coal mine killed 12 people.

CDC and NIOSH Safety and Health Research. *Coal Mining Disasters.* Available at: http://www.cdc.gov/niosh/mining/statistics/discoal.htm. Accessed September 21, 2005.

### January 9, 1928: West Frankfort, Illinois

An explosion in the #18 shaft of a coal mine in the West Frankfort coal mine killed 21 people.

CDC and NIOSH Safety and Health Research. *Coal Mining Disasters.* Available at: http://www.cdc.gov/niosh/mining/statistics/discoal.htm. Accessed September 21, 2005.

### December 20, 1927: Johnston City, Illinois

An explosion in the number one shaft of the Franco coal mine killed seven people.

CDC and NIOSH Safety and Health Research. *Coal Mining Disasters.* Available at: http://www.cdc.gov/niosh/mining/statistics/discoal.htm. Accessed September 21, 2005.

### August 3, 1927: Clay, Kentucky

An explosion in the number seven shaft of the Western Kentucky coal mine killed 15 people.

CDC and NIOSH Safety and Health Research. *Coal Mining Disasters*. Available at: http://www.cdc.gov/niosh/mining/statistics/discoal.htm. Accessed September 21, 2005.

### May 27, 1927: Delagua, Colorado

An explosion at the Delagua coal mine killed seven people.

CDC and NIOSH Safety and Health Research. *Coal Mining Disasters*. Available at: http://www.cdc.gov/niosh/mining/statistics/discoal.htm. Accessed September 21, 2005.

### May 26, 1927: Edwardsville, Pennsylvania

An explosion in the number three shaft of the Woodward coal mine killed seven people.

CDC and NIOSH Safety and Health Research. *Coal Mining Disasters*. Available at: http://www.cdc.gov/niosh/mining/statistics/discoal.htm. Accessed September 21, 2005.

### May 13, 1927: Caples, West Virginia

An explosion in the number three shaft of the Shannon Branch coal mine killed eight people.

CDC and NIOSH Safety and Health Research. *Coal Mining Disasters*. Available at: http://www.cdc.gov/niosh/mining/statistics/discoal.htm. Accessed September 21, 2005.

### April 30, 1927: Everettville, West Virginia

An explosion in the number three shaft of the Federal coal mine killed 97 people.

CDC and NIOSH Safety and Health Research. *Coal Mining Disasters*. Available at: http://www.cdc.gov/niosh/mining/statistics/discoal.htm. Accessed September 21, 2005.

### April 2, 1927: Cokeburg, Pennsylvania

An explosion in the #53 shaft of a coal mine in Cokeburg killed six people.

CDC and NIOSH Safety and Health Research. *Coal Mining Disasters*. Available at: http://www.cdc.gov/niosh/mining/statistics/discoal.htm. Accessed September 21, 2005.

### March 30, 1927: Ledford, Illinois

An explosion in the number two shaft of the Saline coal mine killed eight people.

CDC and NIOSH Safety and Health Research. *Coal Mining Disasters*. Available at: http://www.cdc.gov/niosh/mining/statistics/discoal.htm. Accessed September 21, 2005.

### January 31, 1927: Nortonville, Kentucky

An explosion at the Nortonville Mining coal mine killed five people.

CDC and NIOSH Safety and Health Research. *Coal Mining Disasters*. Available at: http://www.cdc.gov/niosh/mining/statistics/discoal.htm. Accessed September 21, 2005.

### December 9, 1926: Francisco, Indiana

An explosion in the number two shaft of the Francisco coal mine killed 37 people.

CDC and NIOSH Safety and Health Research. *Coal Mining Disasters*. Available at: http://www.cdc.gov/niosh/mining/statistics/discoal.htm. Accessed September 21, 2005.

### November 15, 1926: Moundsville, Pennsylvania

An explosion at the Mound coal mine killed five people.

CDC and NIOSH Safety and Health Research. *Coal Mining Disasters*. Available at: http://www.cdc.gov/niosh/mining/statistics/discoal.htm. Accessed September 21, 2005.

### October 30, 1926: Nanticoke, Pennsylvania

An explosion in the number seven shaft of the Colliery coal mine killed nine people.

CDC and NIOSH Safety and Health Research. *Coal Mining Disasters*. Available at: http://www.cdc.gov/niosh/mining/statistics/discoal.htm. Accessed September 21, 2005.

### October 4, 1926: Rockwood, Tennessee

An explosion at the Rockwood coal mine killed 27 people.

CDC and NIOSH Safety and Health Research. *Coal Mining Disasters*. Available at: http://www.cdc.gov/niosh/mining/statistics/discoal.htm. Accessed September 21, 2005.

### September 3, 1926: Tahona, Oklahoma

An explosion at the Tahona coal mine killed 16 people.

CDC and NIOSH Safety and Health Research. *Coal Mining Disasters*. Available at: http://www.cdc.gov/niosh/mining/statistics/discoal.htm. Accessed September 21, 2005.

### August 26, 1926: Clymer, Pennsylvania

An explosion in the number one shaft of the Clymer coal mine killed 44 people.

CDC and NIOSH Safety and Health Research. *Coal Mining Disasters*. Available at: http://www.cdc.gov/niosh/mining/statistics/discoal.htm. Accessed September 21, 2005.

### July 21, 1926: Moffat, Alabama

An explosion at the Dixie coal mine killed nine people.

CDC and NIOSH Safety and Health Research. *Coal Mining Disasters.* Available at: http://www.cdc.gov/niosh/mining/statistics/discoal.htm. Accessed September 21, 2005.

### July 3, 1926: Kingston, Pennsylvania

An explosion at the Pettebone Colliery coal mine killed seven people.

CDC and NIOSH Safety and Health Research. *Coal Mining Disasters.* Available at: http://www.cdc.gov/niosh/mining/statistics/discoal.htm. Accessed September 21, 2005.

### May 6, 1926: Port Carbon, Pennsylvania

An explosion at the Randolph Colliery coal mine killed five people.

CDC and NIOSH Safety and Health Research. *Coal Mining Disasters.* Available at: http://www.cdc.gov/niosh/mining/statistics/discoal.htm. Accessed September 21, 2005.

### March 8, 1926: Eccles, West Virginia

An explosion in the number five shaft of the Eccles coal mine killed 19 people.

CDC and NIOSH Safety and Health Research. *Coal Mining Disasters.* Available at: http://www.cdc.gov/niosh/mining/statistics/discoal.htm. Accessed September 21, 2005.

### February 16, 1926: Nelson, Kentucky

An explosion at the Nelson coal mine killed eight people.

CDC and NIOSH Safety and Health Research. *Coal Mining Disasters.* Available at: http://www.cdc.gov/niosh/mining/statistics/discoal.htm. Accessed September 21, 2005.

### February 3, 1926: Horning, Pennsylvania

An explosion in the number four shaft of the Horning coal mine killed 20 people.

CDC and NIOSH Safety and Health Research. *Coal Mining Disasters.* Available at: http://www.cdc.gov/niosh/mining/statistics/discoal.htm. Accessed September 21, 2005.

### January 29, 1926: Helena, Alabama

An explosion in the number one shaft of the Mossboro coal mine killed 27 people.

CDC and NIOSH Safety and Health Research. *Coal Mining Disasters.* Available at: http://www.cdc.gov/niosh/mining/statistics/discoal.htm. Accessed September 21, 2005.

### January 29, 1926: West Frankfort, Illinois

An explosion in the number two shaft of the New Orient coal mine killed five people.

CDC and NIOSH Safety and Health Research. *Coal Mining Disasters*. Available at: http://www.cdc.gov/niosh/mining/statistics/discoal.htm. Accessed September 21, 2005.

### January 14, 1926: Farmington, West Virginia
An explosion in the number eight shaft of the Jamison coal mine killed 19 people.

CDC and NIOSH Safety and Health Research. *Coal Mining Disasters*. Available at: http://www.cdc.gov/niosh/mining/statistics/discoal.htm. Accessed September 21, 2005.

### January 13, 1926: Wilburton, Oklahoma
An explosion in the #21 shaft of a coal mine in Wilburton killed 91 people.

CDC and NIOSH Safety and Health Research. *Coal Mining Disasters*. Available at: http://www.cdc.gov/niosh/mining/statistics/discoal.htm. Accessed September 21, 2005.

### December 14, 1925: Tacoma, Washington
An explosion at the Wilkeson coal mine killed five people.

CDC and NIOSH Safety and Health Research. *Coal Mining Disasters*. Available at: http://www.cdc.gov/niosh/mining/statistics/discoal.htm. Accessed September 21, 2005.

### December 10, 1925: Irondale, Alabama
An explosion in the number two shaft of the Overton coal mine killed 53 people.

CDC and NIOSH Safety and Health Research. *Coal Mining Disasters*. Available at: http://www.cdc.gov/niosh/mining/statistics/discoal.htm. Accessed September 21, 2005.

### November 13, 1925: Madisonville, Kentucky
An explosion at the Finley coal mine killed five people.

CDC and NIOSH Safety and Health Research. *Coal Mining Disasters*. Available at: http://www.cdc.gov/niosh/mining/statistics/discoal.htm. Accessed September 21, 2005.

### August 3, 1925: Wilkes-Barre, Pennsylvania
An explosion at the Dorrance coal mine killed ten people.

CDC and NIOSH Safety and Health Research. *Coal Mining Disasters*. Available at: http://www.cdc.gov/niosh/mining/statistics/discoal.htm. Accessed September 21, 2005.

### July 23, 1925: Rockwood, Tennessee
An explosion at the Rockwood coal mine killed ten people.

CDC and NIOSH Safety and Health Research. *Coal Mining Disasters*. Available at: http://www.cdc.gov/niosh/mining/statistics/discoal.htm. Accessed September 21, 2005.

### June 8, 1925: Sturgis, Kentucky

An explosion in the number nine shaft of a coal mine in Sturgis killed 17 people.

CDC and NIOSH Safety and Health Research. *Coal Mining Disasters.* Available at: http://www.cdc.gov/niosh/mining/statistics/discoal.htm. Accessed September 21, 2005.

### May 31, 1925: Piper, Alabama

An explosion in the number two shaft of a coal mine in Piper killed six people.

CDC and NIOSH Safety and Health Research. *Coal Mining Disasters.* Available at: http://www.cdc.gov/niosh/mining/statistics/discoal.htm. Accessed September 21, 2005.

### May 27, 1925: Farmville, North Carolina

An explosion at the Carolina coal mine killed 53 people.

CDC and NIOSH Safety and Health Research. *Coal Mining Disasters.* Available at: http://www.cdc.gov/niosh/mining/statistics/discoal.htm. Accessed September 21, 2005.

### May 22, 1925: Edwardsville, Pennsylvania

An explosion at the Woodward coal mine killed seven people.

CDC and NIOSH Safety and Health Research. *Coal Mining Disasters.* Available at: http://www.cdc.gov/niosh/mining/statistics/discoal.htm. Accessed September 21, 2005.

### April 26, 1925: Sewickley, Pennsylvania

An explosion at the New Slope coal mine killed five people.

CDC and NIOSH Safety and Health Research. *Coal Mining Disasters.* Available at: http://www.cdc.gov/niosh/mining/statistics/discoal.htm. Accessed September 21, 2005.

### April 26, 1925: Millgrove, Pennsylvania

An explosion at the Hutchinson coal mine killed five people.

CDC and NIOSH Safety and Health Research. *Coal Mining Disasters.* Available at: http://www.cdc.gov/niosh/mining/statistics/discoal.htm. Accessed September 21, 2005.

### March 17, 1925: Barrackville, West Virginia

An explosion at the Barrackville coal mine killed 33 people.

CDC and NIOSH Safety and Health Research. *Coal Mining Disasters.* Available at: http://www.cdc.gov/niosh/mining/statistics/discoal.htm. Accessed September 21, 2005.

### February 20, 1925: Sullivan, Indiana

An explosion in the City coal mine killed 52 people.

CDC and NIOSH Safety and Health Research. *Coal Mining Disasters.* Available at: http://www.cdc.gov/niosh/mining/statistics/discoal.htm. Accessed September 21, 2005.

### January 15, 1925: Providence, Kentucky

An explosion in the number one shaft of the Diamond coal mine killed six people.

CDC and NIOSH Safety and Health Research. *Coal Mining Disasters*. Available at: http://www.cdc.gov/niosh/mining/statistics/discoal.htm. Accessed September 21, 2005.

### December 17, 1924: Burnett, Washington

An explosion at the Burnett coal mine killed seven people.

CDC and NIOSH Safety and Health Research. *Coal Mining Disasters*. Available at: http://www.cdc.gov/niosh/mining/statistics/discoal.htm. Accessed September 21, 2005.

### September 21, 1924: Rains, Utah

An explosion in the Rains coal mine killed five people.

CDC and NIOSH Safety and Health Research. *Coal Mining Disasters*. Available at: http://www.cdc.gov/niosh/mining/statistics/discoal.htm. Accessed September 21, 2005.

### September 16, 1924: Sublette, Wyoming

An explosion in the number five shaft of the Sublette coal mine killed 39 people.

CDC and NIOSH Safety and Health Research. *Coal Mining Disasters*. Available at: http://www.cdc.gov/niosh/mining/statistics/discoal.htm. Accessed September 21, 2005.

### July 25, 1924: Brownsville, Pennsylvania

An explosion in the number one shaft of the Gates coal mine killed 10 people.

CDC and NIOSH Safety and Health Research. *Coal Mining Disasters*. Available at: http://www.cdc.gov/niosh/mining/statistics/discoal.htm. Accessed September 21, 2005.

### June 6, 1924: Nanticoke, Pennsylvania

An explosion at the Loomis Collieries coal mine killed 14 people.

CDC and NIOSH Safety and Health Research. *Coal Mining Disasters*. Available at: http://www.cdc.gov/niosh/mining/statistics/discoal.htm. Accessed September 21, 2005.

### April 28, 1924: Benwood, West Virginia

An explosion at the Benwood coal mine killed 119 people.

CDC and NIOSH Safety and Health Research. *Coal Mining Disasters*. Available at: http://www.cdc.gov/niosh/mining/statistics/discoal.htm. Accessed September 21, 2005.

### March 28, 1924: Yukon, West Virginia

An explosion in the number two shaft of the Yukon coal mine killed 26 people.

CDC and NIOSH Safety and Health Research. *Coal Mining Disasters*. Available at: http://www.cdc.gov/niosh/mining/statistics/discoal.htm. Accessed September 21, 2005.

### March 8, 1924: Castle Gate, Utah

An explosion in the number two shaft of a coal mine in Castle Gate killed 172 people.

CDC and NIOSH Safety and Health Research. *Coal Mining Disasters*. Available at: http://www.cdc.gov/niosh/mining/statistics/discoal.htm. Accessed September 21, 2005.

### January 26, 1924: Shanktown, Pennsylvania

An explosion in the #18 shaft of the Lancashire coal mine killed 36 people.

CDC and NIOSH Safety and Health Research. *Coal Mining Disasters*. Available at: http://www.cdc.gov/niosh/mining/statistics/discoal.htm. Accessed September 21, 2005.

### January 25, 1924: Johnston City, Illinois

An explosion at the McClintock coal mine killed 33 people.

CDC and NIOSH Safety and Health Research. *Coal Mining Disasters*. Available at: http://www.cdc.gov/niosh/mining/statistics/discoal.htm. Accessed September 21, 2005.

### December 7, 1923: Happy, Perry County, Kentucky

An explosion at the Black Hawk coal mine killed nine people.

CDC and NIOSH Safety and Health Research. *Coal Mining Disasters*. Available at: http://www.cdc.gov/niosh/mining/statistics/discoal.htm. Accessed September 21, 2005.

### November 6, 1923: Beckley, West Virginia

An explosion at the Glen Rogers coal mine killed 27 people.

CDC and NIOSH Safety and Health Research. *Coal Mining Disasters*. Available at: http://www.cdc.gov/niosh/mining/statistics/discoal.htm. Accessed September 21, 2005.

### August 14, 1923: Kemmerer, Wyoming

An explosion in the number one shaft of the Frontier coal mine killed 99 people.

CDC and NIOSH Safety and Health Research. *Coal Mining Disasters*. Available at: http://www.cdc.gov/niosh/mining/statistics/discoal.htm. Accessed September 21, 2005.

### June 26, 1923: Mount Carmel, Pennsylvania

An explosion at the Richards Colliery coal mine killed five people.

CDC and NIOSH Safety and Health Research. *Coal Mining Disasters*. Available at: http://www.cdc.gov/niosh/mining/statistics/discoal.htm. Accessed September 21, 2005.

### May 5, 1923: Aguilar, Colorado

An explosion at the Southwestern coal mine killed ten people.

CDC and NIOSH Safety and Health Research. *Coal Mining Disasters*. Available at: http://www.cdc.gov/niosh/mining/statistics/discoal.htm. Accessed September 21, 2005.

### March 2, 1923: Arista, West Virginia

An explosion at the Arista coal mine killed ten people.

CDC and NIOSH Safety and Health Research. *Coal Mining Disasters*. Available at: http://www.cdc.gov/niosh/mining/statistics/discoal.htm. Accessed September 21, 2005.

### February 21, 1923: Kaska, Pennsylvania

An explosion at the Alliance coal mine killed five people.

CDC and NIOSH Safety and Health Research. *Coal Mining Disasters*. Available at: http://www.cdc.gov/niosh/mining/statistics/discoal.htm Accessed September 21, 2005.

### February 8, 1923: Dawson, Minnesota

An explosion in the number one shaft of the Stag Canon coal mine killed 120 people.

CDC and NIOSH Safety and Health Research. *Coal Mining Disasters*. Available at: http://www.cdc.gov/niosh/mining/statistics/discoal.htm. Accessed September 21, 2005.

### January 10, 1923: Dolomite, Alabama

An explosion in the number one shaft of the Dolomite coal mine killed five people.

CDC and NIOSH Safety and Health Research. *Coal Mining Disasters*. Available at: http://www.cdc.gov/niosh/mining/statistics/discoal.htm. Accessed September 21, 2005.

### November 25, 1922: Cerillos, New Mexico

An explosion in the number four shaft of a coal mine in Cerillos killed 12 people.

CDC and NIOSH Safety and Health Research. *Coal Mining Disasters*. Available at: http://www.cdc.gov/niosh/mining/statistics/discoal.htm. Accessed September 21, 2005.

### November 22, 1922: Dolomite, Alabama

An explosion in the number three shaft of the Dolomite coal mine killed 90 people.

CDC and NIOSH Safety and Health Research. *Coal Mining Disasters*. Available at: http://www.cdc.gov/niosh/mining/statistics/discoal.htm. Accessed September 21, 2005.

### November 6, 1922: Spangler, Pennsylvania

An explosion in the number one shaft of the Reilly coal mine killed 79 people.

CDC and NIOSH Safety and Health Research. *Coal Mining Disasters*. Available at: http://www.cdc.gov/niosh/mining/statistics/discoal.htm. Accessed September 21, 2005.

### November 5, 1922: Madrid, New Mexico
An explosion in the number four Anthracite Mine killed seven people.

CDC and NIOSH Safety and Health Research. *Coal Mining Disasters*. Available at:
http://www.cdc.gov/niosh/mining/statistics/discoal.htm. Accessed September 21, 2005.

### October 11, 1922: McCurtain, Oklahoma
An explosion in the #11 shaft of the Progressive coal mine killed eight people.

CDC and NIOSH Safety and Health Research. *Coal Mining Disasters*. Available at:
http://www.cdc.gov/niosh/mining/statistics/discoal.htm. Accessed September 21, 2005.

### September 29, 1922: Johnston City, Illinois
An explosion at the Lake Creek coal mine killed five people.

CDC and NIOSH Safety and Health Research. *Coal Mining Disasters*. Available at:
http://www.cdc.gov/niosh/mining/statistics/discoal.htm. Accessed September 21, 2005.

### May 25, 1922: Acmar, Alabama
An explosion in the number three shaft of the Acmar coal mine killed 11
people.

CDC and NIOSH Safety and Health Research. *Coal Mining Disasters*. Available at:
http://www.cdc.gov/niosh/mining/statistics/discoal.htm. Accessed September 21, 2005.

### March 24, 1922: Sopris, Colorado
An explosion in the number two shaft of the Sopris coal mine killed 17
people.

CDC and NIOSH Safety and Health Research. *Coal Mining Disasters*. Available at:
http://www.cdc.gov/niosh/mining/statistics/discoal.htm. Accessed September 21, 2005.

### March 20, 1922: Dilltown, Pennsylvania
An explosion in the number one shaft of the Dilltown coal mine killed five
people.

CDC and NIOSH Safety and Health Research. *Coal Mining Disasters*. Available at:
http://www.cdc.gov/niosh/mining/statistics/discoal.htm. Accessed September 21, 2005.

### February 7, 1922: Pinson Fork, Kentucky
An explosion at the Marietta coal mine killed nine people.

CDC and NIOSH Safety and Health Research. *Coal Mining Disasters*. Available at:
http://www.cdc.gov/niosh/mining/statistics/discoal.htm. Accessed September 21, 2005.

### February 2, 1922: Belle Ellen, Alabama
An explosion in the number two shaft of the Belle Ellen coal mine killed nine
people.

CDC and NIOSH Safety and Health Research. *Coal Mining Disasters.* Available at: http://www.cdc.gov/niosh/mining/statistics/discoal.htm. Accessed September 21, 2005.

### February 2, 1922: Gates, Pennsylvania

An explosion in the number two shaft of the Gates coal mine killed 25 people.

CDC and NIOSH Safety and Health Research. *Coal Mining Disasters.* Available at: http://www.cdc.gov/niosh/mining/statistics/discoal.htm. Accessed September 21, 2005.

### January 30, 1922: Hulen, Kentucky

An explosion at the Layman coal mine killed six people.

CDC and NIOSH Safety and Health Research. *Coal Mining Disasters.* Available at: http://www.cdc.gov/niosh/mining/statistics/discoal.htm. Accessed September 21, 2005.

### August 31, 1921: Harrisburg, Illinois

An explosion at the Harco coal mine killed 12 people.

CDC and NIOSH Safety and Health Research. *Coal Mining Disasters.* Available at: http://www.cdc.gov/niosh/mining/statistics/discoal.htm. Accessed September 21, 2005.

### March 9, 1921: Seek, Pennsylvania

An explosion in the #11 shaft of the Rahn coal mine killed five people.

CDC and NIOSH Safety and Health Research. *Coal Mining Disasters.* Available at: http://www.cdc.gov/niosh/mining/statistics/discoal.htm. Accessed September 21, 2005.

### February 12, 1921: Oak Hill, Colorado

Explosions in the number one and number two shafts of the Moffat coal mine killed five people.

CDC and NIOSH Safety and Health Research. *Coal Mining Disasters.* Available at: http://www.cdc.gov/niosh/mining/statistics/discoal.htm. Accessed September 21, 2005.

### November 23, 1920: Parrish, Alabama

An explosion at the Parrish coal mine killed 12 people.

CDC and NIOSH Safety and Health Research. *Coal Mining Disasters.* Available at: http://www.cdc.gov/niosh/mining/statistics/discoal.htm. Accessed September 21, 2005.

### August 21, 1920: Degnan, Oklahoma

An explosion in the #19 shaft of a coal mine in Degnan killed ten people.

CDC and NIOSH Safety and Health Research. *Coal Mining Disasters.* Available at: http://www.cdc.gov/niosh/mining/statistics/discoal.htm. Accessed September 21, 2005.

### July 19, 1920: Renton, Pennsylvania

An explosion in the number three shaft of the Renton coal mine killed nine people.

CDC and NIOSH Safety and Health Research. *Coal Mining Disasters.* Available at: http://www.cdc.gov/niosh/mining/statistics/discoal.htm. Accessed September 21, 2005.

### June 2, 1920: Cokeburg, Pennsylvania

An explosion at the Ontario coal mine killed six people.

CDC and NIOSH Safety and Health Research. *Coal Mining Disasters.* Available at: http://www.cdc.gov/niosh/mining/statistics/discoal.htm. Accessed September 21, 2005.

### May 3, 1920: Clinton, Indiana

An explosion at the Submarine coal mine killed five people.

CDC and NIOSH Safety and Health Research. *Coal Mining Disasters.* Available at: http://www.cdc.gov/niosh/mining/statistics/discoal.htm. Accessed September 21, 2005.

### April 14, 1920: Dawson, New Mexico

Explosions in the number one and number six shafts of the Stag Canon coal mine killed five people.

CDC and NIOSH Safety and Health Research. *Coal Mining Disasters.* Available at: http://www.cdc.gov/niosh/mining/statistics/discoal.htm. Accessed September 21, 2005.

### 1919–1910

### December 3, 1919: Jacksonville, Indiana

An explosion in the number three shaft of a coal mine in Jacksonville killed six people.

CDC and NIOSH Safety and Health Research. *Coal Mining Disasters.* Available at: http://www.cdc.gov/niosh/mining/statistics/discoal.htm. Accessed September 21, 2005.

### August 18, 1919: La Veta, Colorado

An explosion at the Oakdale coal mine killed 18 people.

CDC and NIOSH Safety and Health Research. *Coal Mining Disasters.* Available at: http://www.cdc.gov/niosh/mining/statistics/discoal.htm. Accessed September 21, 2005.

### August 6, 1919: Wierwood, West Virginia

An explosion at the Wierwood coal mine killed seven people.

CDC and NIOSH Safety and Health Research. *Coal Mining Disasters.* Available at: http://www.cdc.gov/niosh/mining/statistics/discoal.htm. Accessed September 21, 2005.

### July 18, 1919: Kimball, West Virginia

An explosion at the Carswell coal mine killed six people.

CDC and NIOSH Safety and Health Research. *Coal Mining Disasters.* Available at: http://www.cdc.gov/niosh/mining/statistics/discoal.htm. Accessed September 21, 2005.

### July 8, 1919: Lansford, Pennsylvania
An explosion at the Lansford Colliery coal mine killed eight people.

CDC and NIOSH Safety and Health Research. *Coal Mining Disasters.* Available at: http://www.cdc.gov/niosh/mining/statistics/dlscoal.htm. Accessed September 21, 2005.

### June 30, 1919: Alderson, Oklahoma
An explosion in the number five shaft of the Alderson coal mine killed 15 people.

CDC and NIOSH Safety and Health Research. *Coal Mining Disasters.* Available at: http://www.cdc.gov/niosh/mining/statistics/discoal.htm. Accessed September 21, 2005.

### June 5, 1919: Wilkes-Barre, Pennsylvania
Detonation of explosives in tunnel number two of the Baltimore coal mine killed 92 people.

CDC and NIOSH Safety and Health Research. *Coal Mining Disasters.* Available at: http://www.cdc.gov/niosh/mining/statistics/discoal.htm. Accessed September 21, 2005.

### April 29, 1919: Majestic, Alabama
An explosion at the Majestic coal mine killed 22 people.

CDC and NIOSH Safety and Health Research. *Coal Mining Disasters.* Available at: http://www.cdc.gov/niosh/mining/statistics/discoal.htm. Accessed September 21, 2005.

### March 31, 1919: Aguilar, Colorado
An explosion at the Empire coal mine killed 13 people.

CDC and NIOSH Safety and Health Research. *Coal Mining Disasters.* Available at: http://www.cdc.gov/niosh/mining/statistics/discoal.htm. Accessed September 21, 2005.

### September 28, 1918: Royalton, Illinois
An explosion at the North coal mine killed 21 people.

CDC and NIOSH Safety and Health Research. *Coal Mining Disasters.* Available at: http://www.cdc.gov/niosh/mining/statistics/discoal.htm. Accessed September 21, 2005.

### August 28, 1918: Burnett, Washington
An explosion at the Burnett coal mine killed 12 people.

CDC and NIOSH Safety and Health Research. *Coal Mining Disasters.* Available at: http://www.cdc.gov/niosh/mining/statistics/discoal.htm. Accessed September 21, 2005.

*August 7, 1918: Harmarville, Pennsylvania*
An explosion at the Harmar coal mine killed eight people.

CDC and NIOSH Safety and Health Research. *Coal Mining Disasters.* Available at:
http://www.cdc.gov/niosh/mining/statistics/discoal.htm. Accessed September 21, 2005.

*December 20, 1917: Catoosa, Tennessee*
An explosion in the number three shaft of a coal mine in Catoosa killed 11
  people.

CDC and NIOSH Safety and Health Research. *Coal Mining Disasters.* Available at:
http://www.cdc.gov/niosh/mining/statistics/discoal.htm. Accessed September 21, 2005.

*December 15, 1917: Bluefield, West Virginia*
An explosion in the number one shaft of the Yukon coal mine killed 18
  people.

CDC and NIOSH Safety and Health Research. *Coal Mining Disasters.* Available at:
http://www.cdc.gov/niosh/mining/statistics/discoal.htm. Accessed September 21, 2005.

*November 29, 1917: Christopher, Illinois*
An explosion in the #11 shaft of the Old Ben coal mine killed 18 people.

CDC and NIOSH Safety and Health Research. *Coal Mining Disasters.* Available at:
http://www.cdc.gov/niosh/mining/statistics/discoal.htm. Accessed September 21, 2005.

*August 4, 1917: Clay, Kentucky*
An explosion in the number seven shaft of the West Kentucky coal mine killed
  62 people.

CDC and NIOSH Safety and Health Research. *Coal Mining Disasters.* Available at:
http://www.cdc.gov/niosh/mining/statistics/discoal.htm. Accessed September 21, 2005.

*June 13, 1917: Banner, Alabama*
An explosion in the Banner coal mine killed six people.

CDC and NIOSH Safety and Health Research. *Coal Mining Disasters.* Available at:
http://www.cdc.gov/niosh/mining/statistics/discoal.htm. Accessed September 21, 2005.

*June 2, 1917: Herrin, Illinois*
An explosion in the number two shaft of the Rend coal mine killed nine
  people.

CDC and NIOSH Safety and Health Research. *Coal Mining Disasters.* Available at:
http://www.cdc.gov/niosh/mining/statistics/discoal.htm. Accessed September 21, 2005.

*April 27, 1917: Hastings, Colorado*
An explosion at the Hastings coal mine killed 121 people.

CDC and NIOSH Safety and Health Research. *Coal Mining Disasters*. Available at: http://www.cdc.gov/niosh/mining/statistics/discoal.htm. Accessed September 21, 2005.

### March 13, 1917: Henderson, Pennsylvania

An explosion in the number one shaft of the Hendersonville coal mine killed 14 people.

CDC and NIOSH Safety and Health Research. *Coal Mining Disasters*. Available at: http://www.cdc.gov/niosh/mining/statistics/discoal.htm. Accessed September 21, 2005.

### December 13, 1916: Stone City, Kansas

An explosion in the number nine shaft of the Fidelity coal mine killed 20 people.

CDC and NIOSH Safety and Health Research. *Coal Mining Disasters*. Available at: http://www.cdc.gov/niosh/mining/statistics/discoal.htm. Accessed September 21, 2005.

### November 4, 1916: Palos, Alabama

An explosion at the Bessie coal mine killed 30 people.

CDC and NIOSH Safety and Health Research. *Coal Mining Disasters*. Available at: http://www.cdc.gov/niosh/mining/statistics/discoal.htm. Accessed September 21, 2005.

### October 22, 1916: Marvel, Alabama

An explosion at the Roden coal mine killed 18 people.

CDC and NIOSH Safety and Health Research. *Coal Mining Disasters*. Available at: http://www.cdc.gov/niosh/mining/statistics/discoal.htm. Accessed September 21, 2005.

### October 19, 1916: Barrackville, West Virginia

An explosion in the number seven shaft of the Jamison coal mine killed 11 people.

CDC and NIOSH Safety and Health Research. *Coal Mining Disasters*. Available at: http://www.cdc.gov/niosh/mining/statistics/discoal.htm. Accessed September 21, 2005.

### August 8, 1916: Wilkes-Barre, Pennsylvania

An explosion at the Woodward coal mine killed six people.

CDC and NIOSH Safety and Health Research. *Coal Mining Disasters*. Available at: http://www.cdc.gov/niosh/mining/statistics/discoal.htm. Accessed September 21, 2005.

### March 30, 1916: Seward, Pennsylvania

An explosion at the Robindale coal mine killed eight people.

CDC and NIOSH Safety and Health Research. *Coal Mining Disasters*. Available at: http://www.cdc.gov/niosh/mining/statistics/discoal.htm. Accessed September 21, 2005.

### March 28, 1916: Kimball, West Virginia

An explosion at the King coal mine killed ten people.

CDC and NIOSH Safety and Health Research. *Coal Mining Disasters.* Available at: http://www.cdc.gov/niosh/mining/statistics/discoal.htm. Accessed September 21, 2005.

### March 9, 1916: Wilkes-Barre, Pennsylvania

An explosion at the Hollenback coal mine killed six people.

CDC and NIOSH Safety and Health Research. *Coal Mining Disasters.* Available at: http://www.cdc.gov/niosh/mining/statistics/discoal.htm. Accessed September 21, 2005.

### February 29, 1916: Kempton, Maryland

An explosion in the #42 shaft of the David coal mine killed 16 people.

CDC and NIOSH Safety and Health Research. *Coal Mining Disasters.* Available at: http://www.cdc.gov/niosh/mining/statistics/discoal.htm. Accessed September 21, 2005.

### February 11, 1916: Ernest, Pennsylvania

An explosion in the number two shaft of the Ernest coal mine killed 27 people.

CDC and NIOSH Safety and Health Research. *Coal Mining Disasters.* Available at: http://www.cdc.gov/niosh/mining/statistics/discoal.htm. Accessed September 21, 2005.

### February 8, 1916: Plymouth, Pennsylvania

An explosion at the Lance coal mine killed seven people.

CDC and NIOSH Safety and Health Research. *Coal Mining Disasters.* Available at: http://www.cdc.gov/niosh/mining/statistics/discoal.htm. Accessed September 21, 2005.

### November 30, 1915: Boomer, West Virginia

An explosion in the number two shaft of the Boomer coal mine killed 23 people.

CDC and NIOSH Safety and Health Research. *Coal Mining Disasters.* Available at: http://www.cdc.gov/niosh/mining/statistics/discoal.htm. Accessed September 21, 2005.

### November 16, 1915: Ravensdale, Washington

An explosion at the Northwestern coal mine killed 31 people.

CDC and NIOSH Safety and Health Research. *Coal Mining Disasters.* Available at: http://www.cdc.gov/niosh/mining/statistics/discoal.htm. Accessed September 21, 2005.

### August 31, 1915: Boswell, Pennsylvania

An explosion at the Orenda coal mine killed 19 people.

CDC and NIOSH Safety and Health Research. *Coal Mining Disasters.* Available at: http://www.cdc.gov/niosh/mining/statistics/discoal.htm. Accessed September 21, 2005.

### July 27, 1915: Christopher, Illinois

An explosion in the number one shaft of the United Coal mine killed nine people.

CDC and NIOSH Safety and Health Research. *Coal Mining Disasters*. Available at: http://www.cdc.gov/niosh/mining/statistics/discoal.htm. Accessed September 21, 2005.

### May 24, 1915: Johnstown, Pennsylvania

An explosion in the number one shaft of the Smokeless Valley coal mine killed nine people.

CDC and NIOSH Safety and Health Research. *Coal Mining Disasters*. Available at: http://www.cdc.gov/niosh/mining/statistics/discoal.htm. Accessed September 21, 2005.

### April 5, 1915: Panama, Illinois

An explosion at the Shoal Creek coal mine killed 11 people.

CDC and NIOSH Safety and Health Research. *Coal Mining Disasters*. Available at: http://www.cdc.gov/niosh/mining/statistics/discoal.htm. Accessed September 21, 2005.

### March 2, 1915: Layland, West Virginia

An explosion in the number three shaft at the Layland coal mine killed 115 people.

CDC and NIOSH Safety and Health Research. *Coal Mining Disasters*. Available at: http://www.cdc.gov/niosh/mining/statistics/discoal.htm. Accessed September 21, 2005.

### February 18, 1915: Rich Hill, Missouri

An explosion in the number two shaft at the New Home coal mine killed five people.

CDC and NIOSH Safety and Health Research. *Coal Mining Disasters*. Available at: http://www.cdc.gov/niosh/mining/statistics/discoal.htm. Accessed September 21, 2005.

### February 17, 1915: Wilkes-Barre, Pennsylvania

An explosion at the Prospect coal mine killed 13 people.

CDC and NIOSH Safety and Health Research. *Coal Mining Disasters*. Available at: http://www.cdc.gov/niosh/mining/statistics/discoal.htm. Accessed September 21, 2005.

### February 6, 1915: Carlisle, West Virginia

An explosion at the Carlisle coal mine killed 21 people.

CDC and NIOSH Safety and Health Research. *Coal Mining Disasters*. Available at: http://www.cdc.gov/niosh/mining/statistics/discoal.htm. Accessed September 21, 2005.

### October 5, 1914: Mulga, Alabama
An explosion in the Mulga coal mine killed 16 people.

CDC and NIOSH Safety and Health Research. *Coal Mining Disasters.* Available at:
http://www.cdc.gov/niosh/mining/statistics/discoal.htm. Accessed September 21, 2005.

### September 16, 1914: Lansford, Pennsylvania
An explosion in the number four shaft of the Lehigh coal mine killed seven people.

CDC and NIOSH Safety and Health Research. *Coal Mining Disasters.* Available at:
http://www.cdc.gov/niosh/mining/statistics/discoal.htm. Accessed September 21, 2005.

### April 28, 1914: Eccles, West Virginia
Explosions in the number five and six shafts of the Eccles coal mine killed 181
   people.

CDC and NIOSH Safety and Health Research. *Coal Mining Disasters.* Available at:
http://www.cdc.gov/niosh/mining/statistics/discoal.htm. Accessed September 21, 2005.

### January 10, 1914: Rock Castle, Alabama
An explosion at the Rock Castle coal mine killed 12 people.

CDC and NIOSH Safety and Health Research. *Coal Mining Disasters.* Available at:
http://www.cdc.gov/niosh/mining/statistics/discoal.htm. Accessed September 21, 2005.

### December 16, 1913: New Castle, Colorado
An explosion at the Vulcan coal mine killed 37 people.

CDC and NIOSH Safety and Health Research. *Coal Mining Disasters.* Available at:
http://www.cdc.gov/niosh/mining/statistics/discoal.htm. Accessed September 21, 2005.

### November 18, 1913: Acton, Alabama
An explosion in the number two shaft of the Acton coal mine killed 24 people.

CDC and NIOSH Safety and Health Research. *Coal Mining Disasters.* Available at:
http://www.cdc.gov/niosh/mining/statistics/discoal.htm. Accessed September 21, 2005.

### October 22, 1913: Dawson, New Mexico
A coal mine explosion killed 263 people in the number two shaft of the Stag
   Canon.

CDC and NIOSH Safety and Health Research. *Coal Mining Disasters.* Available at:
http://www.cdc.gov/niosh/mining/statistics/discoal.htm. Accessed September 21, 2005.

### August 2, 1913: Tower City, Pennsylvania
An explosion at the East Brookside coal mine killed 20 people.

CDC and NIOSH Safety and Health Research. *Coal Mining Disasters.* Available at:
http://www.cdc.gov/niosh/mining/statistics/discoal.htm. Accessed September 21, 2005.

### May 17, 1913: Belle Valley, Ohio
An explosion at the Noble coal mine killed 15 people.

CDC and NIOSH Safety and Health Research. *Coal Mining Disasters.* Available at: http://www.cdc.gov/niosh/mining/statistics/discoal.htm. Accessed September 21, 2005.

### April 23, 1913: Finleyville, Pennsylvania
An explosion in the Cincinnati coal mine killed 98 people.

CDC and NIOSH Safety and Health Research. *Coal Mining Disasters.* Available at: http://www.cdc.gov/niosh/mining/statistics/discoal.htm. Accessed September 21, 2005.

### February 19, 1913: El Dorado, Illinois
An explosion in the Seagraves coal mine killed five people.

CDC and NIOSH Safety and Health Research. *Coal Mining Disasters.* Available at: http://www.cdc.gov/niosh/mining/statistics/discoal.htm. Accessed September 21, 2005.

### August 13, 1912: Abernaut, Alabama
An explosion in the Abernaut coal mine killed 18 people.

CDC and NIOSH Safety and Health Research. *Coal Mining Disasters.* Available at: http://www.cdc.gov/niosh/mining/statistics/discoal.htm. Accessed September 21, 2005.

### July 16, 1912: Gayton, Virginia
An explosion in the Carbon Hill coal mine killed eight people.

CDC and NIOSH Safety and Health Research. *Coal Mining Disasters.* Available at: http://www.cdc.gov/niosh/mining/statistics/discoal.htm. Accessed September 21, 2005.

### July 11, 1912: Moundsville, West Virginia
An explosion in the Panama coal mine killed eight people.

CDC and NIOSH Safety and Health Research. *Coal Mining Disasters.* Available at: http://www.cdc.gov/niosh/mining/statistics/discoal.htm. Accessed September 21, 2005.

### June 18, 1912: Hastings, Colorado
An explosion in the Hastings coal mine killed 12 people.

CDC and NIOSH Safety and Health Research. *Coal Mining Disasters.* Available at: http://www.cdc.gov/niosh/mining/statistics/discoal.htm. Accessed September 21, 2005.

### April 21, 1912: Madisonville, Kentucky
An explosion in the Coil coal mine killed five people.

CDC and NIOSH Safety and Health Research. *Coal Mining Disasters.* Available at: http://www.cdc.gov/niosh/mining/statistics/discoal.htm. Accessed September 21, 2005.

### March 26, 1912: Jed, West Virginia

An explosion in the Jed coal mine killed 81 people.

CDC and NIOSH Safety and Health Research. *Coal Mining Disasters.* Available at: http://www.cdc.gov/niosh/mining/statistics/discoal.htm. Accessed September 21, 2005.

### March 20, 1912: McCurtain, Oklahoma

An explosion in the number two shaft of the San Bois coal mine killed 73 people.

CDC and NIOSH Safety and Health Research. *Coal Mining Disasters.* Available at: http://www.cdc.gov/niosh/mining/statistics/discoal.htm. Accessed September 21, 2005.

### January 20, 1912: Kemmerer, Wyoming

An explosion in the number four shaft at the Kemmerer coal mine killed six people.

CDC and NIOSH Safety and Health Research. *Coal Mining Disasters.* Available at: http://www.cdc.gov/niosh/mining/statistics/discoal.htm. Accessed September 21, 2005.

### January 19, 1912: Central City, Kentucky

An explosion at the Central coal mine killed five people.

CDC and NIOSH Safety and Health Research. *Coal Mining Disasters.* Available at: http://www.cdc.gov/niosh/mining/statistics/discoal.htm. Accessed September 21, 2005.

### January 16, 1912: Carbon Hill, Virginia

An explosion at the Carbon Hill coal mine killed five people.

CDC and NIOSH Safety and Health Research. *Coal Mining Disasters.* Available at: http://www.cdc.gov/niosh/mining/statistics/discoal.htm. Accessed September 21, 2005.

### January 9, 1912: Plymouth, Pennsylvania

An explosion at the Parrish coal mine killed six people.

CDC and NIOSH Safety and Health Research. *Coal Mining Disasters.* Available at: http://www.cdc.gov/niosh/mining/statistics/discoal.htm. Accessed September 21, 2005.

### December 9, 1911: Briceville, Tennessee

An explosion at the Cross Mountain coal mine killed 84 people.

CDC and NIOSH Safety and Health Research. *Coal Mining Disasters.* Available at: http://www.cdc.gov/niosh/mining/statistics/discoal.htm. Accessed September 21, 2005.

### November 18, 1911: Vivian, West Virginia

An explosion at the Bottom Creek coal mine killed 18 people.

CDC and NIOSH Safety and Health Research. *Coal Mining Disasters.* Available at: http://www.cdc.gov/niosh/mining/statistics/discoal.htm. Accessed September 21, 2005.

### November 9, 1911: Punxatawny, Pennsylvania
An explosion at the Adrian coal mine killed eight people.

CDC and NIOSH Safety and Health Research. *Coal Mining Disasters.* Available at: http://www.cdc.gov/niosh/mining/statistics/discoal.htm. Accessed September 21, 2005.

### October 23, 1911: Harrisburg, Illinois
An explosion in the number nine shaft at the O'Gara coal mine killed eight people.

CDC and NIOSH Safety and Health Research. *Coal Mining Disasters.* Available at: http://www.cdc.gov/niosh/mining/statistics/discoal.htm. Accessed September 21, 2005.

### August 1, 1911: Welch, West Virginia
An explosion at the Standard coal mine killed six people.

CDC and NIOSH Safety and Health Research. *Coal Mining Disasters.* Available at: http://www.cdc.gov/niosh/mining/statistics/discoal.htm. Accessed September 21, 2005.

### July 15, 1911: Sykesville, Pennsylvania
An explosion at the Sykesville coal mine killed 21 people.

CDC and NIOSH Safety and Health Research. *Coal Mining Disasters.* Available at: http://www.cdc.gov/niosh/mining/statistics/discoal.htm. Accessed September 21, 2005.

### May 27, 1911: Shamokin, Pennsylvania
An explosion at the Cameron coal mine killed five people.

CDC and NIOSH Safety and Health Research. *Coal Mining Disasters.* Available at: http://www.cdc.gov/niosh/mining/statistics/discoal.htm. Accessed September 21, 2005.

### April 24, 1911: Elk Garden, West Virginia
An explosion in the #20 shaft of the Ott coal mine killed 23 people.

CDC and NIOSH Safety and Health Research. *Coal Mining Disasters.* Available at: http://www.cdc.gov/niosh/mining/statistics/discoal.htm. Accessed September 21, 2005.

### April 8, 1911: Littleton, Alabama
An explosion at the Banner coal mine killed 128 people.

CDC and NIOSH Safety and Health Research. *Coal Mining Disasters.* Available at: http://www.cdc.gov/niosh/mining/statistics/discoal.htm. Accessed September 21, 2005.

### March 18, 1911: Mineral, Kansas
An explosion in the #16 shaft of a coal mine in Mineral killed five people.

CDC and NIOSH Safety and Health Research. *Coal Mining Disasters.* Available at: http://www.cdc.gov/niosh/mining/statistics/discoal.htm. Accessed September 21, 2005.

### February 9, 1911: Trinidad, Colorado

An explosion at the Cokedale coal mine killed 17 people.

CDC and NIOSH Safety and Health Research. *Coal Mining Disasters.* Available at: http://www.cdc.gov/niosh/mining/statistics/discoal.htm. Accessed September 21, 2005.

### January 20, 1911: Carbon Hill, Virginia

An explosion at the Carbon Hill coal mine killed seven people.

CDC and NIOSH Safety and Health Research. *Coal Mining Disasters.* Available at: http://www.cdc.gov/niosh/mining/statistics/discoal.htm. Accessed September 21, 2005.

### December 14, 1910: Tacoma, Virginia

An explosion at the Greenco coal mine killed eight people.

CDC and NIOSH Safety and Health Research. *Coal Mining Disasters.* Available at: http://www.cdc.gov/niosh/mining/statistics/discoal.htm. Accessed September 21, 2005.

### November 25, 1910: Providence, Kentucky

An explosion in the number three shaft of the Providence coal mine killed ten people.

CDC and NIOSH Safety and Health Research. *Coal Mining Disasters.* Available at: http://www.cdc.gov/niosh/mining/statistics/discoal.htm. Accessed September 21, 2005.

### November 11, 1910: Panama, Illinois

An explosion in the number one shaft of the Shoal Creek coal mine killed six people.

CDC and NIOSH Safety and Health Research. *Coal Mining Disasters.* Available at: http://www.cdc.gov/niosh/mining/statistics/discoal.htm. Accessed September 21, 2005.

### November 8, 1910: Delagua, Colorado

An explosion in the number three shaft of the Victor American coal mine killed 79 people.

CDC and NIOSH Safety and Health Research. *Coal Mining Disasters.* Available at: http://www.cdc.gov/niosh/mining/statistics/discoal.htm. Accessed September 21, 2005.

### November 6, 1910: Black Diamond, Washington

An explosion at the Lawson coal mine killed 16 people.

CDC and NIOSH Safety and Health Research. *Coal Mining Disasters.* Available at: http://www.cdc.gov/niosh/mining/statistics/discoal.htm. Accessed September 21, 2005.

### November 3, 1910: Yolande, Alabama

An explosion in the number one shaft of the Yolande coal mine killed five people.

CDC and NIOSH Safety and Health Research. *Coal Mining Disasters.* Available at: http://www.cdc.gov/niosh/mining/statistics/discoal.htm. Accessed September 21, 2005.

### October 8, 1910: Starksville, Colorado
An explosion at the Starksville coal mine killed 56 people.

CDC and NIOSH Safety and Health Research. *Coal Mining Disasters.* Available at: http://www.cdc.gov/niosh/mining/statistics/discoal.htm. Accessed September 21, 2005.

### May 5, 1910: Palos, Alabama
An explosion in the number three shaft at the Palos coal mine killed 84 people.

CDC and NIOSH Safety and Health Research. *Coal Mining Disasters.* Available at: http://www.cdc.gov/niosh/mining/statistics/discoal.htm. Accessed September 21, 2005.

### April 21, 1910: Amsterdam, Ohio
An explosion at the Amsterdam coal mine killed 15 people.

CDC and NIOSH Safety and Health Research. *Coal Mining Disasters.* Available at: http://www.cdc.gov/niosh/mining/statistics/discoal.htm. Accessed September 21, 2005.

### April 20, 1910: Mulga, Alabama
An explosion at the Mulga coal mine killed 40 people.

CDC and NIOSH Safety and Health Research. *Coal Mining Disasters.* Available at: http://www.cdc.gov/niosh/mining/statistics/discoal.htm. Accessed September 21, 2005.

### March 31, 1910: Wilburton, Oklahoma
An explosion in the number two shaft at the Great Western coal mine killed six people.

CDC and NIOSH Safety and Health Research. *Coal Mining Disasters.* Available at: http://www.cdc.gov/niosh/mining/statistics/discoal.htm. Accessed September 21, 2005.

### March 12, 1910: South Wilkes-Barre, Pennsylvania
An explosion at the South Wilkes-Barre coal mine killed seven people.

CDC and NIOSH Safety and Health Research. *Coal Mining Disasters.* Available at: http://www.cdc.gov/niosh/mining/statistics/discoal.htm. Accessed September 21, 2005.

### February 8, 1910: Stearns, Kentucky
An explosion in the number one shaft of the Barthell coal mine killed six people.

CDC and NIOSH Safety and Health Research. *Coal Mining Disasters.* Available at: http://www.cdc.gov/niosh/mining/statistics/discoal.htm. Accessed September 21, 2005.

### February 5, 1910: Ernest, Pennsylvania
An explosion in the number two shaft of the Ernest coal mine killed 12 people.

CDC and NIOSH Safety and Health Research. *Coal Mining Disasters*. Available at:
http://www.cdc.gov/niosh/mining/statistics/discoal.htm. Accessed September 21, 2005.

### February 1, 1910: Browder, Kentucky
An explosion at the Browder coal mine killed 34 people.

CDC and NIOSH Safety and Health Research. *Coal Mining Disasters*. Available at:
http://www.cdc.gov/niosh/mining/statistics/discoal.htm. Accessed September 21, 2005.

### January 31, 1910: Primero, Colorado
An explosion at the Primero coal mine killed 75 people.

CDC and NIOSH Safety and Health Research. *Coal Mining Disasters*. Available at:
http://www.cdc.gov/niosh/mining/statistics/discoal.htm. Accessed September 21, 2005.

### January 11, 1910: Plymouth, Pennsylvania
An explosion at the Nottingham coal mine killed seven people.

CDC and NIOSH Safety and Health Research. *Coal Mining Disasters*. Available at:
http://www.cdc.gov/niosh/mining/statistics/discoal.htm. Accessed September 21, 2005.

### 1909–1900
### December 23, 1909: Herrin, Illinois
An explosion at the Mine A colliery killed eight people.

CDC and NIOSH Safety and Health Research. *Coal Mining Disasters*. Available at:
http://www.cdc.gov/niosh/mining/statistics/discoal.htm. Accessed September 21, 2005.

### December 11, 1909: Clay, Kentucky
An explosion in the number five shaft of the Baker coal mine killed seven people.

CDC and NIOSH Safety and Health Research. *Coal Mining Disasters*. Available at:
http://www.cdc.gov/niosh/mining/statistics/discoal.htm. Accessed September 21, 2005.

### October 31, 1909: Johnstown, Pennsylvania
An explosion in the number two shaft of the Franklin coal mine killed 13 people.

CDC and NIOSH Safety and Health Research. *Coal Mining Disasters*. Available at:
http://www.cdc.gov/niosh/mining/statistics/discoal.htm. Accessed September 21, 2005.

### October 21, 1909: Hartshorne, Oklahoma
An explosion in the number eight shaft of the Rock Island coal mine killed ten
   people.

CDC and NIOSH Safety and Health Research. *Coal Mining Disasters*. Available at:
http://www.cdc.gov/niosh/mining/statistics/discoal.htm. Accessed September 21, 2005.

### October 3, 1909: Roslyn, Washington

An explosion at the Northwestern coal mine killed ten people.

CDC and NIOSH Safety and Health Research. *Coal Mining Disasters.* Available at: http://www.cdc.gov/niosh/mining/statistics/discoal.htm. Accessed September 21, 2005.

### July 6, 1909: Tollerville, Colorado

An explosion at the Toller coal mine killed nine people.

CDC and NIOSH Safety and Health Research. *Coal Mining Disasters.* Available at: http://www.cdc.gov/niosh/mining/statistics/discoal.htm. Accessed September 21, 2005.

### June 23, 1909: Wehrun, Pennsylvania

An explosion in the number four shaft of the Lackawanna coal mine killed 21 people.

CDC and NIOSH Safety and Health Research. *Coal Mining Disasters.* Available at: http://www.cdc.gov/niosh/mining/statistics/discoal.htm. Accessed September 21, 2005.

### April 9, 1909: Wimber, Pennsylvania

An explosion in the #37 mine shaft of the Eureka coal mine killed seven people.

CDC and NIOSH Safety and Health Research. *Coal Mining Disasters.* Available at: http://www.cdc.gov/niosh/mining/statistics/discoal.htm. Accessed September 21, 2005.

### March 31, 1909: Buery, West Virginia

An explosion at the Echo coal mine killed six people.

CDC and NIOSH Safety and Health Research. *Coal Mining Disasters.* Available at: http://www.cdc.gov/niosh/mining/statistics/discoal.htm. Accessed September 21, 2005.

### March 20, 1909: Evansville, Indiana

An explosion at the Sunnyside coal mine killed six people.

CDC and NIOSH Safety and Health Research. *Coal Mining Disasters.* Available at: http://www.cdc.gov/niosh/mining/statistics/discoal.htm. Accessed September 21, 2005.

### March 2, 1909: Pittston, Pennsylvania

An explosion in the #14 shaft of a coal mine in Pittston killed eight people.

CDC and NIOSH Safety and Health Research. *Coal Mining Disasters.* Available at: http://www.cdc.gov/niosh/mining/statistics/discoal.htm. Accessed September 21, 2005.

### February 2, 1909: Short Creek, Alabama

An explosion at the Short Creek coal mine killed 18 people.

CDC and NIOSH Safety and Health Research. *Coal Mining Disasters.* Available at: http://www.cdc.gov/niosh/mining/statistics/discoal.htm. Accessed September 21, 2005.

### January 25, 1909: Boswell, Pennsylvania

An explosion in the number two shaft of the Orenda coal mine killed five people.

CDC and NIOSH Safety and Health Research. *Coal Mining Disasters.* Available at: http://www.cdc.gov/niosh/mining/statistics/discoal.htm. Accessed September 21, 2005.

### January 19, 1909: Chancellor, California

An explosion at the Stone Canyon coal mine killed six people.

CDC and NIOSH Safety and Health Research. *Coal Mining Disasters.* Available at: http://www.cdc.gov/niosh/mining/statistics/discoal.htm. Accessed September 21, 2005.

### January 12, 1909: Switchback, West Virginia

An explosion at the Lick Branch coal mine killed 67 people.

CDC and NIOSH Safety and Health Research. *Coal Mining Disasters.* Available at: http://www.cdc.gov/niosh/mining/statistics/discoal.htm. Accessed September 21, 2005.

### January 10, 1909: Gayton, Virginia

An explosion at the Carbon Hill coal mine killed six people.

CDC and NIOSH Safety and Health Research. *Coal Mining Disasters.* Available at: http://www.cdc.gov/niosh/mining/statistics/discoal.htm. Accessed September 21, 2005.

### January 10, 1909: Zeigler, Illinois

An explosion at the Zeigler coal mine killed 26 people.

CDC and NIOSH Safety and Health Research. *Coal Mining Disasters.* Available at: http://www.cdc.gov/niosh/mining/statistics/discoal.htm. Accessed September 21, 2005.

### December 29, 1908: Switchback, West Virginia

An explosion at the Lick Branch coal mine killed 50 people.

CDC and NIOSH Safety and Health Research. *Coal Mining Disasters.* Available at: http://www.cdc.gov/niosh/mining/statistics/discoal.htm. Accessed September 21, 2005.

### November 28, 1908: Marianna, Pennsylvania

An explosion at the Rachel & Agnes coal mine killed 154 people.

CDC and NIOSH Safety and Health Research. *Coal Mining Disasters.* Available at: http://www.cdc.gov/niosh/mining/statistics/discoal.htm. Accessed September 21, 2005.

### July 15, 1908: Williamstown, Pennsylvania

An explosion at the Williamstown coal mine killed six people.

CDC and NIOSH Safety and Health Research. *Coal Mining Disasters.* Available at: http://www.cdc.gov/niosh/mining/statistics/discoal.htm. Accessed September 21, 2005.

### May 12, 1908: Wyoming, Pennsylvania
An explosion at the Mount Lookout coal mine killed 12 people.

CDC and NIOSH Safety and Health Research. *Coal Mining Disasters.* Available at: http://www.cdc.gov/niosh/mining/statistics/discoal.htm. Accessed September 21, 2005.

### March 28, 1908: Hanna, Wyoming
An explosion in the number one shaft of the Hanna coal mine killed 59 people.

CDC and NIOSH Safety and Health Research. *Coal Mining Disasters.* Available at: http://www.cdc.gov/niosh/mining/statistics/discoal.htm. Accessed September 21, 2005.

### February 10, 1908: South Carrollton, Kentucky
An explosion at the Moody coal mine killed nine people.

CDC and NIOSH Safety and Health Research. *Coal Mining Disasters.* Available at: http://www.cdc.gov/niosh/mining/statistics/discoal.htm. Accessed September 21, 2005.

### January 30, 1908: Hawk's Nest, West Virginia
An explosion at the Backman coal mine killed nine people.

CDC and NIOSH Safety and Health Research. *Coal Mining Disasters.* Available at: http://www.cdc.gov/niosh/mining/statistics/discoal.htm. Accessed September 21, 2005.

### December 31, 1907: Carthage, New Mexico
An explosion at the Bernal coal mine killed 11 people.

CDC and NIOSH Safety and Health Research. *Coal Mining Disasters.* Available at: http://www.cdc.gov/niosh/mining/statistics/discoal.htm. Accessed September 21, 2005.

### December 19, 1907: Jacobs Creek, Pennsylvania
A gas explosion at the Darr coal mine killed 239 people.

CDC and NIOSH Safety and Health Research. *Coal Mining Disasters.* Available at: http://www.cdc.gov/niosh/mining/statistics/discoal.htm. Accessed September 21, 2005.

### December 16, 1907: Yolande, Alabama
An explosion at the Yolande coal mine killed 57 people.

CDC and NIOSH Safety and Health Research. *Coal Mining Disasters.* Available at: http://www.cdc.gov/niosh/mining/statistics/discoal.htm. Accessed September 21, 2005.

### December 6, 1907: Monongha, West Virginia
An explosion in the Monongha mine killed 361 people.

National Fire Protection Association. *The 20 Deadliest Fires and Explosions in U.S. History.* Available at: http://www.nfpa.org/itemDetail.asp?categoryID=954&itemID= 23340&URL=Research%20&%20Reports/Fire%20statistics/Historical

### December 1, 1907: Fayette City, Pennsylvania
An explosion at the Naomi coal mine killed 34 people.

CDC and NIOSH Safety and Health Research. *Coal Mining Disasters.* Available at:
http://www.cdc.gov/niosh/mining/statistics/discoal.htm. Accessed September 21, 2005.

### June 18, 1907: Priceburg, Pennsylvania
An explosion in the number one shaft of the Johnson coal mine killed seven
    people.

CDC and NIOSH Safety and Health Research. *Coal Mining Disasters.* Available at:
http://www.cdc.gov/niosh/mining/statistics/discoal.htm. Accessed September 21, 2005.

### May 1, 1907: Scarbro, West Virginia
An explosion at the Whipple coal mine killed 16 people.

CDC and NIOSH Safety and Health Research. *Coal Mining Disasters.* Available at:
http://www.cdc.gov/niosh/mining/statistics/discoal.htm. Accessed September 21, 2005.

### April 26, 1907: Black Diamond, Washington
An explosion at the Morgan coal mine killed seven people.

CDC and NIOSH Safety and Health Research. *Coal Mining Disasters.* Available at:
http://www.cdc.gov/niosh/mining/statistics/discoal.htm. Accessed September 21, 2005.

### March 16, 1907: Tacoma, Virginia
An explosion at the Bond & Bruce coal mine killed 11 people.

CDC and NIOSH Safety and Health Research. *Coal Mining Disasters.* Available at:
http://www.cdc.gov/niosh/mining/statistics/discoal.htm. Accessed September 21, 2005.

### March 2, 1907: Taylor, Pennsylvania
An explosion at the Holden coal mine killed seven people.

CDC and NIOSH Safety and Health Research. *Coal Mining Disasters.* Available at:
http://www.cdc.gov/niosh/mining/statistics/discoal.htm. Accessed September 21, 2005.

### February 4, 1907: Thomas, West Virginia
An explosion in the #25 shaft of the Thomas coal mine killed 25 people.

CDC and NIOSH Safety and Health Research. *Coal Mining Disasters.* Available at:
http://www.cdc.gov/niosh/mining/statistics/discoal.htm. Accessed September 21, 2005.

### January 29, 1907: Stuart, West Virginia
An explosion at the Stuart coal mine killed 84 people.

CDC and NIOSH Safety and Health Research. *Coal Mining Disasters.* Available at:
http://www.cdc.gov/niosh/mining/statistics/discoal.htm. Accessed September 21, 2005.

### January 26, 1907: Penco, West Virginia
An explosion at the Lorentz coal mine killed 12 people.

CDC and NIOSH Safety and Health Research. *Coal Mining Disasters.* Available at: http://www.cdc.gov/niosh/mining/statistics/discoal.htm. Accessed September 21, 2005.

### January 23, 1907: Primero, Colorado
An explosion at the Primero coal mine killed 24 people.

CDC and NIOSH Safety and Health Research. *Coal Mining Disasters.* Available at: http://www.cdc.gov/niosh/mining/statistics/discoal.htm. Accessed September 21, 2005.

### January 14, 1907: Clinton, Indiana
An explosion in the number seven shaft of the Deering coal mine killed seven people.

CDC and NIOSH Safety and Health Research. *Coal Mining Disasters.* Available at: http://www.cdc.gov/niosh/mining/statistics/discoal.htm. Accessed September 21, 2005.

### October 24, 1906: Johnstown, Pennsylvania
An explosion at the Rolling Mill coal mine killed seven people.

CDC and NIOSH Safety and Health Research. *Coal Mining Disasters.* Available at: http://www.cdc.gov/niosh/mining/statistics/discoal.htm. Accessed September 21, 2005.

### October 5, 1906: Blossburg, New Mexico
An explosion at the Dutchman coal mine killed ten people.

CDC and NIOSH Safety and Health Research. *Coal Mining Disasters.* Available at: http://www.cdc.gov/niosh/mining/statistics/discoal.htm. Accessed September 21, 2005.

### October 3, 1906: Pocahontas, Virginia
An explosion at the Pocahontas coal mine killed 36 people.

CDC and NIOSH Safety and Health Research. *Coal Mining Disasters.* Available at: http://www.cdc.gov/niosh/mining/statistics/discoal.htm. Accessed September 21, 2005.

### August 6, 1906: Nanticoke, Pennsylvania
An explosion in the number seven shaft of the Susquehanna coal mine killed six people.

CDC and NIOSH Safety and Health Research. *Coal Mining Disasters.* Available at: http://www.cdc.gov/niosh/mining/statistics/discoal.htm. Accessed September 21, 2005.

### April 22, 1906: Tercio, Colorado
An explosion at the Cuatro coal mine killed 18 people.

CDC and NIOSH Safety and Health Research. *Coal Mining Disasters.* Available at: http://www.cdc.gov/niosh/mining/statistics/discoal.htm. Accessed September 21, 2005.

### March 22, 1906: Century, West Virginia
An explosion in the number one shaft of the Century coal mine killed 23 people.

CDC and NIOSH Safety and Health Research. *Coal Mining Disasters.* Available at: http://www.cdc.gov/niosh/mining/statistics/discoal.htm. Accessed September 21, 2005.

### February 27, 1906: Piper, Alabama
An explosion at the Little Cahaba coal mine killed 12 people.

CDC and NIOSH Safety and Health Research. *Coal Mining Disasters.* Available at: http://www.cdc.gov/niosh/mining/statistics/discoal.htm. Accessed September 21, 2005.

### February 19, 1906: Walsenburg, Colorado
An explosion at the Maitland coal mine killed 14 people.

CDC and NIOSH Safety and Health Research. *Coal Mining Disasters.* Available at: http://www.cdc.gov/niosh/mining/statistics/discoal.htm. Accessed September 21, 2005.

### February 8, 1906: Parral, West Virginia
An explosion at the Parral coal mine killed 23 people.

CDC and NIOSH Safety and Health Research. *Coal Mining Disasters.* Available at: http://www.cdc.gov/niosh/mining/statistics/discoal.htm. Accessed September 21, 2005.

### January 24, 1906: Witteville, Oklahoma
An explosion in the number six shaft of the Poteau coal mine killed 14 people.

CDC and NIOSH Safety and Health Research. *Coal Mining Disasters.* Available at: http://www.cdc.gov/niosh/mining/statistics/discoal.htm. Accessed September 21, 2005.

### January 18, 1906: Detroit, West Virginia
An explosion at the Detroit coal mine killed 18 people.

CDC and NIOSH Safety and Health Research. *Coal Mining Disasters.* Available at: http://www.cdc.gov/niosh/mining/statistics/discoal.htm. Accessed September 21, 2005.

### January 4, 1906: Coaldale, West Virginia
An explosion at the Coaldale colliery killed 22 people.

CDC and NIOSH Safety and Health Research. *Coal Mining Disasters.* Available at: http://www.cdc.gov/niosh/mining/statistics/discoal.htm. Accessed September 21, 2005.

### December 2, 1905: Diamondville, Wyoming
An explosion in the number one shaft of the Diamondville coal mine killed 18 people.

CDC and NIOSH Safety and Health Research. *Coal Mining Disasters.* Available at: http://www.cdc.gov/niosh/mining/statistics/discoal.htm. Accessed September 21, 2005.

### November 15, 1905: Bentleyville, Pennsylvania
An explosion at the Braznell coal mine killed seven people.

CDC and NIOSH Safety and Health Research. *Coal Mining Disasters.* Available at:
http://www.cdc.gov/niosh/mining/statistics/discoal.htm. Accessed September 21, 2005.

### November 4, 1905: Vivian, West Virginia
An explosion at the Tidewater coal mine killed seven people.

CDC and NIOSH Safety and Health Research. *Coal Mining Disasters.* Available at:
http://www.cdc.gov/niosh/mining/statistics/discoal.htm. Accessed September 21, 2005.

### October 29, 1905: Monongahela, Pennsylvania
An explosion in the number two shaft at the Hazel Kirk coal mine killed five
    people.

CDC and NIOSH Safety and Health Research. *Coal Mining Disasters.* Available at:
http://www.cdc.gov/niosh/mining/statistics/discoal.htm. Accessed September 21, 2005.

### July 6, 1905: Searight, Pennsylvania
An explosion at the Fuller coal mine killed six people.

CDC and NIOSH Safety and Health Research. *Coal Mining Disasters.* Available at:
http://www.cdc.gov/niosh/mining/statistics/discoal.htm. Accessed September 21, 2005.

### July 5, 1905: Vivian, West Virginia
An explosion at the Tidewater coal mine killed five people.

CDC and NIOSH Safety and Health Research. *Coal Mining Disasters.* Available at:
http://www.cdc.gov/niosh/mining/statistics/discoal.htm. Accessed September 21, 2005.

### April 30, 1905: Wilburton, Oklahoma
An explosion in the #19 shaft of a coal mine in Wilburton killed 13 people.

CDC and NIOSH Safety and Health Research. *Coal Mining Disasters.* Available at:
http://www.cdc.gov/niosh/mining/statistics/discoal.htm. Accessed September 21, 2005.

### April 27, 1905: Du Bois, Pennsylvania
An explosion at the Eleanora coal mine killed 13 people.

CDC and NIOSH Safety and Health Research. *Coal Mining Disasters.* Available at:
http://www.cdc.gov/niosh/mining/statistics/discoal.htm. Accessed September 21, 2005.

### April 20, 1905: Kayford, West Virginia
An explosion at the Cabin Creek coal mine killed six people.

CDC and NIOSH Safety and Health Research. *Coal Mining Disasters.* Available at:
http://www.cdc.gov/niosh/mining/statistics/discoal.htm. Accessed September 21, 2005.

**April 3, 1905: Zeigler, Illinois**

An explosion at the Zeigler coal mine killed 49 people.

CDC and NIOSH Safety and Health Research. *Coal Mining Disasters*. Available at:
http://www.cdc.gov/niosh/mining/statistics/discoal.htm. Accessed September 21, 2005.

**March 22, 1905: Princeton, Idaho**

An explosion at the Oswald coal mine killed nine people.

CDC and NIOSH Safety and Health Research. *Coal Mining Disasters*. Available at:
http://www.cdc.gov/niosh/mining/statistics/discoal.htm. Accessed September 21, 2005.

**March 18, 1905: Red Ash, West Virginia**

Multiple explosions at the Rush Run and Red Ash coal mines killed 24 people.

CDC and NIOSH Safety and Health Research. *Coal Mining Disasters*. Available at:
http://www.cdc.gov/niosh/mining/statistics/discoal.htm. Accessed September 21, 2005.

**February 26, 1905: Wilcoe, West Virginia**

An explosion at the Grapevine coal mine killed six people.

CDC and NIOSH Safety and Health Research. *Coal Mining Disasters*. Available at:
http://www.cdc.gov/niosh/mining/statistics/discoal.htm. Accessed September 21, 2005.

**February 20, 1905: Virginia City, Alabama**

An explosion at the Virginia City coal mine killed 112 people.

CDC and NIOSH Safety and Health Research. *Coal Mining Disasters*. Available at:
http://www.cdc.gov/niosh/mining/statistics/discoal.htm. Accessed September 21, 2005.

**December 7, 1904: Burnett, Washington**

An explosion in the number five shaft of a coal mine in Burnett killed 17 people.

CDC and NIOSH Safety and Health Research. *Coal Mining Disasters*. Available at:
http://www.cdc.gov/niosh/mining/statistics/discoal.htm. Accessed September 21, 2005.

**October 28, 1904: Terico, Colorado**

An explosion at the Terico coal mine killed 19 people.

CDC and NIOSH Safety and Health Research. *Coal Mining Disasters*. Available at:
http://www.cdc.gov/niosh/mining/statistics/discoal.htm. Accessed September 21, 2005.

**May 11, 1904: Herrin, Illinois**

An explosion at the Big Muddy coal mine killed ten people.

CDC and NIOSH Safety and Health Research. *Coal Mining Disasters*. Available at:
http://www.cdc.gov/niosh/mining/statistics/discoal.htm. Accessed September 21, 2005.

### April 20, 1904: Stearns, Kentucky
An explosion in the number five shaft of the Stearns coal mine killed five people.

CDC and NIOSH Safety and Health Research. *Coal Mining Disasters.* Available at: http://www.cdc.gov/niosh/mining/statistics/discoal.htm. Accessed September 21, 2005.

### January 25, 1904: Cheswick, Pennsylvania
An explosion at the Harwick coal mine killed 179 people.

CDC and NIOSH Safety and Health Research. *Coal Mining Disasters.* Available at: http://www.cdc.gov/niosh/mining/statistics/discoal.htm. Accessed September 21, 2005.

### November 21, 1903: Connellsville, Pennsylvania
An explosion at the Ferguson coal mine killed 17 people.

CDC and NIOSH Safety and Health Research. *Coal Mining Disasters.* Available at: http://www.cdc.gov/niosh/mining/statistics/discoal.htm. Accessed September 21, 2005.

### November 20, 1903: Bonanza, Arizona
An explosion in the #20 shaft at the Bonanza coal mine killed 11 people.

CDC and NIOSH Safety and Health Research. *Coal Mining Disasters.* Available at: http://www.cdc.gov/niosh/mining/statistics/discoal.htm. Accessed September 21, 2005.

### June 30, 1903: Hanna, Wyoming
An explosion in the number one shaft at the Hanna coal mine killed 169 people.

CDC and NIOSH Safety and Health Research. *Coal Mining Disasters.* Available at: http://www.cdc.gov/niosh/mining/statistics/discoal.htm. Accessed September 21, 2005.

### June 19, 1903: Bossburg, New Mexico
An explosion in the number three shaft at the Blassburg coal mine killed five people.

CDC and NIOSH Safety and Health Research. *Coal Mining Disasters.* Available at: http://www.cdc.gov/niosh/mining/statistics/discoal.htm. Accessed September 21, 2005.

### April 12, 1903: Carbon, Oklahoma
An explosion at the Central Slope 77 coal mine killed six people.

CDC and NIOSH Safety and Health Research. *Coal Mining Disasters.* Available at: http://www.cdc.gov/niosh/mining/statistics/discoal.htm. Accessed September 21, 2005.

### March 31, 1903: Sandoval, Illinois
An explosion at the Sandoval coal mine killed eight people.

CDC and NIOSH Safety and Health Research. *Coal Mining Disasters.* Available at: http://www.cdc.gov/niosh/mining/statistics/discoal.htm. Accessed September 21, 2005.

### March 23, 1903: Athens, Illinois
An explosion in the number two shaft of the Athens coal mine killed six people.

CDC and NIOSH Safety and Health Research. *Coal Mining Disasters.* Available at: http://www.cdc.gov/niosh/mining/statistics/discoal.htm. Accessed September 21, 2005.

### March 15, 1903: Cardiff, Illinois
An explosion at the Cardiff coal mine killed five people.

CDC and NIOSH Safety and Health Research. *Coal Mining Disasters.* Available at: http://www.cdc.gov/niosh/mining/statistics/discoal.htm. Accessed September 21, 2005.

### November 29, 1902: Shamokin, Pennsylvania
An explosion at the Luke Fidler coal mine killed seven people.

CDC and NIOSH Safety and Health Research. *Coal Mining Disasters.* Available at: http://www.cdc.gov/niosh/mining/statistics/discoal.htm. Accessed September 21, 2005.

### October 1, 1902: Black Diamond, Washington
An explosion at the Lawson coal mine killed 11 people.

CDC and NIOSH Safety and Health Research. *Coal Mining Disasters.* Available at: http://www.cdc.gov/niosh/mining/statistics/discoal.htm. Accessed September 21, 2005.

### September 22, 1902: Stafford, Washington
An explosion at the Stafford coal mine killed six people.

CDC and NIOSH Safety and Health Research. *Coal Mining Disasters.* Available at: http://www.cdc.gov/niosh/mining/statistics/discoal.htm. Accessed September 21, 2005.

### September 15, 1902: Algoma, West Virginia
An explosion in the number seven shaft of the Algoma coal mine killed 17 people.

CDC and NIOSH Safety and Health Research. *Coal Mining Disasters.* Available at: http://www.cdc.gov/niosh/mining/statistics/discoal.htm. Accessed September 21, 2005.

### August 7, 1902: Bowen, Colorado
An explosion at the Bowen coal mine killed 13 people.

CDC and NIOSH Safety and Health Research. *Coal Mining Disasters.* Available at: http://www.cdc.gov/niosh/mining/statistics/discoal.htm. Accessed September 21, 2005.

### July 10, 1902: Johnstown, Pennsylvania
An explosion at the Rolling Mill coal mine killed 112 people.

CDC and NIOSH Safety and Health Research. *Coal Mining Disasters.* Available at: http://www.cdc.gov/niosh/mining/statistics/discoal.htm. Accessed September 21, 2005.

### May 19, 1902: Coal Creek, Tennessee
An explosion at the Fraterville coal mine killed 184 people.

CDC and NIOSH Safety and Health Research. *Coal Mining Disasters*. Available at:
http://www.cdc.gov/niosh/mining/statistics/discoal.htm. Accessed September 21, 2005.

### March 31, 1902: Dayton, Tennessee
An explosion at the Nelson coal mine killed 16 people.

CDC and NIOSH Safety and Health Research. *Coal Mining Disasters*. Available at:
http://www.cdc.gov/niosh/mining/statistics/discoal.htm. Accessed September 21, 2005.

### March 6, 1902: Monongahela, Pennsylvania
An explosion at the Catsburg coal mine killed five people.

CDC and NIOSH Safety and Health Research. *Coal Mining Disasters*. Available at:
http://www.cdc.gov/niosh/mining/statistics/discoal.htm. Accessed September 21, 2005.

### January 24, 1902: Oskaloosa, Iowa
An explosion in the number two shaft of the Lost Creek coal mine killed 20
 people.

CDC and NIOSH Safety and Health Research. *Coal Mining Disasters*. Available at:
http://www.cdc.gov/niosh/mining/statistics/discoal.htm. Accessed September 21, 2005.

### October 26, 1901: Diamondville, Wyoming
An explosion at the Diamondville coal mine killed 22 people.

CDC and NIOSH Safety and Health Research. *Coal Mining Disasters*. Available at:
http://www.cdc.gov/niosh/mining/statistics/discoal.htm. Accessed September 21, 2005.

### October 25, 1901: Plymouth, Pennsylvania
An explosion at the Buttonwood coal mine killed six people.

CDC and NIOSH Safety and Health Research. *Coal Mining Disasters*. Available at:
http://www.cdc.gov/niosh/mining/statistics/discoal.htm. Accessed September 21, 2005.

### September 16, 1901: Spring Gulch, Colorado
An explosion at the Spring Gulch coal mine killed six people.

CDC and NIOSH Safety and Health Research. *Coal Mining Disasters*. Available at:
http://www.cdc.gov/niosh/mining/statistics/discoal.htm. Accessed September 21, 2005.

### June 10, 1901: Port Royal, Pennsylvania
An explosion in the number two shaft at the Port Royal coal mine killed 19
 people.

CDC and NIOSH Safety and Health Research. *Coal Mining Disasters*. Available at:
http://www.cdc.gov/niosh/mining/statistics/discoal.htm. Accessed September 21, 2005.

### May 27, 1901: Dayton, Tennessee
An explosion at the Richland coal mine killed 20 people.

CDC and NIOSH Safety and Health Research. *Coal Mining Disasters.* Available at: http://www.cdc.gov/niosh/mining/statistics/discoal.htm. Accessed September 21, 2005.

### May 15, 1901: Farmington, West Virginia
An explosion at the Chatham coal mine killed ten people.

CDC and NIOSH Safety and Health Research. *Coal Mining Disasters.* Available at: http://www.cdc.gov/niosh/mining/statistics/discoal.htm. Accessed September 21, 2005.

### April 29, 1901: Alderson, Oklahoma
An explosion in the number five shaft of the McAlester coal mine killed six people.

CDC and NIOSH Safety and Health Research. *Coal Mining Disasters.* Available at: http://www.cdc.gov/niosh/mining/statistics/discoal.htm. Accessed September 21, 2005.

### November 9, 1900: Mahanoy City, Pennsylvania
An explosion at the Buck Mountain coal mine killed seven people.

CDC and NIOSH Safety and Health Research. *Coal Mining Disasters.* Available at: http://www.cdc.gov/niosh/mining/statistics/discoal.htm. Accessed September 21, 2005.

### May 23, 1900: Cumnock, North Carolina
An explosion at the Cumnock coal mine killed 23 people.

CDC and NIOSH Safety and Health Research. *Coal Mining Disasters.* Available at: http://www.cdc.gov/niosh/mining/statistics/discoal.htm. Accessed September 21, 2005.

### March 6, 1900: Red Ash, West Virginia
An explosion at the Red Ash coal mine killed 46 people.

CDC and NIOSH Safety and Health Research. *Coal Mining Disasters.* Available at: http://www.cdc.gov/niosh/mining/statistics/discoal.htm. Accessed September 21, 2005.

### 1899–1890
### December 23, 1899: Sumner, Pennsylvania
An explosion at the Sumner coal mine killed 19 people.

CDC and NIOSH Safety and Health Research. *Coal Mining Disasters.* Available at: http://www.cdc.gov/niosh/mining/statistics/discoal.htm. Accessed September 21, 2005.

### December 9, 1899: Carbonado, Washington
An explosion in the number seven shaft at the Carbon Hill coal mine killed 31 people.

CDC and NIOSH Safety and Health Research. *Coal Mining Disasters.* Available at: http://www.cdc.gov/niosh/mining/statistics/discoal.htm. Accessed September 21, 2005.

### July 24, 1899: Grindstone, Pennsylvania
An explosion at the Grindstone coal mine killed five people.

CDC and NIOSH Safety and Health Research. *Coal Mining Disasters.* Available at: http://www.cdc.gov/niosh/mining/statistics/discoal.htm. Accessed September 21, 2005.

### May 23, 1899: Cumnock, North Carolina
An explosion at the Cumnock coal mine killed 23 people.

CDC and NIOSH Safety and Health Research. *Coal Mining Disasters.* Available at: http://www.cdc.gov/niosh/mining/statistics/discoal.htm. Accessed September 21, 2005.

### April 21, 1899: Madrid, New Mexico
An explosion at the Cook & White coal mine killed five people.

CDC and NIOSH Safety and Health Research. *Coal Mining Disasters.* Available at: http://www.cdc.gov/niosh/mining/statistics/discoal.htm. Accessed September 21, 2005.

### February 21, 1899: Blocton, Alabama
An explosion in the number two shaft of the Blocton coal mine killed five people.

CDC and NIOSH Safety and Health Research. *Coal Mining Disasters.* Available at: http://www.cdc.gov/niosh/mining/statistics/discoal.htm. Accessed September 21, 2005.

### September 23, 1898: Brownsville, Pennsylvania
An explosion at the Umpire coal mine killed eight workers.

CDC and NIOSH Safety and Health Research. *Coal Mining Disasters.* Available at: http://www.cdc.gov/niosh/mining/statistics/discoal.htm. Accessed September 21, 2005.

### March 19, 1898: Alabama
An explosion at the number two slope of a coal mine killed six workers.

CDC and NIOSH Safety and Health Research. *Coal Mining Disasters.* Available at: http://www.cdc.gov/niosh/mining/statistics/discoal.htm. Accessed September 21, 2005.

### September 3, 1897: Sunshine, Colorado
An explosion at the Sunshine coal mine killed 12 workers.

CDC and NIOSH Safety and Health Research. *Coal Mining Disasters.* Available at: http://www.cdc.gov/niosh/mining/statistics/discoal.htm. Accessed September 21, 2005.

### March 4, 1897: Huntington, Arkansas

An explosion in the #44 shaft at the Kansas & Texas colliery killed 14 people.

CDC and NIOSH Safety and Health Research. *Coal Mining Disasters*. Available at: http://www.cdc.gov/niosh/mining/statistics/discoal.htm. Accessed September 21, 2005.

### January 4, 1897: Alderson, Oklahoma

An explosion in the number one shaft at the Alderson coal mine killed five people.

CDC and NIOSH Safety and Health Research. *Coal Mining Disasters*. Available at: http://www.cdc.gov/niosh/mining/statistics/discoal.htm. Accessed September 21, 2005.

### December 26, 1896: Princeton, Indiana

An explosion at the Oswald coal mine killed seven people.

CDC and NIOSH Safety and Health Research. *Coal Mining Disasters*. Available at: http://www.cdc.gov/niosh/mining/statistics/discoal.htm. Accessed September 21, 2005.

### October 29, 1896: South Wilkes-Barre, Pennsylvania

An explosion in shaft number three of a coal mine in South Wilkes-Barre, Pennsylvania killed six workers.

CDC and NIOSH Safety and Health Research. *Coal Mining Disasters*. Available at: http://www.cdc.gov/niosh/mining/statistics/discoal.htm. Accessed September 21, 2005.

### March 23, 1896: Du Bois, Pennsylvania

An explosion at the Berwind coal mine killed 13 people.

CDC and NIOSH Safety and Health Research. *Coal Mining Disasters*. Available at: http://www.cdc.gov/niosh/mining/statistics/discoal.htm. Accessed September 21, 2005.

### February 18, 1896: New Castle, Colorado

An explosion at the Vulcan coal mine killed 49 people.

CDC and NIOSH Safety and Health Research. *Coal Mining Disasters*. Available at: http://www.cdc.gov/niosh/mining/statistics/discoal.htm. Accessed September 21, 2005.

### December 20, 1895: Dayton, Tennessee

An explosion at the Nelson coal mine killed 28 people.

CDC and NIOSH Safety and Health Research. *Coal Mining Disasters*. Available at: http://www.cdc.gov/niosh/mining/statistics/discoal.htm. Accessed September 21, 2005.

### December 19, 1895: Cumnock, North Carolina

An explosion at the Cumnock coal mine killed 39 people.

CDC and NIOSH Safety and Health Research. *Coal Mining Disasters*. Available at: http://www.cdc.gov/niosh/mining/statistics/discoal.htm. Accessed September 21, 2005.

### October 7, 1895: Wilkes-Barre, Pennsylvania

An explosion at the Dorrance coal mine killed seven workers.

CDC and NIOSH Safety and Health Research. *Coal Mining Disasters.* Available at:
http://www.cdc.gov/niosh/mining/statistics/discoal.htm. Accessed September 21, 2005.

### April 8, 1895: Lake Whatcom, Washington

An explosion at the Blue Canyon coal mine killed 23 people.

CDC and NIOSH Safety and Health Research. *Coal Mining Disasters.* Available at:
http://www.cdc.gov/niosh/mining/statistics/discoal.htm. Accessed September 21, 2005.

### March 20, 1895: Red Canyon, Wyoming

An explosion at the Red Canyon coal mine killed 60 people.

CDC and NIOSH Safety and Health Research. *Coal Mining Disasters.* Available at:
http://www.cdc.gov/niosh/mining/statistics/discoal.htm. Accessed September 21, 2005.

### February 27, 1895: Madrid, New Mexico

An explosion at the White Ash coal mine killed 24 people.

CDC and NIOSH Safety and Health Research. *Coal Mining Disasters.* Available at:
http://www.cdc.gov/niosh/mining/statistics/discoal.htm. Accessed September 21, 2005.

### February 18, 1895: Mahoney Plane, Pennsylvania

An explosion at the West Bear Ridge coal mine killed five people.

CDC and NIOSH Safety and Health Research. *Coal Mining Disasters.* Available at:
http://www.cdc.gov/niosh/mining/statistics/discoal.htm. Accessed September 21, 2005.

### November 20, 1894: Standard, Washington

An explosion at the Blanche coal mine killed eight people.

CDC and NIOSH Safety and Health Research. *Coal Mining Disasters.* Available at:
http://www.cdc.gov/niosh/mining/statistics/discoal.htm. Accessed September 21, 2005.

### September 21, 1893: Plymouth, Pennsylvania

An explosion in the #11 shaft of the Lance coal mine killed six people.

CDC and NIOSH Safety and Health Research. *Coal Mining Disasters.* Available at:
http://www.cdc.gov/niosh/mining/statistics/discoal.htm. Accessed September 21, 2005.

### June 22, 1893: Nanticoke, Pennsylvania

An explosion in the number one shaft of the Susquehanna coal mine killed
    five people.

CDC and NIOSH Safety and Health Research. *Coal Mining Disasters.* Available at:
http://www.cdc.gov/niosh/mining/statistics/discoal.htm. Accessed September 21, 2005.

### March 13, 1893: Alderson, Oklahoma

An explosion at the Choctaw coal mine killed nine people.

CDC and NIOSH Safety and Health Research. *Coal Mining Disasters*. Available at: http://www.cdc.gov/niosh/mining/statistics/discoal.htm. Accessed September 21, 2005.

### February 14, 1893: Albia, Iowa

An explosion at the Chicago & Iowa colliery killed eight people.

CDC and NIOSH Safety and Health Research. *Coal Mining Disasters*. Available at: http://www.cdc.gov/niosh/mining/statistics/discoal.htm. Accessed September 21, 2005.

### January 10, 1893: King, Colorado

An explosion at the Como coal mine killed 24 people.

CDC and NIOSH Safety and Health Research. *Coal Mining Disasters*. Available at: http://www.cdc.gov/niosh/mining/statistics/discoal.htm. Accessed September 21, 2005.

### July 23, 1892: Pottsville, Pennsylvania

An explosion at the York Farm coal mine killed 15 people.

CDC and NIOSH Safety and Health Research. *Coal Mining Disasters*. Available at: http://www.cdc.gov/niosh/mining/statistics/discoal.htm. Accessed September 21, 2005.

### May 10, 1892: Roslyn, Washington

An explosion at the Roslyn coal mine killed 45 people.

CDC and NIOSH Safety and Health Research. *Coal Mining Disasters*. Available at: http://www.cdc.gov/niosh/mining/statistics/discoal.htm. Accessed September 21, 2005.

### January 7, 1892: Krebs, Oklahoma

An explosion in the #11 shaft at a local colliery killed 100 people.

CDC and NIOSH Safety and Health Research. *Coal Mining Disasters*. Available at: http://www.cdc.gov/niosh/mining/statistics/discoal.htm. Accessed September 21, 2005.

### November 8, 1891: Nanticoke, Pennsylvania

An explosion in the number one shaft at the Susquehanna coal mine killed 12 people.

CDC and NIOSH Safety and Health Research. *Coal Mining Disasters*. Available at: http://www.cdc.gov/niosh/mining/statistics/discoal.htm. Accessed September 21, 2005.

### May 22, 1891: Pratt City, Alabama

An explosion in the number one shaft of the Pratt coal mine killed 11 people.

CDC and NIOSH Safety and Health Research. *Coal Mining Disasters*. Available at: http://www.cdc.gov/niosh/mining/statistics/discoal.htm. Accessed September 21, 2005.

### January 27, 1891: Mount Pleasant, Pennsylvania
An explosion at the Mammouth coal mine killed 109 people.

CDC and NIOSH Safety and Health Research. *Coal Mining Disasters*. Available at:
http://www.cdc.gov/niosh/mining/statistics/discoal.htm. Accessed September 21, 2005.

### May 15, 1890: Ashley, Pennsylvania
An explosion in the number eight shaft of the Jersey coal mine killed 26 people.

CDC and NIOSH Safety and Health Research. *Coal Mining Disasters*. Available at:
http://www.cdc.gov/niosh/mining/statistics/discoal.htm. Accessed September 21, 2005.

### April 2, 1890: Nanticoke, Pennsylvania
An explosion in the number four shaft of the Susquehanna coal mine killed
five people.

CDC and NIOSH Safety and Health Research. *Coal Mining Disasters*. Available at:
http://www.cdc.gov/niosh/mining/statistics/discoal.htm. Accessed September 21, 2005.

### February 1, 1890: Plymouth, Pennsylvania
An explosion at the Nottingham coal mine killed eight people.

CDC and NIOSH Safety and Health Research. *Coal Mining Disasters*. Available at:
http://www.cdc.gov/niosh/mining/statistics/discoal.htm. Accessed September 21, 2005.

### 1889–1880
### November 9, 1888: Frontenac, Kansas
An explosion in the number two shaft of a coal mine in Frontenac killed 40
people.

CDC and NIOSH Safety and Health Research. *Coal Mining Disasters*. Available at:
http://www.cdc.gov/niosh/mining/statistics/discoal.htm. Accessed September 21, 2005.

### November 3, 1888: Westport, Pennsylvania
An explosion at the Kettle Creek coal mine killed 17 people.

CDC and NIOSH Safety and Health Research. *Coal Mining Disasters*. Available at:
http://www.cdc.gov/niosh/mining/statistics/discoal.htm. Accessed September 21, 2005.

### March 29, 1888: Rich Hill, Missouri
An explosion in the number six shaft of the Keith & Perry colliery killed 24
people.

CDC and NIOSH Safety and Health Research. *Coal Mining Disasters*. Available at:
http://www.cdc.gov/niosh/mining/statistics/discoal.htm. Accessed September 21, 2005.

### April 4, 1887: Savanna, Oklahoma

An explosion in the number two shaft of the Old Savanna coal mine killed 18 people.

CDC and NIOSH Safety and Health Research. *Coal Mining Disasters.* Available at: http://www.cdc.gov/niosh/mining/statistics/discoal.htm. Accessed September 21, 2005.

### November 26, 1886: Wilkes-Barre, Pennsylvania

An explosion at the Conyngham coal mine killed 12 people.

CDC and NIOSH Safety and Health Research. *Coal Mining Disasters.* Available at: http://www.cdc.gov/niosh/mining/statistics/discoal.htm. Accessed September 21, 2005.

### August 30, 1886: Scranton, Pennsylvania

An explosion at the Fair Lawn coal mine killed six people.

CDC and NIOSH Safety and Health Research. *Coal Mining Disasters.* Available at: http://www.cdc.gov/niosh/mining/statistics/discoal.htm. Accessed September 21, 2005.

### March 8, 1886: Dunbar, Pennsylvania

An explosion at the Uniondale coal mine killed six people.

CDC and NIOSH Safety and Health Research. *Coal Mining Disasters.* Available at: http://www.cdc.gov/niosh/mining/statistics/discoal.htm. Accessed September 21, 2005.

### January 21, 1886: Newburg, West Virginia

An explosion at the Newburg coal mine killed 39 people.

CDC and NIOSH Safety and Health Research. *Coal Mining Disasters.* Available at: http://www.cdc.gov/niosh/mining/statistics/discoal.htm. Accessed September 21, 2005.

### January 13, 1886: Almy, Wyoming

An explosion of the number four shaft of the Almy coal mine killed 13 people.

CDC and NIOSH Safety and Health Research. *Coal Mining Disasters.* Available at: http://www.cdc.gov/niosh/mining/statistics/discoal.htm. Accessed September 21, 2005.

### August 11, 1885: Mocanaqua, Pennsylvania

A gas explosion at the West End coal mine killed ten people.

CDC and NIOSH Safety and Health Research. *Coal Mining Disasters.* Available at: http://www.cdc.gov/niosh/mining/statistics/discoal.htm. Accessed September 21, 2005.

### October 27, 1884: Uniontown, Pennsylvania

An explosion at the Youngstown coal mine killed 14 people.

CDC and NIOSH Safety and Health Research. *Coal Mining Disasters.* Available at: http://www.cdc.gov/niosh/mining/statistics/discoal.htm. Accessed September 21, 2005.

### March 13, 1884: Pocahontas, Virginia

An explosion at the Laurel coal mine killed 112 people.

CDC and NIOSH Safety and Health Research. *Coal Mining Disasters*. Available at: http://www.cdc.gov/niosh/mining/statistics/discoal.htm. Accessed September 21, 2005.

### February 20, 1884: West Leisenring, Pennsylvania

An explosion at the West Leisenring coal mine killed 19 people.

CDC and NIOSH Safety and Health Research. *Coal Mining Disasters*. Available at: http://www.cdc.gov/niosh/mining/statistics/discoal.htm. Accessed September 21, 2005.

### January 24, 1884: Crested Butte, Colorado

An explosion at the Crested Butte coal mine killed 59 people.

CDC and NIOSH Safety and Health Research. *Coal Mining Disasters*. Available at: http://www.cdc.gov/niosh/mining/statistics/discoal.htm. Accessed September 21, 2005.

### January 9, 1883: Coulterville, Illinois

An explosion at the Coulterville coal mine killed ten people.

CDC and NIOSH Safety and Health Research. *Coal Mining Disasters*. Available at: http://www.cdc.gov/niosh/mining/statistics/discoal.htm. Accessed September 21, 2005.

### May 24, 1882: Shenandoah, Pennsylvania

An explosion at the Kohinoor coal mine killed five people.

CDC and NIOSH Safety and Health Research. *Coal Mining Disasters*. Available at: http://www.cdc.gov/niosh/mining/statistics/discoal.htm. Accessed September 21, 2005.

### February 3, 1882: Coalfield, Virginia

An explosion at the Midlothian coal mine killed 32 people.

CDC and NIOSH Safety and Health Research. *Coal Mining Disasters*. Available at: http://www.cdc.gov/niosh/mining/statistics/discoal.htm. Accessed September 21, 2005.

### March 4, 1881: Almy, Wyoming

An explosion at the Almy coal mine killed 38 people.

CDC and NIOSH Safety and Health Research. *Coal Mining Disasters*. Available at: http://www.cdc.gov/niosh/mining/statistics/discoal.htm. Accessed September 21, 2005.

### February 10, 1881: Robbins, Ohio

An explosion at the Robbins coal mine killed six people.

CDC and NIOSH Safety and Health Research. *Coal Mining Disasters*. Available at: http://www.cdc.gov/niosh/mining/statistics/discoal.htm. Accessed September 21, 2005.

### *May 3, 1880: Shamokin, Pennsylvania*

An explosion at the Lykens Valley coal mine killed five people.

CDC and NIOSH Safety and Health Research. *Coal Mining Disasters.* Available at:
http://www.cdc.gov/niosh/mining/statistics/discoal.htm. Accessed September 21, 2005.

### *March 5, 1880: Nanticoke, Pennsylvania*

An explosion in the number two shaft of the Nanticoke coal mine killed six
people.

CDC and NIOSH Safety and Health Research. *Coal Mining Disasters.* Available at:
http://www.cdc.gov/niosh/mining/statistics/discoal.htm. Accessed September 21, 2005.

### *1879–1870*
### *November 2, 1879: Mill Creek, Pennsylvania*

An explosion at Mill Creek colliery killed five people.

CDC and NIOSH Safety and Health Research. *Coal Mining Disasters.* Available at:
http://www.cdc.gov/niosh/mining/statistics/discoal.htm. Accessed September 21, 2005.

### *May 6, 1879: Audenried, Pennsylvania*

An explosion at Audenried coal mine killed six people.

CDC and NIOSH Safety and Health Research. *Coal Mining Disasters.* Available at:
http://www.cdc.gov/niosh/mining/statistics/discoal.htm. Accessed September 21, 2005.

### *November 21, 1878: Sullivan, Indiana*

An explosion at Sullivan coal mine killed eight people.

CDC and NIOSH Safety and Health Research. *Coal Mining Disasters.* Available at:
http://www.cdc.gov/niosh/mining/statistics/discoal.htm. Accessed September 21, 2005.

### *January 15, 1878: Lundale, Pennsylvania*

An explosion at Potts coal mine killed five people.

CDC and NIOSH Safety and Health Research. *Coal Mining Disasters.* Available at:
http://www.cdc.gov/niosh/mining/statistics/discoal.htm. Accessed September 21, 2005.

### *October 2, 1871: Branch Dale, Pennsylvania*

An explosion at the Otto Red Ash coal mine killed five people.

CDC and NIOSH Safety and Health Research. *Coal Mining Disasters.* Available at:
http://www.cdc.gov/niosh/mining/statistics/discoal.htm. Accessed September 21, 2005.

### *August 14, 1871: Pittston, Pennsylvania*

An explosion at the Eagle Shaft coal mine killed 17 people.

CDC and NIOSH Safety and Health Research. *Coal Mining Disasters*. Available at: http://www.cdc.gov/niosh/mining/statistics/discoal.htm. Accessed September 21, 2005.

### March 22, 1870: Locustdale, Pennsylvania
A coal mine explosion at Potts colliery killed five people.

CDC and NIOSH Safety and Health Research. *Coal Mining Disasters*. Available at: http://www.cdc.gov/niosh/mining/statistics/discoal.htm. Accessed September 21, 2005.

### 1869–1800
### April 3, 1867: Winterpock, Virginia
An explosion at the Bright Hope mine killed 69 people.

CDC and NIOSH Safety and Health Research. *Coal Mining Disasters*. Available at: http://www.cdc.gov/niosh/mining/statistics/discoal.htm. Accessed September 21, 2005.

### 1863: Winterpock, Virginia
An explosion at the Raccoon, Clover Hill mine killed 17 people.

CDC and NIOSH Safety and Health Research. *Coal Mining Disasters*. Available at: http://www.cdc.gov/niosh/mining/statistics/discoal.htm. Accessed September 21, 2005.

### 1859: Winterpock, Virginia
An explosion at the Bright Hope mine killed nine people.

CDC and NIOSH Safety and Health Research. *Coal Mining Disasters*. Available at: http://www.cdc.gov/niosh/mining/statistics/discoal.htm. Accessed September 21, 2005.

### 1855: Coalfield, Virginia
An explosion at Midlothian colliery killed 55 people.

CDC and NIOSH Safety and Health Research. *Coal Mining Disasters*. Available at: http://www.cdc.gov/niosh/mining/statistics/discoal.htm. Accessed September 21, 2005.

### 1854: New Richmond, Virginia
An explosion at Chesterfield colliery killed 19 people.

CDC and NIOSH Safety and Health Research. *Coal Mining Disasters*. Available at: http://www.cdc.gov/niosh/mining/statistics/discoal.htm. Accessed September 21, 2005.

### 1850: Winterpock, Virginia
An explosion at Cox's Pit, Clover Hill colliery killed seven people.

CDC and NIOSH Safety and Health Research. *Coal Mining Disasters*. Available at: http://www.cdc.gov/niosh/mining/statistics/discoal.htm. Accessed September 21, 2005.

### February 1847: Pottsville, Pennsylvania
An explosion at Spencer colliery killed seven people.

CDC and NIOSH Safety and Health Research. *Coal Mining Disasters.* Available at: http://www.cdc.gov/niosh/mining/statistics/discoal.htm. Accessed September 21, 2005.

### June 15, 1844: New Richmond, Virginia
A coal mine explosion at Black Heath colliery killed 11 people.

CDC and NIOSH Safety and Health Research. *Coal Mining Disasters.* Available at: http://www.cdc.gov/niosh/mining/statistics/discoal.htm. Accessed September 21, 2005.

### March 18, 1839: New Richmond, Virginia
An explosion at Black Heath colliery killed 40 people.

CDC and NIOSH Safety and Health Research. *Coal Mining Disasters.* Available at: http://www.cdc.gov/niosh/mining/statistics/discoal.htm. Accessed September 21, 2005.

## Coal Mine Fires

### January 19, 2006: Melville, West Virginia
A conveyor belt caught fire at the Alma number one mine, which separated two miners from their 12-member crew. The two men died. This fire occurred less than a month after another West Virginia mine experienced an explosion that killed 12 miners. Both mining disasters have prompted officials to introduce legislation that would focus on emergency response for underground mining operations.

U.S. Department of Labor, Mine Safety and Health Administration. *Aracoma Alma Mine #1 Information Single Source Page.* Available at: http://www.msha.gov/Aracoma/AlmaMine.asp

### December 19, 1984: Orangeville, Utah
A fire at Emory Mining Company's Wilberg coal mine killed 27 people.

CDC and NIOSH Safety and Health Research. *Coal Mining Disasters.* Available at: http://www.cdc.gov/niosh/mining/statistics/discoal.htm. Accessed September 21, 2005.

### March 8, 1960: Pine Creek, West Virginia
A fire in the #22 shaft of a local coal mine killed 18 people.

CDC and NIOSH Safety and Health Research. *Coal Mining Disasters.* Available at: http://www.cdc.gov/niosh/mining/statistics/discoal.htm. Accessed September 21, 2005.

### November 4, 1948: Kitzmiller, Maryland
A fire in the number one shaft of the Milt coal mine killed five people.

CDC and NIOSH Safety and Health Research. *Coal Mining Disasters*. Available at:
http://www.cdc.gov/niosh/mining/statistics/discoal.htm. Accessed September 21, 2005.

### July 5, 1944: Powhatan, Ohio
A fire at the Powhatan coal mine killed 66 people.

CDC and NIOSH Safety and Health Research. *Coal Mining Disasters*. Available at:
http://www.cdc.gov/niosh/mining/statistics/discoal.htm. Accessed September 21, 2005.

### June 7, 1944: Clarksville, Pennsylvania
A fire at the Emerald coal mine killed six people.

CDC and NIOSH Safety and Health Research. *Coal Mining Disasters*. Available at:
http://www.cdc.gov/niosh/mining/statistics/discoal.htm. Accessed September 21, 2005.

### August 1, 1936: Dowell, Illinois
A fire at the Kathleen coal mine killed nine people.

CDC and NIOSH Safety and Health Research. *Coal Mining Disasters*. Available at:
http://www.cdc.gov/niosh/mining/statistics/discoal.htm. Accessed September 21, 2005.

### May 11, 1935: Barrackville, West Virginia
A fire in the #41 shaft of a colliery in Barrackville killed five people.

CDC and NIOSH Safety and Health Research. *Coal Mining Disasters*. Available at:
http://www.cdc.gov/niosh/mining/statistics/discoal.htm. Accessed September 21, 2005.

### December 22, 1925: Bellaire, Ohio
A fire at the Webb coal mine killed nine people.

CDC and NIOSH Safety and Health Research. *Coal Mining Disasters*. Available at:
http://www.cdc.gov/niosh/mining/statistics/discoal.htm. Accessed September 21, 2005.

### December 13, 1921: Morrison, Colorado
A fire at the Satanic coal mine killed six people.

CDC and NIOSH Safety and Health Research. *Coal Mining Disasters*. Available at:
http://www.cdc.gov/niosh/mining/statistics/discoal.htm. Accessed September 21, 2005.

### February 23, 1921: Dowell, Illinois
A fire at the Kathleen coal mine killed seven people.

CDC and NIOSH Safety and Health Research. *Coal Mining Disasters*. Available at:
http://www.cdc.gov/niosh/mining/statistics/discoal.htm. Accessed September 21, 2005.

### November 16, 1920: Earlington, Kentucky

A fire at the Arnold coal mine killed six people.

CDC and NIOSH Safety and Health Research. *Coal Mining Disasters*. Available at: http://www.cdc.gov/niosh/mining/statistics/discoal.htm. Accessed September 21, 2005.

### October 29, 1919: Amsterdam, Ohio

A fire in the number two shaft of a colliery in Amsterdam killed 20 people.

CDC and NIOSH Safety and Health Research. *Coal Mining Disasters*. Available at: http://www.cdc.gov/niosh/mining/statistics/discoal.htm. Accessed September 21, 2005.

### October 8, 1894: Shamokin, Pennsylvania

A fire in the Luke Fidler coal mine killed five people.

CDC and NIOSH Safety and Health Research. *Coal Mining Disasters*. Available at: http://www.cdc.gov/niosh/mining/statistics/discoal.htm. Accessed September 21, 2005.

### August 24, 1894: Franklin, Washington

A fire in the Franklin coal mine killed 37 people.

CDC and NIOSH Safety and Health Research. *Coal Mining Disasters*. Available at: http://www.cdc.gov/niosh/mining/statistics/discoal.htm. Accessed September 21, 2005.

### April 1, 1893: Shamokin, Pennsylvania

A fire at the Neilson coal mine killed ten people.

CDC and NIOSH Safety and Health Research. *Coal Mining Disasters*. Available at: http://www.cdc.gov/niosh/mining/statistics/discoal.htm. Accessed September 21, 2005.

### March 3, 1890: Wilkes-Barre, Pennsylvania

A fire in the number three shaft of a south Wilkes-Barre coal mine killed eight people.

CDC and NIOSH Safety and Health Research. *Coal Mining Disasters*. Available at: http://www.cdc.gov/niosh/mining/statistics/discoal.htm. Accessed September 21, 2005.

### August 21, 1884: Shamokin, Pennsylvania

A fire at the Buck Ridge colliery killed seven people.

CDC and NIOSH Safety and Health Research. *Coal Mining Disasters*. Available at: http://www.cdc.gov/niosh/mining/statistics/discoal.htm. Accessed September 21, 2005.

### May 9, 1877: Wadesville, Pennsylvania

A fire at a Wadesville coal mine killed seven people.

CDC and NIOSH Safety and Health Research. *Coal Mining Disasters*. Available at: http://www.cdc.gov/niosh/mining/statistics/discoal.htm. Accessed September 21, 2005.

### July 24, 1876: Nortonville, California
A fire at the Black Diamond coal mine killed six people.

CDC and NIOSH Safety and Health Research. *Coal Mining Disasters.* Available at: http://www.cdc.gov/niosh/mining/statistics/discoal.htm. Accessed September 21, 2005.

### May 20, 1876: Coalfield, Virginia
A fire at the Midlothian coal mine killed eight people.

CDC and NIOSH Safety and Health Research. *Coal Mining Disasters.* Available at: http://www.cdc.gov/niosh/mining/statistics/discoal.htm. Accessed September 21, 2005.

### June 10, 1873: Shamokin, Pennsylvania
A coal mine fire at the Henry Clay mine killed ten people.

CDC and NIOSH Safety and Health Research. *Coal Mining Disasters.* Available at: http://www.cdc.gov/niosh/mining/statistics/discoal.htm. Accessed September 21, 2005.

### July 1872: Portage County, Ohio
A fire at the Atwater Slope coal mine killed ten people.

CDC and NIOSH Safety and Health Research. *Coal Mining Disasters.* Available at: http://www.cdc.gov/niosh/mining/statistics/discoal.htm. Accessed September 21, 2005.

### September 6, 1869: Plymouth, Pennsylvania
One hundred ten miners were killed in a mine-shaft fire at the Avondale mine. The fire blocked their escape route and only source of air.

CDC and NIOSH Safety and Health Research. *Coal Mining Disasters.* Available at: http://www.cdc.gov/niosh/mining/statistics/discoal.htm. Accessed September 21, 2005.

U.S. Department of Labor, Mine Safety and Health Administration. District 1 – Coal Mine Safety & Health Fatality Information. *Historical Coal Mine Disasters in Anthracite Region.* Available at: http://www.msha.gov/District/Dist_01/Reports/Avondale/page01.htm.

## Copper Explosions and/or Mine Fires
### March 31, 1954: Santa Rita, New Mexico
A powder truck explosion at the Kennecott Copper Company killed five people.

CDC and NIOSH Safety and Health Research. *Coal Mining Disasters.* Available at: http://www.cdc.gov/niosh/mining/statistics/discoal.htm. Accessed September 21, 2005.

### January 5, 1943: Ducktown, Tennessee
An explosion at the Boyd Mine killed nine people.

CDC and NIOSH Safety and Health Research. *Coal Mining Disasters.* Available at: http://www.cdc.gov/niosh/mining/statistics/discoal.htm. Accessed September 21, 2005.

### June 8, 1917: Butte, Montana
A fire at the Granite Mountain copper mine killed 163 people.

CDC and NIOSH Safety and Health Research. *Coal Mining Disasters.* Available at: http://www.cdc.gov/niosh/mining/statistics/discoal.htm. Accessed September 21, 2005.

### May 12, 1905: Butte, Montana
The detonation of explosive materials at the Cora copper mine killed seven people.

CDC and NIOSH Safety and Health Research. *Coal Mining Disasters.* Available at: http://www.cdc.gov/niosh/mining/statistics/discoal.htm. Accessed September 21, 2005.

### April 11, 1896: Butte, Montana
A powder explosion at the St. Lawrence copper mine killed six workers.

CDC and NIOSH Safety and Health Research. *Coal Mining Disasters.* Available at: http://www.cdc.gov/niosh/mining/statistics/discoal.htm. Accessed September 21, 2005.

### April 21, 1893: Butte, Montana
A fire in the number two shaft of the Silver Bow copper mine killed nine people.

CDC and NIOSH Safety and Health Research. *Coal Mining Disasters.* Available at: http://www.cdc.gov/niosh/mining/statistics/discoal.htm. Accessed September 21, 2005.

### November 23, 1889: Butte, Montana
A fire at the Neversweat-St. Lawrence copper mine killed six people.

CDC and NIOSH Safety and Health Research. *Coal Mining Disasters.* Available at: http://www.cdc.gov/niosh/mining/statistics/discoal.htm. Accessed September 21, 2005.

### February 16, 1881: Belmont, Montana
A fire from a blacksmith forge at the Belmont copper mine killed six people.

CDC and NIOSH Safety and Health Research. *Coal Mining Disasters.* Available at: http://www.cdc.gov/niosh/mining/statistics/discoal.htm. Accessed September 21, 2005.

## Dynamite and Powder Explosions
### August 31, 1938: Asheville, North Carolina
Detonation of dynamite at the Asheville granite quarry caused an explosion that killed five people.

CDC and NIOSH Safety and Health Research. *Coal Mining Disasters.* Available at: http://www.cdc.gov/niosh/mining/statistics/discoal.htm. Accessed September 21, 2005.

### June 27, 1918: Virginia, Minnesota
A powder explosion at the Silver iron pit killed 18 people.

CDC and NIOSH Safety and Health Research. *Coal Mining Disasters.* Available at: http://www.cdc.gov/niosh/mining/statistics/discoal.htm. Accessed September 21, 2005.

### July 17, 1917: Trident, Montana
A powder explosion at the Three Forks gypsum killed eight people.

CDC and NIOSH Safety and Health Research. *Coal Mining Disasters.* Available at: http://www.cdc.gov/niosh/mining/statistics/discoal.htm. Accessed September 21, 2005.

### October 19, 1915: Butte, Montana
A dynamite explosion at the Granite Mountain Shaft copper mine killed 16 people.

CDC and NIOSH Safety and Health Research. *Coal Mining Disasters.* Available at: http://www.cdc.gov/niosh/mining/statistics/discoal.htm. Accessed September 21, 2005.

### July 7, 1912: Ely, Nevada
A dynamite explosion at the Eureka Pit copper mine killed ten people.

CDC and NIOSH Safety and Health Research. *Coal Mining Disasters.* Available at: http://www.cdc.gov/niosh/mining/statistics/discoal.htm. Accessed September 21, 2005.

### January 18, 1911: Radersburg, Montana
Detonation of explosive powder at the Keating gold mine killed six people.

CDC and NIOSH Safety and Health Research. *Coal Mining Disasters.* Available at: http://www.cdc.gov/niosh/mining/statistics/discoal.htm. Accessed September 21, 2005.

### March 2, 1910: Treadwell, Alaska
Detonation of explosive powder at the Alaska-Mexican gold mine killed 37 people.

CDC and NIOSH Safety and Health Research. *Coal Mining Disasters.* Available at: http://www.cdc.gov/niosh/mining/statistics/discoal.htm. Accessed September 21, 2005.

### June 4, 1901: Iron Mountain, Michigan
A dynamite explosion at the Chapin iron mine killed eight people.

CDC and NIOSH Safety and Health Research. *Coal Mining Disasters.* Available at: http://www.cdc.gov/niosh/mining/statistics/discoal.htm. Accessed September 21, 2005.

### *May 1, 1900: Scofield, Utah*

An explosion of blasting powder in the winter quarters of a coal mine killed 200 people.

CDC and NIOSH Safety and Health Research. *Coal Mining Disasters.* Available at: http://www.cdc.gov/niosh/mining/statistics/discoal.htm. Accessed September 21, 2005.

### *April 11, 1896: Butte, Montana*

A powder explosion at the St. Lawrence copper mine killed six workers.

CDC and NIOSH Safety and Health Research. *Coal Mining Disasters.* Available at: http://www.cdc.gov/niosh/mining/statistics/discoal.htm. Accessed September 21, 2005.

### *September 26, 1895: Leadville, Colorado*

A dynamite explosion at the Belgian gold mine killed six workers.

CDC and NIOSH Safety and Health Research. *Coal Mining Disasters.* Available at: http://www.cdc.gov/niosh/mining/statistics/discoal.htm. Accessed September 21, 2005.

### *July 17, 1894: Stockton, Pennsylvania*

An explosion of dynamite killed eight people in the East Sugar Loaf coal mine.

CDC and NIOSH Safety and Health Research. *Coal Mining Disasters.* Available at: http://www.cdc.gov/niosh/mining/statistics/discoal.htm. Accessed September 21, 2005.

### *November 14, 1889: Silver Cliff, Colorado*

An explosion of dynamite at the Bull Domingo gold and silver mine killed ten people.

CDC and NIOSH Safety and Health Research. *Coal Mining Disasters.* Available at: http://www.cdc.gov/niosh/mining/statistics/discoal.htm. Accessed September 21, 2005.

### *February 13, 1874: Phoenix, Michigan*

An explosion of dynamite at a copper mine killed six people.

CDC and NIOSH Safety and Health Research. *Coal Mining Disasters.* Available at: http://www.cdc.gov/niosh/mining/statistics/discoal.htm. Accessed September 21, 2005.

## Ethylene Explosions

### *August 19, 2004: Ontario, California*

Four employees of the Sterigenics facility suffered minor injuries from an explosion that occurred inside an ethylene oxide sterilization chamber. The facility was rendered unusable.

EXPLOSIVE AND FIRE EVENTS **233**

U.S. Chemical Safety and Hazard Investigation Board. CSB investigation information page. *Sterigenics Ethylene Oxide Explosion: Ontario, CA, August 19, 2004.* Available at: http://www.csb.gov/index.cfm?folder=current_investigations&page=info&INV_ID=49

### October 23, 1989: Pasadena, Texas

A series of explosions and an ensuing fire killed 23 workers at a plastics manufacturing plant that was owned by Phillips Petroleum Company. More than 80 others were injured. The presumed cause was an ethylene leak.

United States Fire Administration, Federal Emergency Management Agency. *Phillips Petroleum Chemical Plant Explosion and Fire Pasadena, Texas.* Technical Report Series: Report 035 of Major Fire Investigation Project. U.S. Fire Administration National Fire Data Center; 1987. Available at: http://www.interfire.org/res_file/pdf/Tr-035.pdf

## Explosions, Miscellaneous

### May 11, 2004: Glasgow, Scotland, United Kingdom

The Stockline Plastics plant of ICL Plastics plc exploded, killing nine and injuring more than 40 people.

Scottish Environmental Protection Agency. Press Release 2004. Explosion at Stockline Plastics Ltd., Glasgow. Available at: http://sepa.org.uk/news/releases/view.asp?id=64&y=2004

Parliamentary Information Management Services. Early day Motion 778. Public Inquiry into ICL/Stockline Explosion, Glasgow. Available at: http://edmi.parliament.uk/EDMi/EDMDetails.aspx?EDMID=29092%09%09%09%09%09%09%09&SESSION=875

### January 27, 2002: Lagos, Nigeria

Multiple explosions at a military depot triggered a stampede from the adjacent neighborhoods. More than 600 people died.

Africare. News Release, 2003. *Africare Assists Victims of Nigeria Explosions.* Available at: http://www.africare.org/news/news_release/nigerianbombing.html

### April 2002: Gazipur, Bangladesh

One person died and seven others were injured when an explosion occurred at the Globe Insecticide Limited factory. The plant produced mainly antimosquito insecticides.

Workplace Disasters.Factory blast kills one, injures seven. *Hazards and Workers' Health International Newsletter.* Available at: http://www.hazards.org/disasters/

### January 28, 1986: Cape Canaveral, Florida

A few seconds after liftoff, the NASA space shuttle *Challenger* exploded, killing seven astronauts onboard.

Young MA. In: Catastrophes used as reference points in the manual. *The Community Crisis Response Team Training Manual.* 2nd ed. U.S. Department of Justice, Office for Victims of Crime and National Organization for Victims Assistance (NOVA). Available at: http://www.ojp.usdoj.gov/ovc/publications/infores/crt/appendd.htm

### October 31, 1963: Indianapolis, Indiana

An explosion at the Indiana State Fairgrounds killed 81 people and injured almost 400 people.

Young MA. In: Catastrophes used as reference points in the manual. *The Community Crisis Response Team Training Manual.* 2nd ed. U.S. Department of Justice, Office for Victims of Crime and National Organization for Victims Assistance (NOVA). Available at: http://www.ojp.usdoj.gov/ovc/publications/infores/crt/appendd.htm

### May 26, 1954: Quonset Point, Rhode Island

An explosion and ensuing fire aboard the aircraft carrier *USS Bennington* killed 103 members of the crew.

United States Navy. A Brief History of U.S. Navy Aircraft Carriers. Part IV—Korea and the 1950s From: *United States Naval Aviation, 1910–1995* [Naval Historical Center]. *Dictionary of American Naval Fighting Ships.* Available at: http://www.navy.mil/navydata/ships/carriers/cv-hist4.html

### March 31, 1954: Santa Rita, New Mexico

A powder-truck explosion at the Kennecott Copper Company killed five people.

CDC and NIOSH Safety and Health Research. *Coal Mining Disasters.* Available at: http://www.cdc.gov/niosh/mining/statistics/discoal.htm. Accessed September 21, 2005.

### November 5, 1953: Bonanza, Utah

A dust explosion at the American Gilsonite Company killed eight people. The company processed gilsonite, a form of natural asphalt.

CDC and NIOSH Safety and Health Research. *Coal Mining Disasters.* Available at: http://www.cdc.gov/niosh/mining/statistics/discoal.htm. Accessed September 21, 2005.

### February 19, 1937: Walkermine, California

Detonation of explosives at the Walker copper quarry killed six people.

CDC and NIOSH Safety and Health Research. *Coal Mining Disasters.* Available at: http://www.cdc.gov/niosh/mining/statistics/discoal.htm. Accessed September 21, 2005.

### November 30, 1936: Delta, Pennsylvania

Detonation of explosives at the Funkhouser slate quarry killed nine people.

CDC and NIOSH Safety and Health Research. *Coal Mining Disasters.* Available at: http://www.cdc.gov/niosh/mining/statistics/discoal.htm. Accessed September 21, 2005.

### November 12, 1934: Avalon, California

Detonation of explosives at the Rohl Connolly granite quarry killed nine people.

CDC and NIOSH Safety and Health Research. *Coal Mining Disasters.* Available at: http://www.cdc.gov/niosh/mining/statistics/discoal.htm. Accessed September 21, 2005.

### May 17, 1930: Union, West Virginia

Detonation of explosives at the Terry & Butterskill rock quarry killed six people.

CDC and NIOSH Safety and Health Research. *Coal Mining Disasters.* Available at: http://www.cdc.gov/niosh/mining/statistics/discoal.htm. Accessed September 21, 2005.

### April 19, 1920: Ormrod, Pennsylvania

Detonation of explosives at the Lehigh limestone quarry killed six people.

CDC and NIOSH Safety and Health Research. *Coal Mining Disasters.* Available at: http://www.cdc.gov/niosh/mining/statistics/discoal.htm. Accessed September 21, 2005.

### April 27, 1865: Mississippi River

An explosion and fire aboard the *SS Sultana* steamship killed 1,547 people.

National Fire Protection Association. *The 20 Deadliest Fires and Explosions in U.S. History.* Available at: http://www.nfpa.org/itemDetail.asp?categoryID=954&itemID=23340&URL=Research%20&%20Reports/Fire%20statistics/Historical

## Factory Fires

### May 24, 2002: India

A fire at the Agra shoe factory killed at least 36 workers and injured ten others.

Workplace Disasters. Shoe factory fire kills 36. *Hazards and Workers' Health International Newsletter.* Available at: http://www.hazards.org/disasters/

### May 10, 1993: Bangkok, Thailand

One of the world's deadliest factory fires killed at least 187 workers of a doll factory and injured approximately 500 others.

Symonds P. *Industrial Inferno: The Story of the Thai Toy Factory.* Oak Park, MI: Mehring Books; 1997.

*March 25, 1911: New York City, New York*

A fire in the Asch Building killed 146 of the 500 employees of the Triangle Shirtwaist Factory. Most of the victims were young female immigrants.

Sione P, ed. *The Triangle Factory Fire Online Exhibit.* Cornell University ILR School. Available at: http://www.ilr.cornell.edu/trianglefire/

## Fertilizer Explosion

*February 2004: Neishabour, Iran*

Railroad cars that were loaded with fertilizer, petrol, and sulfur products derailed and exploded, killing more than 320 people and devastating five local villages.

CNN.com World. *Iran Train Blast Toll Now 309.* February 19, 2004. Available at: http://www.cnn.com/2004/WORLD/meast/02/19/iran.train/

## Fires, Miscellaneous

*August 2005: Paris, France*

A fire in a Paris apartment building killed at least 17 people and injured 30 others. Many of the victims were asphyxiated while they slept. At least six of the victims were children. The building, which housed many African immigrants, was reported to be in mediocre-to-poor condition.

CNN.com World. *Cause of Paris Death Blaze Probed.* August 26, 2005. Available at: http://www.cnn.com/2005/WORLD/europe/08/25/paris.fire/

*April 15, 2005: Paris, France*

A fire at the Paris Opera hotel resulted in the deaths of 24 residents, many of whom were children. At the time of the fire, the 32-room hotel was overcrowded. Authorities believe that the fire may have started accidentally when a night watchman's girlfriend lit candles on the floor for a romantic setting.

CNN.com World. *Cause of Paris Death Blaze Probed.* August 26, 2005. Available at: http://www.cnn.com/2005/WORLD/europe/08/25/paris.fire/

*December 30, 2004: Buenos Aires, Argentina*

A fire at the Cromagnon Republic club killed 180 people.

National Fire Protection Association. *Public Assembly and Nightclub Fires: The 10 Deadliest Foreign (outside the U.S.) Nightclub Fires since 1970.* Available at: http:// www.nfpa.org/itemDetail.asp?categoryID=851&itemID=21090&URL= Research%20&%20Reports/Fact%20sheets/Safety%20in%20other%20occupancies/ Nightclubs/assembly%20occupancies/Public%20assembly%20and%20nightclub%20fires

### August 1, 2004: Asunción, Paraguay
A fast-moving fire in a crowded supermarket killed 399 people. Survivors
of the inferno reported that the market doors were locked, slowing escape.

*Paraguay Inferno Survivors: Doors Were Shut.* China Daily. Available at: http://www.
chinadaily.com.cn/english/doc/2004-08/03/content_357105.htm

### February 18, 2003: Daegu, South Korea
An arsonist started a fire in the subway by igniting a box filled with gasoline.
the fire raced through two trains, killing at least 120 people and injuring
more than 140 commuters.

*Arsonist Kills 120 on S Korea Tube.* The Guardian. February 18, 2003. Available at:
http://www.guardian.co.uk/korea/article/0,897925,00.html

### December 1, 2002: Caracas, Venezuela
A fire at the La Goajira nightclub killed 47 people.

National Fire Protection Association. *Public Assembly and Nightclub Fires: The 10 Deadliest Foreign (outside the U.S.) Nightclub Fires since 1970.* Available at: http://www.nfpa.
org/itemDetail.asp?categoryID=851&itemID=21090&URL=Research%20&%20Reports/
Fact%20sheets/Safety%20in%20other%20occupancies/Nightclubs/
assembly%20occupancies/Public%20assembly%20and%20nightclub%20fires

### October 30, 2002: Ho Chi Minh City, Vietnam
A fire believed to have started in a disco nightclub spread to a restaurant
where a wedding reception was being held. Sixty-one people died. Most of
the victims were attending the wedding reception.

National Fire Protection Association. *Public Assembly and Nightclub Fires. The 10 Deadliest Foreign (outside the U.S.) Nightclub Fires since 1970.* Available at: http://www.nfpa.
org/itemDetail.asp?categoryID=851&itemID=21090&URL=Research%20&%20Reports/
Fact%20sheets/Safety%20in%20other%20occupancies/Nightclubs/
assembly%20occupancies/Public%20assembly%20and%20nightclub%20fires

### May 1, 2002: Brazoria County, Texas
A fire broke out at Third Coast Industries, a facility that blended and packaged
motor oils and other automotive products. The plant was not
designed to prevent the spread of fire, which ultimately consumed
1.2 million gallons of combustible and flammable liquids. The facility
was destroyed, 100 local residents were evacuated, a local school was
closed, and significant environmental clean-up was required.

U.S. Chemical Safety and Hazard Investigation Board. CSB investigation information
page. *Third Coast Industries Petroleum Products Facility Fire: Brazoria County, TX, May
1, 2002.* Available at: http://www.csb.gov/index.cfm?folder=completed_investigations
&page=info&INV_ID=30

### February 19, 2002: Cairo, Egypt

An overcrowded train en route to Luxor caught on fire from a gas canister on board. The conductor did not stop for an additional $2\frac{1}{2}$ miles, and approximately 360 people died.

CNN.com. *Major Train Disasters since 1900.* Available at: http://www.cnn.com/2004/ WORLD/meast/02/18/iran.train.disaster.ap/.

### February 2, 2001: Chesterton, Indiana

A fire at the Bethlehem Steel Corporation's Burns Harbor mill killed two people. Four millwrights were injured. At the time of the fire, workers were trying to remove a slip blind and a cracked valve from a coke-oven gas line that led to a decommissioned furnace. During the process, flammable liquid was released and ignited.

U.S. Chemical Safety and Hazard Investigation Board. CSB investigation information page. *Bethlehem Steel Corporation Gas Condensate Fire: Chesterton, IN, February 2, 2001.* Available at: http://www.csb.gov/index.cfm?folder=completed_investigations &page=info&INV_ID=19

### December 25, 2000: Luoyang, China

A shopping-plaza fire killed 309 people, most of whom were attending a Christmas party at an unlicensed disco.

National Fire Protection Association. *Public Assembly and Nightclub Fires. The 10 Deadliest Foreign (outside the U.S.) Nightclub Fires since 1970.* Available at: http://www.nfpa. org/itemDetail.asp?categoryID=851&itemID=21090&URL=Research%20&%20Reports/ Fact%20sheets/Safety%20in%20other%20occupancies/Nightclubs/ assembly%20occupancies/Public%20assembly%20and%20nightclub%20fires

### December 3, 1998: Manila, Philippines

A fire at the Catholic Bahay Kalinga orphanage killed at least 28 people.

CNN.com Asia-Pacific. *Fire Kills 28 at Manila Orphanage.* December 3, 1998. Available at: http://www.cnn.com/WORLD/asiapcf/9812/03/philippines.orphanage.02/index. html

### October 28, 1998: Gothenburg, Sweden

A fire rapidly spread through a dance hall, killing 63 people. It is thought that overcrowding, combustible storage, and the absence of a fire alarm system contributed to the fire's rapid spread and death toll.

National Fire Protection Association. Fire Investigations Department. *Fire Investigation Summary: Dance Hall Fire.* Available at: http://www.nfpa.org/assets/files/PDF/ gothenburg.pdf

### May 15, 1998: Jakarta, Indonesia

Hundreds of rioting looters died after being trapped in burning shopping malls.

*Days of Rage. May 15, 1998.* The NewsHour with Jim Lehrer transcript. Online News-Hour at PBS.org. Available at: http://www.pbs.org/newshour/bb/asia/jan-june98/indonesia_5-15.html

### March 26, 1998: Mombasa, Kenya

A school fire killed 24 teenaged girls while they were in their dormitory.

BBC News Africa. *Kenya Fire Kills 24 Teenagers.* March 26, 1998. Available at: http://news.bbc.co.uk/1/hi/world/africa/70253.stm

### March 19, 1996: Quezon City, Philippines

A fire at a local nightclub killed at least 149 people. Most of the victims were young partygoers who were celebrating the end of the school term.

Emergency Disaster Management, Inc. *Hazards and Disasters: Technological Events: Fire and Explosion: Entertainment Center/Restaurant/Nightclub/Discotheque Fires.* Available at: http://www.emergency-management.net/disco_fires.htm

### April 25, 1995: Urumqi, China

A fire at a karaoke club in the Xinjiang province killed 51 people.

National Fire Protection Association. *Public Assembly and Nightclub Fires: The 10 Deadliest Foreign (outside the U.S.) Nightclub Fires since 1970.* Available at: http://www.nfpa.org/itemDetail.asp?categoryID=851&itemID=21090&URL=Research%20&%20Reports/Fact%20sheets/Safety%20in%20other%20occupancies/Nightclubs/assembly%20occupancies/Public%20assembly%20and%20nightclub%20fires

### February 15, 1995: Taichung, Taiwan

A fire at the Weierkang Club killed 64 people. The site was a three-story structure containing a nightclub, restaurant, and karaoke bar.

National Fire Protection Association. *Public Assembly and Nightclub Fires: The 10 Deadliest Foreign (outside the U.S.) Nightclub Fires since 1970.* Available at: http://www.nfpa.org/itemDetail.asp?categoryID=851&itemID=21090&URL=Research%20&%20Reports/Fact%20sheets/Safety%20in%20other%20occupancies/Nightclubs/assembly%20occupancies/Public%20assembly%20and%20nightclub%20fires

### December 17, 1983: Madrid, Spain

A fire at the Alcala 20 disco killed 81 people.

National Fire Protection Association. *Public Assembly and Nightclub Fires: The 10 Deadliest Foreign (outside the U.S.) Nightclub Fires since 1970.* Available at: http://www.nfpa.org/itemDetail.asp?categoryID=851&itemID=21090&URL=Research%20&%20Reports/Fact%20sheets/Safety%20in%20other%20occupancies/Nightclubs/assembly%20occupancies/Public%20assembly%20and%20nightclub%20fires

### February 14, 1981: Dublin, Ireland, United Kingdom
A fire at the Stardust Night Club killed 48 people. When a reconstructed scenario was performed to determine why and how the fire spread so quickly, it was found that many toxic chemicals were produced in the atmosphere during the fire. It was presumed that the guests in the nightclub fire inhaled these chemicals. High concentrations of carbon monoxide, HCN, and HCl were all recorded in the reconstruction. Death was so rapid that the guests were unable to find an exit.

Davies JWL. Toxic chemicals versus lung tissue—an aspect of inhalation injury revisited. The Everett Idris Evans Memorial Lecture—1986. *J Burn Care Rehabil* 1986; 7(3):213–222.

### November 21, 1980: Las Vegas, Nevada
The MGM Grand Hotel and Casino experienced a raging fire that originated in the deli and quickly spread throughout the casino. Smoke filled the 26-story building and 85 people died. It was found that many of the people located on the upper floors died of inhaled products of combustion.

Clark County Fire Department. *The MGM Grand Hotel Fire Investigation Report.* Available at: http://www.co.clark.nv.us/fire/mgm_doc.htm

Cohen MA, Guzzardi LJ, et al. Inhalation of products of combustion. *Ann Emerg Med* 1983; 12:628–632.

Young MA. In: Catastrophes used as reference points in the manual. *The Community Crisis Response Team Training Manual.* 2nd ed. U.S. Department of Justice, Office for Victims of Crime and National Organization for Victims Assistance (NOVA). Available at: http://www.ojp.usdoj.gov/ovc/publications/infores/crt/appendd.htm

### August 20, 1978: Abadan, Iran
Arsonists set fire to a crowded theater, killing nearly 400 people.

National Fire Protection Association. *The 20 Deadliest Single-Building or Complex Fires and Explosions in U.S. History.* Available at: http://www.nfpa.org/itemDetail.asp?categoryID=954&itemID=23343&URL=Research%20&%20Reports/Fire%20statistics/Historical

### May 28, 1977: Southgate, Kentucky
A fire at the Beverly Hills Supper Club killed 165 people.

Young MA. In: Catastrophes used as reference points in the manual. *The Community Crisis Response Team Training Manual.* 2nd ed. U.S. Department of Justice, Office for Victims of Crime and National Organization for Victims Assistance (NOVA). Available at: http://www.ojp.usdoj.gov/ovc/publications/infores/crt/appendd.htm

### January 10, 1973: Isle of Mann, Scotland, United Kingdom

A fire at a Isle of Mann resort killed 50 people. Smoke and toxic gases were thought to be the predominant factor in the victims' deaths.

Einhorn IN. Physiological and toxicological aspects of smoke produced during the combustion of polymeric materials. *Environ Health Perspect* 1975, 11:163–189.

### May 2, 1972: Kellogg, Idaho

A fire at the Sunshine Mining Company killed 91 people. It is believed that smoke and toxic gases were a predominant factor in the deaths of the miners.

CDC and NIOSH Safety and Health Research. *Coal Mining Disasters.* Available at: http://www.cdc.gov/niosh/mining/statistics/discoal.htm. Accessed September 21, 2005.

Einhorn IN. Physiological and toxicological aspects of smoke produced during the combustion of polymeric materials. *Environ Health Perspect* 1975; 11:163–189.

### November 20, 1971: St. Laurent du Pont, France

A fire at Club Cinq killed 143 people.

National Fire Protection Association. *Public Assembly and Nightclub Fires: The 10 Deadliest Foreign (outside the U.S.) Nightclub Fires since 1970.* Available at: http://www.nfpa. org/itemDetail.asp?categoryID=851&itemID=21090&URL=Research%20&%20Reports/ Fact%20sheets/Safety%20in%20other%20occupancies/Nightclubs/ assembly%20occupancies/Public%20assembly%20and%20nightclub%20fires

### September 15, 1971: Salt Lake City, Utah

A fire in the Lil-Haven Nursing Home resulted in the deaths of six patients. The fire lasted about 10 minutes, and none of the victims showed signs of body burns. There was also no outward evidence of a fire, except for slight smoke damage under the roof. Smoke and soot patterns revealed signs of a fast-moving fire, and the fatalities were attributed to smoke and toxic gases.

Einhorn IN. Physiological and toxicological aspects of smoke produced during the combustion of polymeric materials. *Environ Health Perspect* 1975; 11:163–189.

### 1970: Marietta, Ohio

A fire at the Harmar House Nursing Home killed 22 elderly residents. Smoke and toxic gases were thought to be associated with the victims' deaths.

Einhorn IN. Physiological and toxicological aspects of smoke produced during the combustion of polymeric materials. *Environ Health Perspect* 1975; 11:163–189.

### March 6, 1968: Calumet, Louisiana

A fire at the Cargill Salt Mine killed 21 people.

CDC and NIOSH Safety and Health Research. *Coal Mining Disasters.* Available at: http://www.cdc.gov/niosh/mining/statistics/discoal.htm. Accessed September 21, 2005.

### July 29, 1967: North Vietnam
A fire on the *USS Forrestal* killed 134 people.

Freeman GA. *Sailors to the End: The Deadly Fire on the USS Forrestal and the Heroes Who Fought It.* New York: HarperCollins; 2002.

### November 1965: Salt Lake City, Utah
The crash of a United Airlines Boeing 727 jetliner at the Salt Lake City Airport killed 43 of the 91 passengers onboard. Smoke and toxic gases were thought to be associated with the victims' deaths. The fumes inside the cabin may have included burning polymeric materials (fibers, coatings, elastomers, foams). The Civil Aeronautics Board found the incident to be a "survivable crash with no fatalities on impact."

Einhorn IN. Physiological and toxicological aspects of smoke produced during the combustion of polymeric materials. *Environ Health Perspect* 1975; 11:163–189.

### November 23, 1963: Fitchville, Ohio
A fire at the Golden Age Nursing home killed 63 people.

National Fire Protection Association. *Deadliest Fires in U.S. Facilities for Older Adults since 1950.* Available at: http://www.nfpa.org/itemDetail.asp?categoryID=954&itemID=20732&URL=Research%20&%20Reports/Fire%20statistics/Historical&cookie%5Ftest=1

### December 1, 1958: Chicago, Illinois
A fire broke out at the base of a stair well at the Roman Catholic grade school Our Lady of the Angels, resulting in the deaths of 90 students and three nuns. An additional 77 victims were seriously injured when smoke, heat, and fire cut off escape routes.

Babcock CI. The Chicago school fire. *The Quarterly, National Fire Protection Association*; 1959. Available at: http://www.nfpa.org/assets/files/PDF/Research/LadyOfAngels.pdf

### July 16, 1950: Lark, Utah
A fire at a lead and zinc smelting plant killed five people.

CDC and NIOSH Safety and Health Research. *Coal Mining Disasters.* Available at: http://www.cdc.gov/niosh/mining/statistics/discoal.htm. Accessed September 21, 2005.

### April 5, 1949: Effingham, Illinois
A fire burned the St. Anthony's Hospital and killed 77 people.

Kacich T. The News-Gazette. *Hot Type: 150 Years of the Best Local Stories from the News-Gazette.* Sports-Publishing LLC; 2002: p. 182–183.

### December 7, 1946: Atlanta, Georgia
A fire in the Winecoff Hotel killed 119 people.

National Fire Protection Association. *The 20 Deadliest Single-Building or Complex Fires and Explosions in U.S. History.* Available at: http://www.nfpa.org/itemDetail.asp?categoryID=954&itemID=23343&URL=Research%20&%20Reports/Fire%20statistics/Historical

### July 6, 1944: Hartford, Connecticut

A fire broke out during a performance of the Ringling Bros. and Barnum & Bailey circus. As a result of the fire, 168 people died and 487 were injured. The flames moved rapidly along the tent canvas because it had been water-proofed with a mixture of gasoline and paraffin.

Kimball WY. Hartford Circus holocaust. *The Quarterly, National Fire Protection Association.* 1944. Available at: http://www.nfpa.org/assets/files/PDF/Hartfordcircus.pdf.

Hartford History. *The Circus Fire.* Available at: http://www.hartfordhistory.net/circus.html

### April 23, 1940: Natchez, Mississippi

A fire at the Rhythm Club dance hall killed 207 people.

National Fire Protection Association. *The 20 deadliest single-building or complex fires and explosions in U.S. history.* Available at: http://www.nfpa.org/itemDetail.asp?categoryID=954&itemID=23343&URL=Res

### April 21, 1930: Columbus, Ohio

A fire broke out in the Ohio State Penitentiary and killed 320 inmates.

National Fire Protection Association. *The 20 Deadliest Fires and Explosions in U.S. History.* Available at: http://www.nfpa.org/itemDetail.asp?categoryID=954&itemID=23340&URL=Research%20&%20Reports/Fire%20statistics/Historical

### March 4, 1908: Collinwood, Ohio

A fire at the Lakeview Grammar School killed 175 people, prompting the revision of school fire codes.

National Fire Protection Association. *The 20 Deadliest Single-Building or Complex Fires and Explosions in U.S. History.* Available at: http://www.nfpa.org/itemDetail.asp?categoryID=954&itemID=23343&URL=Research%20&%20Reports/Fire%20statistics/Historical

### January 12, 1908: Boyertown, Pennsylvania

One hundred seventy people attending a church-sponsored stage performance died in a fire at the Rhodes Opera House.

National Fire Protection Association. *The 20 Deadliest Single-Building or Complex Fires and Explosions in U.S. History.* Available at: http://www.nfpa.org/itemDetail.asp?categoryID=954&itemID=23343&URL=Research%20&%20Reports/Fire%20statistics/Historical

### June 15, 1904: New York City, New York

A fire aboard the *General Slocum* excursion steamship killed 1,030 people.

National Fire Protection Association. *The 20 Deadliest Fires and Explosions in U.S. History.* Available at: http://www.nfpa.org/itemDetail.asp?categoryID=954&itemID=23340&URL=Research%20&%20Reports/Fire%20statistics/Historical

### December 30, 1903: Chicago, Illinois

A fire at the Iroquois Theatre killed 602 people and injured 250 others. The fire may have been started by an open-arc spotlight touching a border drop. Most of the victims died from smoke inhalation or burns. Others were trampled in the panic.

A tragedy remembered. *National Fire Protection Association Journal* 1995; p. 75–79. Available at: http://www.nfpa.org/assets/files/PDF/iroquois.pdf

### June 30, 1900: Hoboken, New Jersey

A fire on the *North German Lloyd* steamship erupted, killing 326 people.

National Fire Protection Association. *The 20 Deadliest Fires and Explosions in U.S. History.* Available at: http://www.nfpa.org/itemDetail.asp?categoryID=954&itemID=23340&URL=Research%20&%20Reports/Fire%20statistics/Historical

### December 5, 1876: Brooklyn, New York

A fire in Conway's Theater killed 285 people.

National Fire Protection Association. *The 20 Deadliest Single-Building or Complex Fires and Explosions in U.S. History.* Available at: http://www.nfpa.org/itemDetail.asp?categoryID=954&itemID=23343&URL=Res

### October 8, 1871: Chicago, Illinois

A fire began in or near Patrick and Catherine O'Leary's barn in the southwestern section of Chicago. The fire, which was intensified by high winds, burned out of control for more than 24 hours. Rain finally extinguished the fire days later. Three and a half square miles of the city were destroyed and about 250 to 300 people died. Another 98,500 people were left homeless.

Chicago Public Library. *Chicago Timeline: 1871 The Great Fire.* Available at: http://www.chipublib.org/004chicago/timeline/greatfire.html

Chicago Historical Society and Academic Technologies of Northwestern University. *The Great Chicago Fire.* Available at: http://www.chicagohs.org/fire/intro/

### December 26, 1811: Richmond, Virginia

A fire at the Richmond Theater killed 160 people.

National Fire Protection Association. *The 20 Deadliest Single-Building or Complex Fires and Explosions in U.S. History.* Available at: http://www.nfpa.org/itemDetail.asp?categoryID=954&itemID=23343&URL=Res

### September 2, 1666: London, England, United Kingdom
The "Great Fire of London" destroyed a large proportion of London, including St. Paul's Cathedral. It is confirmed that six people died in the fire, which began in the shop of Thomas Farynor, the King's baker, in Pudding Lane.

London Brigade. *The Great of London.* Last update February 23, 2005. Available at: http://www.london-.gov.uk/about_us/our_history/the_great__of_london.asp

Pepys S. *The Diary of Samuel Pepys.* Le Gallienne R, ed. New York: Modern Library, Random House; 2001.

## Fireworks Explosion

### May 13, 2000: Enschede, Netherlands
A fireworks depot exploded, killing 20 people and injuring 589 others. It was estimated that 100 tons of fireworks material exploded, which destroyed 400 local residences.

Grimes RL, Nugteren A, Pettersson P, Zondag H, Post P, ed. *Disaster Ritual: Explorations of an Emerging Ritual Repertoire (Liturgia Condenda, 15).* 2003, Peeter, Bondgenotenlaan, Leuven.

CNN.com World. *Rescuers Search for More Victims from Deadly Dutch Fireworks Explosion.* May 13, 2000. Available at: http://archives.cnn.com/2000/WORLD/europe/05/13/netherlands.explosion.02/

## Fuel Explosion

### December 8, 1963: Elkton, Maryland
A jetliner was struck by lightning, causing three fuel tanks to explode. As a result, 81 people died. This has been the only documented case of a lightning-caused plane crash.

Uman MA. *All About Lightning.* Mineola, NY: Dover Publications Inc; 1986; p. 30.

## Gasoline Explosions

### January 25, 2005: Perth Amboy, New Jersey
Three workers were killed from a gas explosion at the Acetylene Service Company plant, where acetylene was produced, repackaged, and distributed for welding. The explosion originated near six large storage tanks that received liquid waste from the acetylene-generating system.

U.S. Chemical Safety and Hazard Investigation Board. CSB investigation information page. *Acetylene Service Company Gas Explosion: Perth Amboy, NJ, January 25, 2005.* Available at: http://www.csb.gov/index.cfm?folder=current_investigations&page=info&INV_ID=51

### April 8, 2004: Gallup, New Mexico
Highly flammable gasoline components were released and ignited from the Giant Industries Ciniza refinery when maintenance workers removed a malfunctioning pump from the hydrofluoric acid (HF) alkylation unit. A shut-off valve was not secured, leading to the release and subsequent explosions. Four workers were seriously injured.

U.S. Chemical Safety and Hazard Investigation Board. CSB investigation information page. *Giant Industries Refinery Explosions and Fire: Gallup, NM, April 8, 2004.* Available at: http://www.csb.gov/index.cfm?folder=completed_investigations&page=info& INV_ID=47

### January 25, 1999: Taylor, British Columbia, Canada
The town of Taylor was evacuated after a series of gas explosions at the Solex Gas Liquids plant. Fifteen people, mostly firefighters, were injured.

Public Safety and Emergency Preparedness Canada. *Canadian Disaster Database.* Available at: http://www.psepc-sppcc.gc.ca/red/em/cdd/search-em.asp. Accessed September 21, 2005.

### November 21, 1996: San Juan, Puerto Rico
An explosion occurred in a six-story building that was thought to be the result of leaking gas. Thirty-three people were killed and 69 people were injured.

National Transportation Safety Board. Pipeline Accident Report: San Juan Gas Company. PB97-916501; NTSB/PAR-97/01. Available at: http://www.ntsb.gov/ Publictn/1997/PAR9701.pdf

### July 6, 1988: North Sea (off of Scottish Coast)
Liquefied flammable gas escaped from a line on the *Piper Alpha* oil rig and ignited, causing an explosion that killed 167 people.

SafetyLine Institute of WorkSafe Western Australia. *The Piper Alpha Disaster.* Available at: http://www.safetyline.wa.gov.au/institute/level1/course6/lecture98/l98_02.asp

### 1984: Cubatao, Brazil
An explosion of a gasoline pipeline killed approximately 89 people and forced the evacuation of an additional 2,500 residents.

*UNEP-APELL Disasters Database.* Available at: http://www.uneptie.org/pc/apell/ disasters/disasters.html. Accessed September 21, 2005.

### November 19, 1984: St. J. Ixhuatepec, Mexico
An explosion of a gasoline (LPG) storage tank killed 500 people, injured at least 2,500, and forced the evacuation of more than 200,000 residents.

*UNEP-APELL Disasters Database.* Available at: http://www.uneptie.org/pc/apell/ disasters/disasters.html. Accessed September 21, 2005.

Health and Safety Executive (HYSE), Control of Major Accident Hazards (COMAH). Safety Report Assessment Guidance: Case Studies. *PEMEX LPG Terminal, Mexico City, Mexico. 19 November 1984.* Available at: http://www.hse.gov.uk/comah/stragtech/ casepemex84.htm

### 1983: Nile River, Egypt
There was an explosion during the transport of LPG gasoline, injuring 44 and killing 317 people.

*UNEP-APELL Disasters Database.* Available at: http://www.uneptie.org/pc/apell/ disasters/disasters.html. Accessed September 21, 2005.

### June 8, 1979: Franklin, Louisiana
A gas explosion at the Belle Isle Mine killed five people.

CDC and NIOSH Safety and Health Research. *Coal Mining Disasters.* Available at: http://www.cdc.gov/niosh/mining/statistics/discoal.htm. Accessed September 21, 2005.

### August 28, 1963: Moab, Utah
A gas explosion at the Texas Gulf Sulfur Company killed 18 people.

CDC and NIOSH Safety and Health Research. *Coal Mining Disasters.* Available at: http://www.cdc.gov/niosh/mining/statistics/discoal.htm. Accessed September 21, 2005.

### March 18, 1937: New London, Texas
A gas explosion at the Consolidated High School killed 294 schoolchildren and teachers. The explosion likely occurred as a result of leaking gas under the building. The arc of an electric switch in a training room ignited the explosion when a teacher plugged a connection into a wall socket located near an open door.

Smith HO. The London, Texas, school disaster. *The Quarterly, National Fire Protection Association* 1937; 30(4). Available at: http://www.nfpa.org/assets/files/PDF/Research/ LondonTexasSchool.pdf

### April 15, 1920: Delcambro, Louisiana
A gas explosion at the Jefferson Island salt mine killed six people.

CDC and NIOSH Safety and Health Research. *Coal Mining Disasters.* Available at: http://www.cdc.gov/niosh/mining/statistics/discoal.htm. Accessed September 21, 2005.

### November 28, 1910: Durant, Oklahoma
A gas explosion at the Jumbo asphalt mine killed 13 people.

CDC and NIOSH Safety and Health Research. *Coal Mining Disasters.* Available at: http://www.cdc.gov/niosh/mining/statistics/discoal.htm. Accessed September 21, 2005.

## Gold Mine Fires

### October 30, 1952: Herron, Michigan
A shaft explosion at Herron, Alpena Enterprises killed five people.

CDC and NIOSH Safety and Health Research. *Coal Mining Disasters.* Available at: http://www.cdc.gov/niosh/mining/statistics/discoal.htm. Accessed September 21, 2005.

### July 14, 1930: Placer County, California
A fire at the Glenn gold mine killed five people.

CDC and NIOSH Safety and Health Research. *Coal Mining Disasters.* Available at: http://www.cdc.gov/niosh/mining/statistics/discoal.htm. Accessed September 21, 2005.

### August 27, 1922: Jackson, California
A fire at the Argonaut gold mine killed 47 people.

CDC and NIOSH Safety and Health Research. *Coal Mining Disasters.* Available at: http://www.cdc.gov/niosh/mining/statistics/discoal.htm. Accessed September 21, 2005.

### September 20, 1873: Gold Hill, Nevada
A fire in the blacksmith forge at the Yellow Jacket gold mine killed six people.

CDC and NIOSH Safety and Health Research. *Coal Mining Disasters.* Available at: http://www.cdc.gov/niosh/mining/statistics/discoal.htm. Accessed September 21, 2005.

### April 8, 1873: Gold Hill, Nevada
A timber fire at the Kentucky-Yellow Jacket gold mine killed 37 people.

CDC and NIOSH Safety and Health Research. *Coal Mining Disasters.* Available at: http://www.cdc.gov/niosh/mining/statistics/discoal.htm. Accessed September 21, 2005.

## Gunpowder Explosions and/or Fires

### April 6, 1968: Virginia
Forty-one people were killed when stocks of gunpowder at a sporting-goods store exploded.

Martin M. *City Explosion Lives on in RHS Classroom.* Palladium-Item. April 6, 2005. Available at: http://www.pal-item.com/apps/pbcs.dll/article?AID=/20050406/NEWS01/504060304/1008.

### April 3, 1856: Rhodes, Greece
Gunpowder that had been left in the Palace of the Grand Masters exploded, blowing the top level off the church and resulting in the deaths of about 4,000 residents.

Metcalf K, Juris B. *A Short History of Rhodes.* Presented at: 9th Greek Australian Legal and Medical Conference: 2003; Rhodes, Greece. Available at: http://www.lmconference.com.au/papers/2003/kmetcalf.html

### August 18, 1769: Brescia, Italy
About one sixth of the town of Brescia was devastated when lightning struck the tower of Church of San Nazaire. Fire from the lightning strike ignited 20,000 pounds of gunpowder that were being held in the church. A massive explosion resulted, killing approximately 3,000 residents.

Krider EP. *Lightning and Gunpowder in the 18th Century.* Institute of Atmospheric Physics, The University of Arizona. Available at: www.meteohistory.org/2004polling_preprints/docs/abstracts/krider_abstract.pdf

## Hydrocarbon Explosions and/or Fires
### January 13, 2003: Rosharon, Texas
A vapor-cloud fire erupted at BLSR Operating Limited's oil field waste-disposal facility when two vacuum trucks were delivering flammable waste. Hydrocarbon vapor was released as the trucks were being unloaded, which sparked a vapor-cloud fire. Three people were fatally burned, and four other workers sustained serious burns.

U.S. Chemical Safety and Hazard Investigation Board. *Investigation Report: Vapor Cloud Deflagration and Fire.* Report No. 2003-06-I-TX. Washington, DC: CSB Investigation Board; 2003. Available at: http://www.csb.gov/completed_investigations/docs/BLSRFinalInvestigationReport.pdf

### April 22, 1992: Guadalajara, Mexico
An explosion caused by hydrocarbon oil and gas in the city sewers injured more than 1,500 people and killed 206 city residents.

*UNEP-APELL Disasters Database.* Available at: http://www.uneptie.org/pc/apell/disasters/disasters.html. Accessed September 21, 2005.

## Hydroxylamine Explosion
### February 19, 1999: Allentown, Pennsylvania
A process vessel containing hundreds of pounds of hydroxylamine exploded at Concept Sciences Incorporated's production facility while employees were distilling an aqueous solution of hydroxylamine and potassium

sulfate. Five people were killed, and two others survived with moderate to serious injuries. Four people in a nearby building were injured as well.

U.S. Chemical Safety and Hazard Investigation Board. CSB investigation information page. *Concept Sciences Hydroxylamine Explosion: Allentown, PA, February 19, 1999.* Available at: http://www.csb.gov/index.cfm?folder=completed_investigations& page=info&INV_ID=32

## Molasses Flood and Explosion

### January 15, 1919: Boston, Massachusetts

A tank of molasses exploded, killing 21 people and crumpling the steel support of an elevated train. The explosion may have been caused by a combination of fermentation, sudden rise in temperature, and inadequate storage tank. Buildings were knocked off their foundations or buried under two million gallons of molasses. Prior to the explosion, the owner of the tank, US Industrial Alcohol, dealt with warnings of structural problems by painting the tank brown to mask leaking molasses.

Mason J. The Molasses Disaster of January 15, 1919. *Yankee Magazine* January 1965: p. 52–53, 109–111.

Park E. Without Warning, Molasses in January Surged Over Boston. *Smithsonian* November 1983; 14(8):213–230.

Puleo S. *Dark Tide: The Great Boston Molasses Flood of 1919.* Boston: Beacon Press; 2003.

## Munitions Explosions

### August 1956: Cali, Colombia

Seven army ammunition trucks exploded, reportedly killing 1,100 people.

National Fire Protection Agency. *Important Dates in Fire History.* Available at: http://www.nfpa.org/itemDetail.asp?categoryID=954&itemID=23375&URL= Research%20&%20Reports/Fire%20statistics/Historical&cookie%5Ftest=1

### July 17, 1944: Port Chicago, California

Three hundred twenty-two people were killed when ships carrying ammunition collided, resulting in a major explosion.

National Fire Protection Association. *The 20 Deadliest Fires and Explosions in U.S. History.* Available at: http://www.nfpa.org/itemDetail.asp?categoryID=954&itemID= 23340&URL=Research%20&%20Reports/Fire%20statistics/Historical

### December 6, 1917: Halifax, Nova Scotia, Canada

A Belgian steamer collided with *Mont Blanc,* an ammunition ship carrying
more than 2,500 tons of explosive materials. The resulting explosion lev-
eled part of Halifax and killed approximately 1,600 people.

Etkin D, Hague CE, Brooks GR, eds. *An Assessment of Natural Hazards and Disasters in
Canada.* Norwell, MA: Springer/Kluwer; 2003: p. 443.

### April 10, 1917: Eddystone, Pennsylvania

An explosion in the Eddystone Ammunition Company plant killed 133 workers.

National Fire Protection Association. *The 20 Deadliest Single-Building or Complex Fires
and Explosions in U.S. History.* Available at: http://www.nfpa.org/itemDetail.asp?
categoryID=954&itemID=23343&URL=Research%20&%20Reports/Fire%20statistics/
Historical

## Natural Gas Explosions

### July 30, 2004: Ghislenghien, Belgium

A natural gas pipeline exploded, killing at least ten people and injuring 100 to
200 others. The blast occurred after construction workers pierced an underground gas line. Two nearby factories caught fire. The blast was seen
and felt several miles away.

CNN.com International Edition. *Deadly gas explosion rocks Belgium.* July 30, 2004.
Available at: http://edition.cnn.com/2004/WORLD/europe/07/30/belgium.gas.blast/
index.html

### 1989: Acha Ufa, Russia

An explosion of a liquefied, natural-gas pipeline killed approximately 500 to
575 people when two Trans-Siberian Railroad trains were engulfed by fire.

United Nations Economic and Social Council, Economic Commission for Europe
Committee on Environmental Policy: Draft Chapter on Technological and Natural
Hazards. September 20, 2002.

## Nitric Oxide Explosion

### September 21, 2003: Miami Township, Ohio

An underground distillation tower at the Isotec chemical manufacturing plant
was destroyed by a violent explosion that ruptured a carbon monoxide gas
pipe, forcing the evacuation of 2,000 nearby residents. The Isotec plant produced rare forms of oxygen and nitrogen utilized in medicine and research.

U.S. Chemical Safety and Hazard Investigation Board. CSB investigation information
page. *Isotec/Sigma Aldrich Nitric Oxide Explosion: Miami Township, OH, September 21,
2003.* Available at: http://www.csb.gov/index.cfm?folder=completed_investigations
&page=info&INV_ID=43

## Nitrogen Dioxide and Hydrogen Cyanide Fire

### *1929: Cleveland, Ohio*

A fire in the radiology department of the Cleveland Clinic caused 125 casualties. The fire consumed 50,000 nitrocellulose x-ray films. Ninety-seven workers died immediately, and 26 delayed fatalities may have been a result of nitrogen dioxide-induced pulmonary changes.

Gregory KL, Malinoski VF, et al. Cleveland Clinic Fire Survivorship Study, 1929–1965. *Arch Environ Health* 1969; 18:508–515.

## Oil Explosions and/or Fires

### *August 9, 1999: Calgary, Alberta, Canada*

A series of explosions at Hub Oil, an oil recycling plant in Calgary, ignited a fire that forced the evacuation of 2,000 local residents. The fire released toxic, oily smoke into the environment.

Public Safety and Emergency Preparedness Canada. *Canadian Disaster Database.* Available at: http://www.psepc-sppcc.gc.ca/red/em/cdd/search-em.asp. Accessed September 21, 2005.

### *1998: Jesse, Nigeria*

An oil pipeline exploded, killing more than 500 people instantly. Hundreds more were severely burned. The resulting fire spread to nearby villages, engulfing Moosqar and Oghara and killing sleeping farmers and residents. Authorities believe the pipeline was intentionally punctured.

*Nigerian pipeline blast kills hundreds.* The Michigan Daily. October 20, 1998. Available at: http://www.pub.umich.edu/daily/1998/oct/10-20-98/news/news13.html

## Overpressurization Explosions and/or Fires

### *March 23, 2005: Texas City, Texas*

Fifteen workers were killed and 100 others injured as a result of a massive explosion at the BP Texas City refinery. The blast originated in the plant's isomerization unit. Many of the victims were located near an atmospheric vent stack when the explosions occurred. A distillation tower overpressurized once it became flooded with hydrocarbons and resulted in a geyserlike release.

U.S. Chemical Safety and Hazard Investigation Board. CSB investigation information page. *BP America Refinery Explosion: Texas City, TX, March 23, 2005.* Available at: http://www.csb.gov/index.cfm?folder=current_investigations&page=info&INV_ID=52

### April 11, 2003: Louisville, Kentucky

One worker was killed at the D.D. Williamson food additive plant. A process vessel became overpressurized and catastrophically failed. The failure released aqueous ammonia, and caused extensive physical damage.

U.S. Chemical Safety and Hazard Investigation Board. CSB investigation information page. *D.D. Williamson & Co. Catastrophic Vessel Failure: Louisville, KY, April 11, 2003.* Available at: http://www.csb.gov/index.cfm?folder=completed_investigations&page=info&INV_ID=36

### March 4, 1998: Pitkin, Louisiana

A major vessel failed and fire erupted on the Temple 22-1 Common Point Separation Facility owned by Sonta Exploration Co. The vessel ruptured from overpressurization during start-up. This released flammable material that then ignited, killing four workers and significantly damaging the property.

U.S. Safety and Hazard Investigation Board. CSB investigation information page. *Son at Exploration Co. Catastrophic Vessel Overpressurization: Pitkin, LA, March 4, 1998.* Available at: http://www.csb.gov/index.cfm?folder=completed_investigations&page=index

## Petroleum Fire

### February 23, 1999: Martinez, California

A petroleum fire in the crude unit at Tosco Corporation's Avon refinery occurred when workers attempted to replace piping attached to a fractionator tower while the process unit was in operation. Naptha was released onto the hot fractionator and ignited. The flames engulfed five workers; four were killed and one sustained serious injury.

U.S. Chemical Safety and Hazard Investigation Board. CSB investigation information page. *Tosco Avon Refinery Petroleum Naphtha Fire: Martinez, CA, February 23, 1999.* Available at: http://www.csb.gov/index.cfm?folder=completed_investigations&page=info&INV_ID=22

## Phenolic Resin Explosion

### February 20, 2003: Corbin, Kentucky

An explosion and fire at the CTA Acoustics manufacturing plant fatally injured seven workers. The plant produced fiberglass insulation for the automotive industry. Accumulation of resin dust in a production area likely ignited from a malfunctioning oven. The resin was a phenolic binder used to produce fiberglass mats.

U.S. Chemical Safety and Hazard Investigation Board. CSB investigation information page. *CTA Acoustics Dust Explosion and Fire: Corbin, KY, February 20, 2003.* Available at: http://www.csb.gov/index.cfm?folder=completed_investigations&page=info&INV_ID=35

## Plastics Explosions and/or Fires

### April 23, 2004: Illiopolis, Illinois

An explosion in a PVC production unit at Formosa Plastics occurred after the release of highly flammable vinyl chloride, which ignited. A water deluge system, designed to flood the work area with water in case of vinyl chloride release, failed to operate. Five workers were killed, and others seriously injured. The explosion also forced evacuation of the local community.

U.S. Chemical Safety and Hazard Investigation Board. CSB News Release. *CSB Investigation of Formosa Accident Continues; Agency Analyzes Evidence Determining Root Causes.* Available at: http://www.csb.gov/index.cfm?folder=news_releases&page=news&NEWS_ID=215

### January 29, 2003: Kinston, North Carolina

An explosion and fire at the West Pharmaceutical Services plant killed six workers and injured dozens more. The explosion was fueled by a fine plastic powder that accumulated over a suspended ceiling located in the manufacturing area of the plant. The plant was destroyed, putting hundreds of people out of work.

U.S. Chemical Safety and Hazard Investigation Board. CSB investigation information page. *West Pharmaceutical Services Dust Explosion and Fire: Kinston, NC, January 29, 2003.* Available at: http://www.csb.gov/index.cfm?folder=completed_investigations&page=info&INV_ID=34

### March 13, 2001: Augusta, Georgia

Three workers were killed when they opened a pressurized process vessel containing hot plastic at the BP Amoco Polymers plant. The partially unbolted cover blew off the vessel, which expelled hot plastic and caused the workers' deaths. Nearby tubing subsequently broke from the force of the release, and hot fluid ignited a fire.

U.S. Chemical Safety and Hazard Investigation Board. CSB investigation information page. *BP Amoco Thermal Decomposition Incident: Augusta, GA, March 13, 2001.* Available at: http://www.csb.gov/index.cfm?folder=completed_investigations&page=info&INV_ID=2

### January 6, 1970: Washington, DC, Navy Yard

A copy-machine fire started on the sixth floor of an office building. The machine was made of plastic and Teflon parts; the fire was quickly put out. The responding firefighters carried masks with them to the scene, but since the smoke and fire were not excessive, the masks were not used. The firefighters reported constricting tightness in their chests, accompanied by a burning sensation. Dyspnea persisted for 24 hours, at which time a 33-year-old firefighter fainted and later died. A Washington, DC, clinical study investigating exposure to thermal degradation of polyvinyl chloride (PVC) from 1970 to 1975 showed that 170 people exposed one to four times to these products showed signs of acute toxicity within a few hours of exposure. These include pain in the anterior aspect of the chest, neck/throat pain, dyspnea, headache, dizziness, and irregular pulse. Degradation of PVC products results in the formation of at least 75 potentially toxic compounds, including hydrogen chloride.

Dyer RF, Esch VH. Polyvinyl chloride toxicity in fires. Hydrogen chloride toxicity in fire fighters. *JAMA* 1976; 235(4):393–397.

## Propane Explosions

### April 9, 1998: Albert City, Iowa

An 18,000-gallon propane tank exploded at the Herrig Brothers farm, killing two volunteer firefighters and injuring seven other emergency personnel.

U.S. Chemical Safety and Hazard Investigation Board. CSB investigation information page. *Herrig Brothers Farm Propane Tank Explosion: Albert City, IA, April 9, 1998* Available at: http://www.csb.gov/index.cfm?folder=completed_investigations&page=info&INV_ID=31

### December 21, 1992: St. John's, Canada

A major fire sparked a series of propane-tank explosions and forced 500 people to evacuate.

Public Safety and Emergency Preparedness Canada. *Canadian Disaster Database.* Available at: http://www.psepc-sppcc.gc.ca/red/em/cdd/search-em.asp. Accessed September 21, 2005.

## Pyrotechnic Fire

### February 20, 2003: West Warwick, Rhode Island

More than 300 people were attending a rock concert at The Station nightclub. As the band opened, sparks from a pyrotechnic display ignited the walls and ceiling. A fire ensued, spread at a high velocity, and cut the crowd off from the front exit. One hundred people died and more than 200 were injured.

Dunbar JA. The Rhode Island nightclub fire: the story from the perspective of an on-duty ED nurse. *J Emerg Nurs* 2004; 30;464–466.

## Quarry Explosions

### August 31, 1938: Asheville, North Carolina

Detonation of dynamite at the Asheville Quarry caused an explosion that killed five people.

CDC and NIOSH Safety and Health Research. *Coal Mining Disasters.* Available at: http://www.cdc.gov/niosh/mining/statistics/discoal.htm. Accessed September 21, 2005.

### February 19, 1937: Walkermine, California
Detonation of explosives at the Walker copper quarry killed six people.

CDC and NIOSH Safety and Health Research. *Coal Mining Disasters.* Available at: http://www.cdc.gov/niosh/mining/statistics/discoal.htm. Accessed September 21, 2005.

### November 30, 1936: Delta, Pennsylvania
Detonation of explosives at the Funkhouser slate quarry killed nine people.

CDC and NIOSH Safety and Health Research. *Coal Mining Disasters.* Available at: http://www.cdc.gov/niosh/mining/statistics/discoal.htm. Accessed September 21, 2005.

### November 12, 1934: Avalon, California
Detonation of explosives at the Rohl Connolly granite quarry killed nine people.

CDC and NIOSH Safety and Health Research. *Coal Mining Disasters.* Available at: http://www.cdc.gov/niosh/mining/statistics/discoal.htm. Accessed September 21, 2005.

### February 27, 1922: Strawplains, Tennessee
An explosion at the Holston marble quarry killed nine people.

CDC and NIOSH Safety and Health Research. *Coal Mining Disasters.* Available at: http://www.cdc.gov/niosh/mining/statistics/discoal.htm. Accessed September 21, 2005.

### May 17, 1930: Union, West Virginia
Detonation of explosives at the Terry & Butterskill rock quarry killed six people.

CDC and NIOSH Safety and Health Research. *Coal Mining Disasters.* Available at: http://www.cdc.gov/niosh/mining/statistics/discoal.htm. Accessed September 21, 2005.

### August 13, 1920: Pounding Mills, Virginia
Detonation of explosive materials at the Pounding Mills rock quarry killed nine people.

CDC and NIOSH Safety and Health Research. *Coal Mining Disasters.* Available at: http://www.cdc.gov/niosh/mining/statistics/discoal.htm. Accessed September 21, 2005.

### April 19, 1920: Ormrod, Pennsylvania
Detonation of explosives at the Lehigh limestone quarry killed six people.

CDC and NIOSH Safety and Health Research. *Coal Mining Disasters.* Available at: http://www.cdc.gov/niosh/mining/statistics/discoal.htm. Accessed September 21, 2005.

### June 2, 1910: West Coplay, Pennsylvania
An explosion at the Lehigh limestone quarry killed eight people.

CDC and NIOSH Safety and Health Research. *Coal Mining Disasters.* Available at: http://www.cdc.gov/niosh/mining/statistics/discoal.htm. Accessed September 21, 2005.

### June 1, 1910: Devils Slide, Utah
An explosion at the Union limestone quarry killed 25 people.

CDC and NIOSH Safety and Health Research. *Coal Mining Disasters.* Available at: http://www.cdc.gov/niosh/mining/statistics/discoal.htm. Accessed September 21, 2005.

### April 13, 1910: Nazareth, Pennsylvania
An explosion at a limestone quarry killed 11 people.

CDC and NIOSH Safety and Health Research. *Coal Mining Disasters.* Available at: http://www.cdc.gov/niosh/mining/statistics/discoal.htm. Accessed September 21, 2005.

## Terrorist Explosions

### July 7, 2005: London, England, United Kingdom
A series of coordinated terrorist bombs detonated, targeting the transport system of the city. At least 54 people were killed and approximately 700 injured. Three bombs exploded on underground subway trains and one on a double-decker bus.

Lockey DJ, MacKenzie R, Redhead J, et al. London bombings July 2005: the immediate pre-hospital medical response. *Resuscitation* 2005; 66(2):ix–xii.

### February 9, 2005: Madrid, Spain
A car bomb exploded several hundred meters from Madrid's convention center, injuring 43 people. The explosion occurred hours before the Spanish king and queen and visiting Mexican president were to inaugurate an art fair. Basque separatists took responsibility. The car was reported to have been packed with 66 pounds of explosives.

Goodman A. *Madrid Car Bomb: 43 Injured.* CNN.com World. February 9, 2005. Available at: http://www.cnn.com/2005/WORLD/europe/02/09/spain.blast/index.html

### January 30, 2005: Madrid, Spain
A bomb exploded in the resort Hotel Port Denia located in southwest Spain, injuring one person. A telephone warning was placed from the Basque separatist group ETA. The bomb was detonated in the resort's courtyard. The hotel was immediately evacuated before the explosion, which occurred two days before a Parliament debate on independence for the Basque region.

Goodman A. *Explosion Targets Spanish Hotel.* CNN.com World; January 30, 2005. Available at: http://www.cnn.com/2005/WORLD/europe/01/30/spain.blast/index.html

### January 19, 2005: Baghdad, Iraq
At least 26 people died after a series of explosions occurred in and around
  Baghdad. A group led by Al-Qaeda ally Abu Musab al-Zarqawi took responsibility for a truck-bomb explosion outside the Australian embassy, as
  well as three other suicide bombings in Iraq. The other three bombings occurred at police stations in eastern Baghdad, in a central Haifa street, and
  at a U.S. convoy near the international airport in Baghdad.

Guardian Unlimited Special Reports. *26 Killed in Baghdad Blasts.* January 19, 2005.
Available at: http://www.guardian.co.uk/Iraq/Story/0,2763,1393695,00.html

### September 9, 2004: Jakarta, Indonesia
A car bomb exploded outside the Australian embassy in Jakarta, killing nine
  people and injuring 182 others. Unknown suicide attackers detonated a
  Daihatsu van that was filled with explosives and fertilizer outside the embassy building.

Bowden R. *Jakarta Embassy Bombing Re-Focuses Election Campaigns.* Worldpress.org;
September 13, 2004. Available at: http://www.worldpress.org/Asia/1936.cfm

### August 5, 2004: Jakarta, Indonesia
Jakarta's Marriott hotel exploded, killing 12 people and injuring 150 others,
  when a suicide bomber detonated explosives. The same group, Jemaah
  Islamiyah was blamed for the 2002 nightclub blasts in Bali.

CNN.com World. *Malaysian Held over Marriott Blast.* March 1, 2004. Available at:
http://www.cnn.com/2004/WORLD/asiapcf/03/01/marriott.arrest/index.html.

### March 11, 2004: Madrid, Spain
A series of ten coordinated bombings occurred on the commuter-railroad system in Madrid. The explosions happened during rush hour, when four
  trains experienced on-board explosions. One hundred ninety-one people
  died and more than 1,800 people were injured. An additional three bombs
  were deactivated, and all the devices were thought to have been concealed
  in backpacks. Evidence pointed to the involvement of extremist Islamic
  groups, not the ETA Basque group as originally thought.

de Ceballos JP, Turegano-Fuentes F, Perez-Diaz D, et al. 11 March 2004: The terrorist
bomb explosions in Madrid, Spain—an analysis of the logistics, injuries sustained and
clinical management of casualties treated at the closest hospital. *Crit Care* 2005; 9(1):
104–111.

### December 31, 2003: Baghdad, Iraq
Eight people died and 35 were wounded when a car bomb exploded outside a
  Baghdad restaurant.

United States Army. *Timeline of Terrorism: 2004–2000.* Last updated January 18, 2006.
Available at: http://www.army.mil/terrorism/2004-2000/index.html

### November 20, 2003: Istanbul, Turkey
A car bomb exploded outside the British Consulate, killing 30 people, including the consul general. Four hundred fifty others were injured.

U.S. Department of State, Office of the Coordinator for Counterterrorism. *Patterns of Global Terrorism. Appendix A: Chronology of Significant International Terrorist Incidents, 2003.* Washington, DC: Office of the Coordinator for Counterterrorism; 2004. Available at: http://www.globalsecurity.org/security/library/report/2004/pgt_2003/pgt_2003_33773pf.htm

### November 15, 2003: Bogotá, Colombia
Grenades exploded in both the Bogotá Beer Company and Palos De Moguer Bar, killing one and wounding 72 people.

U.S. Department of State, Office of the Coordinator for Counterterrorism. *Patterns of Global Terrorism. Appendix A: Chronology of Significant International Terrorist Incidents, 2003.* Washington, DC: Office of the Coordinator for Counterterrorism; 2004. Available at: http://www.globalsecurity.org/security/library/report/2004/pgt_2003/pgt_2003_33773pf.htm

### November 15, 2003: Istanbul, Turkey
Sixteen people died and 240 others were injured at the Never Shalom synagogue after a car bomb exploded. Another explosion at the Beth Israel synagogue killed four and wounded 60 people.

U.S. Department of State, Office of the Coordinator for Counterterrorism. *Patterns of Global Terrorism. Appendix A: Chronology of Significant International Terrorist Incidents, 2003.* Washington, DC: Office of the Coordinator for Counterterrorism; 2004. Available at: http://www.globalsecurity.org/security/library/report/2004/pgt_2003/pgt_2003_33773pf.htm

### October 12, 2003: Baghdad, Iraq
Six people died and 32 were wounded when two car bombs exploded outside the Baghdad Hotel.

United States Army. *Timeline of Terrorism: 2004–2000.* Last updated January 18, 2006. Available at:http://www.army.mil/terrorism/2004-2000/index.html

### August 25, 2003: Mumbai, India
Two explosions occurred at the Mumba Devi temple and the historical site Gateway of India. The bombs killed 40 and injured 120 people.

U.S. Department of State, Office of the Coordinator for Counterterrorism. *Patterns of Global Terrorism. Appendix A: Chronology of Significant International Terrorist Incidents, 2003.* Washington, DC: Office of the Coordinator for Counterterrorism; 2004. Available at: http://www.globalsecurity.org/security/library/report/2004/pgt_2003/pgt_2003_33773pf.htm

### August 19, 2003: Baghdad, Iraq

A truck bomb exploded outside the Canal Hotel, which housed the United
Nations headquarters in Iraq. Twenty-three people died, including three
U.S. citizens. One hundred others were wounded in the attack.

U.S. Department of State, Office of the Coordinator for Counterterrorism. *Patterns of Global Terrorism. Appendix A: Chronology of Significant International Terrorist Incidents, 2003.* Washington, DC: Office of the Coordinator for Counterterrorism; 2004. Available at: http://www.globalsecurity.org/security/library/report/2004/pgt_2003/pgt_2003_33773pf.htm

### August 2, 2003: Baghdad, Iraq

A car bomb exploded outside the Jordanian Embassy. Nineteen people died
and 50 others were wounded.

U.S. Department of State, Office of the Coordinator for Counterterrorism. *Patterns of Global Terrorism. Appendix A: Chronology of Significant International Terrorist Incidents, 2003.* Washington, DC: Office of the Coordinator for Counterterrorism; 2004. Available at: http://www.globalsecurity.org/security/library/report/2004/pgt_2003/pgt_2003_33773pf.htm

### July 23, 2003: Katra, India

An explosion near a Hindu temple killed six people. The explosion was suspected to be linked to extremist groups located in India.

U.S. Department of State, Office of the Coordinator for Counterterrorism. *Patterns of Global Terrorism. Appendix A: Chronology of Significant International Terrorist Incidents, 2003.* Washington, DC: Office of the Coordinator for Counterterrorism; 2004. Available at: http://www.globalsecurity.org/security/library/report/2004/pgt_2003/pgt_2003_33773pf.htm

### June 7, 2003: Kabul, Afghanistan

A taxi filled with explosives deliberately hit a bus that was taking German
peacekeeping personnel to the airport. Five people on the bus died and 29
were injured.

U.S. Department of State, Office of the Coordinator for Counterterrorism. *Patterns of Global Terrorism. Appendix A: Chronology of Significant International Terrorist Incidents, 2003.* Washington, DC: Office of the Coordinator for Counterterrorism; 2004. Available at: http://www.globalsecurity.org/security/library/report/2004/pgt_2003/pgt_2003_33773pf.htm

## *May 19, 2003: Jerusalem, Israel*
A suicide bomber attacked a commuter bus, killing seven people and wounding 26 others in the explosion. The bomber had been disguised as an Orthodox Jew. Islamic Resistance Movement (HAMAS) claimed responsibility for the bombing.

U.S. Department of State, Office of the Coordinator for Counterterrorism. *Patterns of Global Terrorism. Appendix A: Chronology of Significant International Terrorist Incidents, 2003*. Washington. DC: Office of the Coordinator for Counterterrorism; 2004. Available at: http://www.globalsecurity.org/security/library/report/2004/pgt_2003/pgt_2003_33773pf.htm

## *May 16, 2003: Casablanca, Morocco*
Five bombs exploded within minutes of each other, occurring at a Jewish cemetery and community center, a restaurant and hotel, and the Belgian consulate. Thirty-three people died and 101 were injured. The Salafiya Jihadiya extremist group claimed responsibility for the orchestrated attacks.

U.S. Department of State, Office of the Coordinator for Counterterrorism. *Patterns of Global Terrorism. Appendix A: Chronology of Significant International Terrorist Incidents, 2003*. Washington, DC: Office of the Coordinator for Counterterrorism; 2004. Available at: http://www.globalsecurity.org/security/library/report/2004/pgt_2003/pgt_2003_33773pf.htm

## *May 12, 2003: Riyadh, Saudi Arabia*
Thirty people were killed at various western and international housing complexes in three separate suicide-bombing attacks.

U.S. Department of State, Office of the Coordinator for Counterterrorism. *Patterns of Global Terrorism. Appendix A: Chronology of Significant International Terrorist Incidents, 2003*. Washington, DC: Office of the Coordinator for Counterterrorism; 2004. Available at: http://www.globalsecurity.org/security/library/report/2004/pgt_2003/pgt_2003_33773pf.htm

## *April 30, 2003: Tel Aviv, Israel*
Suicide bombers from the Islamic Resistance Movement (HAMAS) and Al-Aqsa Martyrs Brigade attacked a pub near the US Embassy, and the resulting explosion killed three Israelis and injured 64 others.

U.S. Department of State, Office of the Coordinator for Counterterrorism. *Patterns of Global Terrorism. Appendix A: Chronology of Significant International Terrorist Incidents, 2003*. Washington, DC: Office of the Coordinator for Counterterrorism; 2004. Available at: http://www.globalsecurity.org/security/library/report/2004/pgt_2003/pgt_2003_33773pf.htm

### April 24, 2003: Kefar Saba, Israel

A suicide bomber from the Al-Aqsa Martyrs Brigade attacked a busy train station, and the resulting explosion killed a security guard. Eleven other people were injured.

U.S. Department of State, Office of the Coordinator for Counterterrorism. *Patterns of Global Terrorism. Appendix A: Chronology of Significant International Terrorist Incidents, 2003*. Washington, DC: Office of the Coordinator for Counterterrorism; 2004. Available at: http://www.globalsecurity.org/security/library/report/2004/pgt_2003/pgt_2003_33773pf.htm

### April 22, 2003: Kashmir, India

A bomb exploded at a dairy facility in Gulshanpora Batagund. Six people were killed and 12 injured.

U.S. Department of State, Office of the Coordinator for Counterterrorism. *Patterns of Global Terrorism. Appendix A: Chronology of Significant International Terrorist Incidents, 2003*. Washington, DC: Office of the Coordinator for Counterterrorism; 2004. Available at: http://www.globalsecurity.org/security/library/report/2004/pgt_2003/pgt_2003_33773pf.htm

### April 2, 2003: Davao, Philippines

An explosion on a passenger wharf killed 16 people and injured 55 others. The ammonium-nitrate bomb was believed to be detonated by members of the Jemaah Islamiyah. Suspects told officials they were also involved in the bombing of the Davao airport.

U.S. Department of State, Office of the Coordinator for Counterterrorism. *Patterns of Global Terrorism. Appendix A: Chronology of Significant International Terrorist Incidents, 2003*. Washington, DC: Office of the Coordinator for Counterterrorism; 2004. Available at: http://www.globalsecurity.org/security/library/report/2004/pgt_2003/pgt_2003_33773pf.htm

### March 26, 2003: Kashmir, India

An oil tanker exploded outside a Narwal fuel storage facility and was engulfed by flames. The bomb killed one person and wounded six others.

U.S. Department of State, Office of the Coordinator for Counterterrorism. *Patterns of Global Terrorism. Appendix A: Chronology of Significant International Terrorist Incidents, 2003*. Washington, DC: Office of the Coordinator for Counterterrorism; 2004. Available at: http://www.globalsecurity.org/security/library/report/2004/pgt_2003/pgt_2003_33773pf.htm

### March 20, 2003: Sidon, Lebanon

An explosion that ripped through an apartment complex killed two people and injured nine others. The bomb, consisting of approximately two kilograms of TNT, was detonated on the steps of a first-floor stairway and damaged three apartments and several cars in the surrounding area. It was thought that the attackers were targeting a Dutch woman who lived in the complex with her Lebanese husband.

U.S. Department of State, Office of the Coordinator for Counterterrorism. *Patterns of Global Terrorism. Appendix A: Chronology of Significant International Terrorist Incidents, 2003*. Washington, DC: Office of the Coordinator for Counterterrorism; 2004. Available at: http://www.globalsecurity.org/security/library/report/2004/pgt_2003/pgt_2003_33773pf.htm

### March 13, 2003: Kashmir, India
An explosion on a bus killed four people at a bus terminal in Rajouri.

U.S. Department of State, Office of the Coordinator for Counterterrorism. *Patterns of Global Terrorism. Appendix A: Chronology of Significant International Terrorist Incidents, 2003*. Washington, DC: Office of the Coordinator for Counterterrorism; 2004. Available at: http://www.globalsecurity.org/security/library/report/2004/pgt_2003/pgt_2003_33773pf.htm

### March 11, 2003: Kashmir, India
A bomb exploded in a Rajouri candy store. Two people were killed and nine others wounded.

U.S. Department of State, Office of the Coordinator for Counterterrorism. *Patterns of Global Terrorism. Appendix A: Chronology of Significant International Terrorist Incidents, 2003*. Washington, DC: Office of the Coordinator for Counterterrorism; 2004. Available at: http://www.globalsecurity.org/security/library/report/2004/pgt_2003/pgt_2003_33773pf.htm

### March 5, 2003: Haifa, Israel
Fifteen people died and 40 were wounded after a suicide bombing occurred on a commuter bus.

United States Army. *Timeline of Terrorism: 2004–2000*. Last updated January 18, 2006. Available at: http://www.army.mil/terrorism/2004-2000/index.html

### March 4, 2003: Davao, Philippines
A bomb exploded in an airport terminal, killing 21 people and wounding 149 others.

U.S. Department of State, Office of the Coordinator for Counterterrorism. Patterns of Global Terrorism. *Appendix A: Chronology of Significant International Terrorist Incidents, 2003*. Washington, DC: Office of the Coordinator for Counterterrorism; 2004. Available at: http://www.globalsecurity.org/security/library/report/2004/pgt_2003/pgt_2003_33773pf.htm

### February 25, 2003: Caracas, Venezuela

Four people were wounded when two bombs were detonated within minutes of each other, damaging the Spanish and Colombian embassies.

U.S. Department of State, Office of the Coordinator for Counterterrorism. Patterns of Global Terrorism. Appendix A: *Chronology of Significant International Terrorist Incidents, 2003*. Washington, DC: Office of the Coordinator for Counterterrorism; 2004. Available at: http://www.globalsecurity.org/security/library/report/2004/pgt_2003/pgt_2003_33773pf.htm

### October 12, 2002: Kuta, Bali

An electronically triggered bomb exploded in Paddy's bar, forcing the injured into the streets. About 10-15 seconds later, a second car bomb exploded in front of the Sari Club. Two hundred two people were killed, with the majority being Australian citizens.

Australian Government; Attorney-General's Department; Emergency Management Australia. *EMA Disasters Database*. Available at: http://www.ema.gov.au/ema/emadisasters.nsf/0/aa511e8a1fc9399fca256d670018f528?OpenDocument

### July 31, 2002: Jerusalem, Israel

Nine people died and 87 were injured when a hidden bomb exploded at the Frank Sinatra International Student Center of the Hebrew University. The dead and wounded included several nationalities. The Islamic Resistance Movement (HAMAS) claimed responsibility for the attack.

United States Army. *Timeline of Terrorism: 2004–2000*. Last updated January 18, 2006. Available at: http://www.army.mil/terrorism/2004-2000/index.html

### June 14, 2002: Karachi, Pakistan

An al-Qaeda-linked car bomb exploded outside the US Consulate. Eleven people were killed and 51 people wounded as a result of the explosion.

United States Army. *Timeline of Terrorism: 2004–2000*. Last updated January 18, 2006. Available at: http://www.army.mil/terrorism/2004-2000/index.html

### March 20, 2002: Lima, Peru

Nine people died and 32 were wounded after a car bomb exploded outside a shopping center located near the US Embassy.

United States Army. *Timeline of Terrorism: 2004–2000*. Last updated January 18, 2006. Available at: http://www.army.mil/terrorism/2004-2000/index.html

### September 11, 2001: New York City, New York; Washington, DC; and Pennsylvania

Terrorists destroyed the World Trade Center by flying hijacked Boeing 767 airplanes into each of the towers. Each plane released approximately 10,000 gallons of jet fuel into the buildings, causing the temperature to reach 14,000°F. The south tower collapsed 57 minutes after being hit; the north tower collapsed 29 minutes later. Of the estimated 1,450 people who were in the tower above the planes' entry, only four escaped. The official death toll in New York reached 2,752. A third hijacked plane crashed into the Pentagon, and a fourth, believed to be heading for a Washington, DC target, crashed into a field in Pennsylvania. The combined attacks killed a total of 3,025 US citizens. Many foreign nationals were also killed.

Kirschenbaum L, Keene A, O'Neill P, Westfal R, Astiz ME. The experience at St. Vincent's Hospital, Manhattan, on September 11, 2001: Preparedness, response, and lessons learned. *Crit Care Med* 2005; 33(1 Suppl):S48–S52.

United States Army. *Timeline of Terrorism: 2004–2000*. Last updated January 18, 2006. Available at: http://www.army.mil/terrorism/2004-2000/index.html

### October 12, 2000: Aden, Yemen

US Navy destroyer *USS Cole* was extensively damaged when a small boat, loaded with explosive material, blew up alongside the destroyer. Seventeen sailors died in this terrorist attack.

U.S. Department of State; USINFO; International Security—Response to Terrorism. *Attack on USS Cole*. Available at: http://usinfo.state.gov/is/international_security/terrorism/uss_cole.html

### October 18, 1998: Colombia

Seventy-one people were killed and 100 others injured when a bomb exploded on the Ocensa pipeline. The National Liberation Army (ELN) planted the bomb on the pipeline that was owned by companies from several countries.

United States Army. *Timeline of Terrorism: 1999–1990*. Last updated January 18, 2006. Available at: http://www.army.mil/terrorism/1999-1990/index.html

### August 7, 1998: Kenya, Tanzania

Two truck bombs exploded at the U.S. Embassies in Nairobi, Kenya and Dar es Salaam, Tanzania. The explosions resulted in 257 deaths and more than 5,000 injuries. Most of the victims were African civilians.

United States Department of State. International Information Programs: Response to Terrorism. *U.S. Embassy Bombings*. Available at: http://usinfo.state.gov/is/international_security/terrorism/embassy_bombings.html

#### September 4, 1997: Jerusalem, Israel

Bombs exploded in the Ben Yehuda shopping center. The bombs killed eight people and wounded 200 others. The suicide bombers were members of the Islamic Resistance Movement (HAMAS) who committed suicide in the attacks.

United States Army. *Timeline of Terrorism: 1999–1990.* Last updated January 18, 2006. Available at: http://www.army.mil/terrorism/1999-1990/index.html

#### December 3, 1996: Paris, France

Four people were killed and 86 injured when a bomb exploded aboard a subway train as it pulled into the Port Royal station.

United States Army. *Timeline of Terrorism: 1999–1990.* Last updated January 18, 2006. Available at: http://www.army.mil/terrorism/1999-1990/index.html

#### June 25, 1996: Dhahran, Saudi Arabia

A truck bomb exploded on the northern perimeter of the American portion of the Khobar Towers housing complex. The bomb killed 19 servicemen and injured hundreds of others. The injured included civilians of different nationalities.

The Library of Congress. Federal Research Division: Terrorism and Crime Studies. *Khobar Towers.* Last updated August 2, 2005. Available at: http://www.loc.gov/rr/frd/khobar.htm

#### February 9, 1996: London, England, United Kingdom

The Irish Republican Army (IRA) planted a bomb in London. The bomb exploded and killed two people and injured 100 others.

United States Army. *Timeline of Terrorism: 1999–1990.* Last updated January 18, 2006. Available at: http://www.army.mil/terrorism/1999-1990/index.html

#### November 13, 1995: Riyadh, Saudi Arabia

One US citizen and several foreign national governmental employees were killed in a bomb explosion planted by the Islamic Movement of Change.

United States Army. *Timeline of Terrorism: 1999-1990.* Last updated January 18, 2006. Available at: http://www.army.mil/terrorism/1999-1990/index.html.

#### April 19, 1995: Oklahoma City, Oklahoma

A truck bomb that exploded outside the Alfred P. Murrah Federal Building killed 168 people. An additional 759 people sustained injuries. Many of the fatalities occurred in the collapse zone of the structure. Timothy McVeigh and Terry Nichols were charged with the antigovernment bombing.

United States Army. *Timeline of Terrorism: 1999–1990.* Last updated January 18, 2006. Available at: http://www.army.mil/terrorism/1999-1990/index.html

Teague DC. Mass casualties in the Oklahoma City bombing. *Clin Orthop Relat Res* 2004; (422):77–81.

### February 26, 1993: New York City, New York
A nitrogen bomb weighing more than 1,000 pounds detonated in the parking garage of the World Trade Center, causing what would be considered a 16-alarm fire. The explosion killed six people and injured 1,042 others.

Aguilera K. *Financial History. Wall St. Reacts to Catastrophe, Moves Toward Recovery.* Available at: http://www.financialhistory.org/fh/2002/74-1.htm

Parachini JV. The World Trade Center Bombers (1993). In: *Toxic terror: assessing terrorist use of chemical and biological weapons.* Tucker JB, ed. Cambridge: MIT Press; 2000; pp. 185–206.

Anti-Defamation League. The Joint Terrorism Task Force. *The World Trade Center Bombing.* Available at: http://www.adl.org/learn/jttf/wtcb_jttf.asp

### December 21, 1988: Lockerbie, Scotland, United Kingdom
In August 2003, Libya formally admitted that it was responsible for the bombing of the Pan-Am Boeing 747 Flight 103 that was en route to New York. The plane exploded in air and crashed into this Scottish town. All 259 passengers on board died.

United States Army. *Timeline of Terrorism: 1989–1980.* Last updated January 18, 2006. Available at: http://www.army.mil/terrorism/1989-1980/index.html

### April 5, 1986: West Berlin, Germany
A disco explosion killed two US soldiers and injured 79 American servicemen. Libyans were responsible for the bombing.

United States Army. *Timeline of Terrorism: 1989–1980.* Last updated January 18, 2006. Available at: http://www.army.mil/terrorism/1989-1980/index.html

### December 18, 1985: Rome, Italy and Vienna, Austria
Terrorist gunmen attacked the ticket counters at both European airports, killing a total of 16 people and wounding 75 others.

United States Army. *Timeline of Terrorism: 1989–1980.* Last updated January 18, 2006. Available at: http://www.army.mil/terrorism/1989-1980/index.html

### June 23, 1985: Ireland, United Kingdom
Air India Flight 182 exploded in the air, due to a terrorist bomb. Three hundred twenty-nine people were killed.

Young MA. In: Catastrophes used as reference points in the manual. *The Community Crisis Response Team Training Manual.* 2nd ed. U.S. Department of Justice, Office for Victims of Crime and National Organization for Victims Assistance (NOVA). Available at: http://www.ojp.usdoj.gov/ovc/publications/infores/crt/appendd.htm

### October 23, 1983: Beirut, Lebanon

A truck bomb exploded near the US military barracks compound, killing 242 Marines. In addition, 58 French paratroopers who were part of the United Nations peacekeeping effort were killed in a second bombing. The Islamic Jihad took responsibility for the simultaneous attacks.

United States Army. *Timeline of Terrorism: 1989–1980.* Last updated January 18, 2006. Available at: http://www.army.mil/terrorism/1989-1980/index.html

### April 18, 1983: Beirut, Lebanon

The Islamic Jihad took responsibility for a suicide truck-bomb explosion outside the US Embassy. The explosion killed 63 people and injured 120 others. Seventeen of the victims were American.

United States Army. *Timeline of Terrorism: 1989–1980.* Last updated January 18, 2006. Available at: http://www.army.mil/terrorism/1989-1980/index/html

### January 1975: New York City, New York

The Puerto Rican nationalist group FALN claimed responsibility for a bomb that killed four and injured more than 50 others in Fraunces Tavern restaurant. The police tied the attack to 13 other bombings.

Aguilera K. *Financial History. Wall St. Reacts to Catastrophe, Moves Toward Recovery.* Available at: http://www.financialhistory.org/fh/2002/74-1.htm

### September 16, 1920: New York City, New York

A TNT bomb was planted in an unattended horse-drawn wagon and exploded on Wall Street opposite the House of Morgan. It killed 38 people and injured hundreds of others. Bolshevist or anarchist terrorists were believed to be responsible.

Aguilera K. *Financial History. Wall St. Reacts to Catastrophe, Moves Toward Recovery.* Available at: http://www.financialhistory.org/fh/2002/74-1.htm

# INDEX

Ethylene explosions, 232–233
Ethylene glycol, 33
2-Ethylhexanol, 33
Europe
    cholera outbreaks (1826–1837), 124
    diphtheria epidemics (1576), 86
    leprosy (1179), 99
    lethal gases used in concentration camps
        (1940s), 17
    occupational exposures to cotton dust
        (1700s), 82
    phosgene gas use in World War I
        (1914–1918), 18
    TOCP-contaminated drug (1930s), 72
    TOCP-contaminated extract of Jamaican
        ginger plant (1930–1931), 72
    yellow phosphorous poisoning (1800s), 61

**F**
Factory fires, 235–236
"Fen-phen" diet regimen (1997), 26
Fentanyl, 3-methylfentanyl, 34
Fentanyl-laced heroin, 33
Fertilizer explosion, 236
*Filoviridae*, 101
Fires, 236–245. *See also* specific types of fires
Fireworks explosions
    at fireworks facility (Beijing, 2003), 158
    Netherlands (2000), 245
    phosphorus poisoning from (1999),
        60–61
Flanagan, Catherine, 9
Florida
    anthrax exposure (2001), 78
    carbon monoxide poisoning from
        portable generators (Hurricane
        Katrina, 2005), 14–15
    *Challenger* space shuttle explodes (Cape
        Canaveral, 1986), 234
    ciguatera fish poisoning (Miami, 1982),
        81
    liquid chlorine released from punctured
        rail tank car (Youngstown, 1978),
        22
    Norwalk-like virus infection (1998), 106
    thallium poisoning by neighbor (1988),
        69
    typhoid fever (1998–1999), 115

Fluoride, 34–35
Fluoride and arsenic, 35
Fonofos, 55
France
    ammonium nitrate explosions
        (Toulouse, 2001), 155
    arsenical neuropathy from wine and
        bread (1828), 10
    bubonic plague (Marseilles, 1720), 129
    Charles V dies of typhus (1552), 112
    chlorine gas released by Germans
        (Ypres, 1915–1918), 17
    copper sulfate exposure (1969), 25
    diphtheria epidemics (1576), 86
    dysentery outbreak among soldiers
        (1346), 87
    ergot alkaloids cause deaths of 40,000
        people (Aquitaine, 994 AD), 90
    ergot fungus in rye crop (Pont-Saint-
        Esprit, 1951), 89
    fire at Club Cinq (St. Laurent du Pont,
        1971), 241
    fire at Paris Opera Hotel (2005), 236
    fire in Paris apartment building (2005),
        236
    hexachlorophene-contaminated
        disinfectant (1971–1972), 36
    organotin compound causes oral
        intoxication (1954), 57
    radioactive thorium waste found
        (Pargny sur Saulx, 1997), 143
    salt placed into cooling contour by
        saboteurs (Blayais reactor, 1995),
        151
    terrorist explosions on subway train
        (Paris, 1996), 266
    triethyltin iodide contamination of oral
        antibiotic (1954), 71
*Francisella tularensis*, 92
Franklin expedition (1846), 43
"Frozen addicts," 51
Fuel explosion, 245

**G**
Gabon, Ebola hemorrhagic fever (1997), 88
Gas blast, liquefied natural gas (LNG),
    35–36
Gasoline explosions, 245–247

gas explosion at Texas Gulf Sulfur Co. (Moab, 1963), 247
quarry explosions (Devil's Slide, 1910), 257

**V**

Vaccination, tuberculosis outbreak following (Lubeck, 1930), 122
Vanadium, 72
*Variola major,* 101, 116, 119–120
Venezuela
  fire at La Goajira nightclub (Caracas, 2002), 237
  terrorist explosions (Caracas, 2003), 264
Venom, scorpion, 123
Vermont
  *campylobacter jejuni* in water supply (Bennington, 1978), 81
  Legionnaires' disease traced to air conditioning system (Waterbury, 2002), 98–99
*Vibrio cholerae,* 123–125
*Vibrio cholerae* O1 El Tor, 125
*Vibrio parahemolyticus,* 125
*Vibrio vulnificus,* 125, 126
Vietnam
  dengue hemorrhagic fever (1998), 85
  dicoumarin-type anticoagulant in talc (1981), 73
  dioxin exposure from Agent Orange (1962–1971), 30
  fire at wedding reception (Ho Chi Minh City, 2002), 237
  neurotoxicity from ingesting RDX powder (1960–1970), 38
  SARS appears in (Hanoi, 2003), 118
Vinyl chloride, 72
  monomer, 73
Virginia
  chlordecone (Kepone) exposure (James River, 1973–1975), 23
  coal mine explosions (1884–1850), 223, 225
  coal mine explosions (1909–1906), 206, 208, 209
  ine explosions (1912–1910), 99–200, 202

coal mine explosions (1946–1932), 168, 173, 175, 176
coal mine explosions (1992), 162
Daconil exposure (Arlington, 1982), 26
detonation of explosive materials at rock quarry (Pounding Mills, 1920), 160
fire at the Richmond Theater (1811), 244
gunpowder explodes at sporting-goods store (1968), 248
hydrocarbons, exposure to (2004), 39
norovirus infection in youth encampment (2001), 104–105
Vitamin $B_6$, 126
Volcanic gas, 73

**W**

Wales, phenol spills into local water supply (1974–1991), 58
Warfarin, 73
Washington, DC
  exposure to thermal degradation of polyvinyl chloride (PVC) (Navy Yard, 1970), 254–255
  group A rotavirus transmitted by food (2000), 113
  isoniazid therapy, illness and deaths from (1970), 43
  quinine-adulterated heroin (1979–1982), 63
  terrorist plane crashes into the Pentagon (Sept. 11, 2001), 265
Washington State
  coal mine explosions (1899–1892), 216–217, 219, 220
  coal mine explosions (1909–1902), 205, 208, 212, 214
  coal mine explosions (1910), 202
  coal mine explosions (1918–1915), 193, 196
  coal mine explosions (1925–1924), 185, 187
  coal mine explosions (1930), 178
  coal mine fire (Franklin, 1894), 228
  cyanide poisoning from Sudafed (1991), 25